Handbook of
Food Allergies

IMMUNOLOGY SERIES
NOEL R. ROSE

Professor and Chairman
Department of Immunology and
* Infectious Diseases*
The Johns Hopkins University
School of Hygiene and Public Health
Baltimore, Maryland

1. Mechanisms in Allergy: Reagin-Mediated Hypersensitivity
   Edited by Lawrence Goodfriend, Alec Sehon, and Robert P. Orange

2. Immunopathology: Methods and Techniques
   Edited by Theodore P. Zacharia and Sidney S. Breese, Jr.

3. Immunity and Cancer in Man: An Introduction
   Edited by Arnold E. Reif

4. *Bordetella pertussis:* Immunological and Other Biological Activities
   J.J. Munoz and R.K. Bergman

5. The Lymphocyte: Structure and Function (in two parts)
   Edited by John J. Marchalonis

6. Immunology of Receptors
   Edited by B. Cinader

7. Immediate Hypersensitivity: Modern Concepts and Development
   Edited by Michael K. Bach

8. Theoretical Immunology
   Edited by George I. Bell, Alan S. Perelson, and George H. Pimbley, Jr.

9. Immunodiagnosis of Cancer (in two parts)
   Edited by Ronald B. Herberman and K. Robert McIntire

10. Immunologically Mediated Renal Diseases: Criteria for Diagnosis and
    Treatment
    Edited by Robert T. McCluskey and Giuseppe A. Andres

11. Clinical Immunotherapy
    Edited by Albert F. LoBuglio

12. Mechanisms of Immunity to Virus-Induced Tumors
    Edited by John W. Blasecki

13. Manual of Macrophage Methodology: Collection, Characterization,
    and Function
    Edited by Herbert B. Herscowitz, Howard T. Holden, Joseph A.
    Bellanti, and Abdul Ghaffar

14. Suppressor Cells in Human Disease
    Edited by James S. Goodwin

15. Immunological Aspects of Aging
    Edited by Diego Segre and Lester Smith

16. Cellular and Molecular Mechanisms of Immunologic Tolerance
Edited by Tomáš Hraba and Milan Hašek

17. Immune Regulation: Evolution and Biological Significance
Edited by Laurens N. Ruben and M. Eric Gershwin

18. Tumor Immunity in Prognosis: The Role of Mononuclear Cell Infiltration
Edited by Stephen Haskill

19. Immunopharmacology and the Regulation of Leukocyte Function
Edited by David R. Webb

20. Pathogenesis and Immunology of Treponemal Infection
Edited by Ronald F. Schell and Daniel M. Musher

21. Macrophage-Mediated Antibody-Dependent Cellular Cytotoxicity
Edited by Hillel S. Koren

22. Molecular Immunology: A Textbook
Edited by M. Zouhair Atassi, Carel J. van Oss, and Darryl R. Absolom

23. Monoclonal Antibodies and Cancer
Edited by George L. Wright, Jr.

24. Stress, Immunity, and Aging
Edited by Edwin L. Cooper

25. Immune Modulation Agents and Their Mechanisms
Edited by Richard L. Fenichel and Michael A. Chirigos

26. Mononuclear Phagocyte Biology
Edited by Alvin Volkman

27. The Lactoperoxidase System: Chemistry and Biological Significance
Edited by Kenneth M. Pruitt and Jorma O. Tenovuo

28. Introduction to Medical Immunology
Edited by Gabriel Virella, Jean-Michel Goust, H. Hugh Fudenberg, and Christian C. Patrick

29. Handbook of Food Allergies
Edited by James C. Breneman

30. Human Hybridomas: Diagnostic and Therapeutic Applications
Edited by Anthony J. Strelkauskas

31. Complications of Organ Transplantation
Edited by Luis H. Toledo-Pereyra

Other Volumes in Preparation

Aging and the Immune Response: Cellular and Humoral Aspects
Edited by Edmond A. Goidl
Monoclonal Antibodies: Hybridoma Techniques
Edited by Lawrence B. Schook

Handbook of
Food Allergies

edited by

James C. Breneman

Midwest Immunology Center, Inc.
Galesburg, Michigan

Marcel Dekker, Inc.   **New York and Basel**

ISBN 0-8247-7558-9

MARCEL DEKKER, INC.
270 Madison Avenue, New York, New York 10016

Current printing (last digit):
10 9 8 7 6 5 4 3 2 1

PRINTED IN THE UNITED STATES OF AMERICA

Preface

This book is addressed to those physicians who have suspected that we are what we eat!

Throughout recent medical history thousands of physicians have been told by millions of patients that certain foods produce certain symptoms. The physician's usual role was to discredit these anecdotal reports because there existed no measurable proof of a causal relationship. Certain physicians, however, became believers if only because of the sheer number of such reports. It is to these open-minded physicians that some vindication is now due. As the new medical science of food allergy develops, additional mysterious symptoms and disease processes will be explained. The unraveling of these enigmas supports not only these curious yet believing physicians but, more important, their patients, who will be the ultimate recipients of the benefits.

The discovery of IgE was the first step in credibility. IgE testing so convincingly confirmed the numerous clinical observations of food allergy that few now question its reality. More recent testing methods have shown involvement of other immune structures in the production of food allergy symptoms.

Until 20 years ago most proof of food allergy was dependent on anecdotal sources. In the past two decades proof has been dependent on evidence from elimination-diet technique. Now the evidence comes from the laboratory, thus qualifying food allergy as a newly quantifiable medical science.

The rather poor status of food allergy as a science among the other branches of medicine was probably well deserved. Massive amounts of misinformation and self-interest promotion contributed to distrust by physicians. Most diagnostic procedures lacked sensitivity and reliability, and therefore any treatment based on these inaccurate tests yielded poor results. Also, after decades of poor results, patients also began to distrust food allergists.

In 1970 the American College of Allergists embarked upon an effort to transform the *cult* of food allergy into the *science* of food allergy. Since 1974 the Food Allergy Symposia have convened the world leaders in this science, resulting in the exchange and progressive accumulation of scientific data about food allergy. In 1980 the president of the American College of Allergists (Solomon Klotz, M.D.) decreed that food allergy had achieved the status of "the newest medical science."

It is the purpose of this book to present this up-to-date accumulation of data. To do this, world leaders in the field have been solicited to prepare chapters in the areas of food intolerance where they are recognized authorities. Authors were given free rein to present all the knowledge and facts in their particular spheres.

Authors were also admonished to be conservative lest speculative statements might later be disproven—and again threaten the credibility of all food allergy science. These admonitions were well presented by Franz Joseph Gall: "Men who enjoy a great name should, more than others, guard themselves against spreading hazardous ideas, for, however erroneous they may be, they will be repeated for centuries."

Handbook of Food Allergies therefore represents the current views of these world leaders in the science of food allergy. Because the science is in its infancy, caution has been exercised; overoptimism has been curbed and unbridled enthusiasm has been discouraged. An effort has been made to present the truth, the whole truth, and nothing but the truth as these authors know it.

James C. Breneman

Introduction

In the field of food allergy there has been little agreement. Even definition of the term is somewhat unsettled; however, a consensus is usually achieved with the definition "an immune reaction causing a morbid response to ingestants." This definition is dependent on the doubtful theory that all immune reactions to food cause symptoms, a theory for which there is little proof. It would be naive to assume that food allergy reactions take place only in tissue capable of producing perceptible symptoms. In all likelihood, the majority of food allergy reactions are silent, insidious, and chronic because they take place in tissue (or organs) that do not perceive discomfort (pain or pruritus) or obvious dysfunction of a major organ.

Most of our organs and tissue are incapable of manifesting symptoms of discomfort or dysfunction. Blood vessel walls, brain tissue, hepatic tissue, splenic tissue, renal tissue, and pancreatic tissue are examples of tissues that do not hurt, or itch, or readily display obvious malfunction. Chronic immune insults, therefore, can go on daily with no recognizable food allergy symptoms. Only after years of low-grade tissue destruction are these recognized as being due to aging.

These so-called delayed food reactions were once difficult to diagnose. They appeared so long after the ingestion of the guilty food that neither patient nor physician could see the cause-and-effect association. Unlike the immediate (IgE) reactions to foods, which showed very obvious cause-and-effect association and had a satisfactory diagnostic test (intradermal aqueous injection and RAST), the delayed (occult) type had very vague symptom-ingestion history, no satisfactory diagnostic tests, and a plethora of promoters ready to take advantage of the resulting ignorance. Patients knew they felt bad and unscrupulous physicians and promoters exploited the opportunity. The patient continued to suffer—as did the credibility of the food allergist.

It was not until the International Food Allergy Symposia were begun in 1974 that food scientists were given a stage from which to present their work. Food allergy began to assume the stature of a medical science. For so many decades the term "food allergist" smacked of quackery. Now it is respectable to be a food allergist. Now the promotors of unscientific material are being replaced by ethical food scientists. Finally, the ultimate goal is being achieved: real benefit for our patients.

Food allergy lagged 50 to 100 years behind inhalant allergy. There are several reasons for this. Inhalant allergy had a simple, inexpensive, yet accurate diagnostic test, the skin test. This resulted in the establishment of effective therapy, immunotherapy.

Ingestant allergy (food allergy) had no such simple diagnostic test; the cult was riddled with misinformation; no effective treatment could result since no accurate diagnosis could be made. Disgruntled patients and disenchanted physicians shunned or ignored the problem. For all of these reasons, academicians avoided trying to interest medical students in the problem.

Fortunately, three events in the past two decades have changed the picture and vaulted food allergy into a position of unusual prominence in a very short time: (1) discovery of IgE by Johansson and the Ishizakas (1966), (2) Gell-Coombs' classification of immune (allergic) reactions (1963), and (3) inauguration of the International Food Allergy Symposia (1974).

The first two breakthroughs showed the potential complexity of immune reactions and, especially, the possible variation of food allergy manifestations and mechanisms. The third event gave scientific physicians an opportunity to discuss and, free from ridicule, build their information banks on food allergy.

Some differences of opinion will be noted as one reads the text. Since even experts disagree, opposing sides are presented herein to show the many controversies that still exist. At the present rate of advance in the science of food allergy, these controversies will certainly soon be resolved.

Contents

Preface   iii

Introduction   v

Contributors   ix

1. Immunology of Food Allergy   1
   James C. Breneman

2. Immunology of Food Antigens   13
   Michael J. Sweeney and Solomon D. Klotz

3. Gastroenterology of Food Hypersensitivity   37
   Aubrey J. Katz

4. Pediatric Food Allergy   55
   Sami L. Bahna and Mohan D. Gandhi

5. Food Allergy in Adults   71
   Vinay K. Jain and R. K. Chandra

6. Diseases Produced or Affected by Food Intolerance   83
   Jean A. Monro

7. Migraine and Allergy 99
   Jean A. Monro

8. Arthritis and Food Allergy 115
   Richard S. Panush, Lawrence P. Endo, and Ella M. Webster

9. Non-IgE-Mediated and Delayed Adverse Reactions to Food
   or Additives 125
   William T. Kniker and L. Maria Rodriguez

10. Laboratory Tests for Food Hypersensitivity 163
    Robert J. Dockhorn

11. Today's Approved Diagnostic and Treatment Methods 181
    Cecil Collins-Williams and Laurent V. Constantin

12. Unproven and Unapproved Methods of Diagnosis and Treatment 211
    John A. Anderson

13. Maintaining Patient Compliance During an Elimination Diet 233
    Eileen Rhude Yoder

14. Prophylaxis of Food Allergy 261
    Douglas E. Johnstone

15. New and Promising Treatments 271
    Robert N. Hamburger and Gary A. Cohen

Index 279

Contributors

John A. Anderson, M.D. Chairman, Department of Pediatrics, and Head, Division of Allergy and Clinical Immunology, Henry Ford Hospital, Detroit, Michigan

Sami L. Bahna, M.D., Ph.D. Professor of Pediatrics and Chief, Section of Allergy and Immunology, Department of Pediatrics, Louisiana State University School of Medicine, New Orleans, Louisiana

James C. Breneman, M.D., Diplomate ABAI President, Midwest Immunology Center, Inc., Galesburg, Michigan

R. K. Chandra, M.D., F.R.C.P.(C) Professor, Departments of Pediatrics, Medicine, and Biochemistry, Janeway Child Health Centre, Memorial University of Newfoundland, St. John's, Newfoundland, Canada

Gary A. Cohen, M.D. Assisstant Clinical Professor, Department of Pediatrics, University of California – San Diego, La Jolla, California

Cecil Collins-Williams, M.D., F.R.C.P.(C)[*] Professor, Department of Paediatrics, University of Toronto, Toronto, Ontario, Canada

[*]Present affiliation: Professor Emeritus, Department of Paediatrics, University of Toronto, Toronto, Ontario, Canada

Laurent V. Constantin, M.D., F.R.C.P.(C)[*]   Fellow, Division of Allergy, The Hospital for Sick Children, Toronto, Ontario, Canada

Robert J. Dockhorn, M.D.   Clinical Professor, Departments of Pediatrics and Medicine, University of Missouri School of Medicine, Kansas City, Missouri

Lawrence P. Endo, M.D.   Postdoctoral Fellow, Division of Clinical Immunology, Rheumatology, and Allergy, Department of Medicine, College of Medicine, University of Florida, Gainesville, Florida

Mohan D. Gandhi, M.D.   Clinical Assistant Professor of Pediatrics, Section of Allergy and Immunology, Department of Pediatrics, Louisiana State University School of Medicine, New Orleans, Louisiana

Robert N. Hamburger, M.D.   Professor and Head, Pediatric Immunology and Allergy Division, Department of Pediatrics, University of California – San Diego, La Jolla, California

Vinay K. Jain, M.B., B.S.   Postdoctoral Fellow, The Health Sciences Center, Memorial University of Newfoundland, St. John's, Newfoundland, Canada

Douglas E. Johnstone, M.D.   Clinical Professor, Department of Pediatrics, University of Rochester School of Medicine and Dentistry, Rochester, New York

Aubrey J. Katz, M.D.   Assistant Clinical Professor, Harvard Medical School, and Associate in Medicine (Gastroenterology), Department of Pediatrics, The Children's Hospital, Boston, Massachusetts

Solomon D. Klotz, M.D., Diplomate ABAI,   Senior Director, Allergy/Immunology Research Laboratory of Central Florida, and Adjunct Professor, Department of Biology, University of Central Florida, Orlando, Florida

William T. Kniker, M.D.   Chief, Division of Clinical Immunology, and Professor, Departments of Pediatrics and Microbiology, University of Texas Health Science Center, San Antonio, Texas

Jean A. Monro, M.D.   Medical Director, Department of Allergy and Environmental Medicine, The Nightingale Hospital, London, England

---

Present affiliation: Vice-president, Medical Affairs, A. H. Robins Canada, Mississauga, Ontario, Canada

Richard S. Panush, M.D. Professor and Chief, Division of Clinical Immunology, Rheumatology, and Allergy, Department of Medicine, College of Medicine, University of Florida, and Chief, Clinical Immunology Section, Medical and Research Services, Veterans Administration Medical Center, Gainesville, Florida

L. Maria Rodriguez, R.D. Division of Clinical Immunology, Department of Pediatrics, University of Texas Health Science Center, San Antonio, Texas

Michael J. Sweeney, Ph.D. Director, Allergy/Immunology Research Laboratory of Central Florida, and Professor, Department of Laboratory Sciences, University of Central Florida, Orlando, Florida

Ella M. Webster, M.D. Postdoctoral Fellow, Division of Clinical Immunology, Rheumatology, and Allergy, Department of Medicine, College of Medicine, University of Florida, Gainesville, Florida

Eileen Rhude Yoder, Ph.D. President, Medical Diet Systems, Inc., Orland Park, Illinois

Handbook of
Food Allergies

1
Immunology of Food Allergy

JAMES C. BRENEMAN
Midwest Immunology Center, Inc., Galesburg, Michigan

DIFFERENCES FROM INHALANT ALLERGY*

To understand ingestant (food) allergy clearly, it is most helpful to observe the dynamic contrasts that exist between inhalant and ingestant allergies.

The types of antigens in inhalant allergies are primarily dusts, pollens, and epidermals (water-soluble fractions). In contrast, the antigens of ingestant allergy are very complex and both water and fat soluble. The number of antigens in inhalant allergy is usually 150 or less (except for hypersensitivity pneumonitis). The number of antigens in ingestant allergy is much greater, 6000, 400 of which are nutrient foodstuffs.

Reaction time in an inhalant allergy is usually immediate or within a few seconds, but the bolus of food allergy can be in the gastrointestinal tract from 3 to 5 days. The allergens of inhalant allergy are stable: simple and unchanging (i.e., undergo no great change to induce reaction). The reverse is true of an ingestant allergen: a complex bolus of food, changing constantly under assault by digestants, bacteria, and toxins, and constantly releasing new, potential antigens.

In inhalant allergies, the exposed mucosal surface is a few square inches of respiratory tract; however, for ingestant allergy, it is 20 ft of bowel, or 1 acre of exposed surface. The mucosa-antigen contact time for inhalant allergy is a few seconds, compared with the 3–5 days it takes an ingestant antigen to make its transit through the bowel. The timing of symptoms for inhalant allergies is immediate to no longer than 20 min. Timing of symptoms for ingestant allergy

*This information was taken from J. C. Breneman, *Basics of Food Allergy*, 2nd ed., pp. 19 and 20 [1].

1

can be immediate or take up to 5 days to determine. The allergic mechanism involved in inhalant allergy is IgE, immediate, or type I only (except hypersensitivity pneumonitis). The allergic mechanisms in ingestant allergy include all four types of allergic reactions or even a combination of several reactions. Systems involved in an inhalant allergic reaction are mostly respiratory as opposed to the involvement of any tissue, organ or system − even the whole patient − during an ingestant allergic response.

The prevalent antigen in inhalant allergy is ragweed. However, it is interesting to note that cow's milk is the "ragweed" of food allergy. Clinical testing for an inhalant allergy can now be accurately determined by good, diagnostic, skin tests and the radio allergosorbent test (RAST). Most laboratory tests, however, prove impractical for ingestant allergy (except Type I involvement).

Even the disease status of ingestant allergy is at variance with that of inhalant allergy. Inhalant allergy is a clinically established and recognized disease, but there are yet areas of doubt in the scope of ingestant allergy disease. Though areas of challenge still exist, many mysterious syndromes are now being exposed as ingestant (food) allergic responses. For inhalant allergies, infection is the main confusing complication. In the ingestant allergies, however, confusing digestive, enzymatic, absorptive, neoplastic, mechanical, and chemical factors may complicate the picture, as well as specific foods intolerance: gluten, lactose, tyramine, alcohol, and others.

Treatment for inhalant allergies is now unified and simplified through conventional immunotherapy. Treatment, however, for a patient suffering from ingestant allergy is very complicated and individualized. Alcohol can complicate absorption. Gluten produces types I and III allergy. The white of an egg can bypass antibodies to release mediators.

DELAYED AND IMMEDIATE FOOD ALLERGY DIFFERENCES*

Immediate (obvious) food allergy is usually easily recognizable to patients. These allergic reactions can be obvious, acute, or even life threatening. Violent responses of this nature can manifest themselves in acute hives, laryngeal edema, and asphyxia. Death, though rare, is possible. This patient rarely, therefore, needs a physician to point out such a sensitivity − it is "obvious."

Delayed food allergy (occult), on the other hand, includes all non-IgE immune reactions to ingestants. It is much more prevalent. This allergic response frequently produces vague, chronic, low-grade symptoms, such as failure to thrive, chronic (migraine) headaches, chronic indigestion, recurrent abdominal pain,

*This information was taken from J. C. Breneman, *Basics of Food Allergy,* 2nd ed., pp. 20–22 [1].

fatigue, "biliousness," nocturnal enuresis, joint symptoms, apthous ulcers, seizures, and chronic respiratory symptoms, which are often mistakenly diagnosed as infections. Delayed food allergy is responsible for incalculable human morbidity. It is the least recognized (thus called "occult") and therefore the least treated disease in the United States.

An obvious (immediate) food allergy response is an all-or-none reaction; the delayed (occult) is dose related, not quantitative. The obvious reaction is immediate, within 1–60 min., but the delayed reaction can take up to 5 days to manifest itself. The immediate, obvious reaction is mediated by IgE (possibly IgG_4 and IgD are also involved). The delayed, occult reaction involves Gell-Coombs types II, III, and IV immune reactions. Occult reactions are very prevalent, but the immediate or obvious reactions are less common. An intradermal skin test can diagnose the obvious reactions, but its use would produce unreliable information for the occult responses. Obvious food reactions could prove fatal, but there is no threat of mortality with an occult food allergy reaction. The severity of an immediate food allergy reaction is predictable and reproducible: one of shock. The severity of an occult reaction is cyclic; morbidity is low grade and chronic. Usually an immediate-type reaction involves only one shock organ. An occult reaction, by contrast, is a systemic malaise.

The immediate food allergy is usually permanent, but the occult usually diminishes with prolonged avoidance of the antigen. Immediate food allergy patients respond to antihistamines (H_1 type) cromolyn, and corticosteroids, but occult reaction sufferers receive benefit from neither antihistamines nor cromolyn. The success of treating occult allergic reactions with corticosteroids varies.

INCIDENCE OF FOOD ALLERGY

Elimination diet-challenge techniques can establish the incidence of ingestant intolerance but not the incidence of immune reaction to foods. Some nonimmune reactions to foods include those to caffeine in coffee; lactose in milk; bacterial, viral, and parasitic food poisoning; digestive diseases, such as gallbladder disease and pancreatic diseases; and idiosyncratic reactions.

Accurate diagnosis of food allergy has been wanting. Diagnostic inaccuracies have made incidence estimates difficult. Probably less than 10% of all immune immune reactions to food are of type I and therefore diagnosable by accurate laboratory tests. This leaves 90% as delayed, or occult, and relatively undiagnosable by simple, accurate laboratory tests. Any estimates of incidence, therefore, are guesses. Seat-of-the-pants estimates from food allergists around the United States fix incidences in a range from ¼ to 60% or from 625,000 to 150,000,000 persons. A realistic estimate would place the incidence of both immediate and delayed food allergy in the United States between 10 and 20%, or from 25,000,000 to 50,000,000 persons. Most of these are unknown food allergy sufferers. This great reservoir of morbidity would be treatable if there existed a simple, yet accurate, method to diagnose delayed-type reactions to food. Hope seems on the horizon. Dockhorn's chapter on laboratory diagnosis addresses in vitro and in vivo tests for delayed (occult) reaction to foods. If these new tests continue to look promising, perhaps allergists will be able to uncover this sea of undiagnosed delayed reactors and therefore treat them appropriately.

As soon as diagnosis is facilitated, treatment seems to follow with predictable ease. Avoidance of the food allergen seems rather a primitive treatment for this day and age. Pharmaceutical research will, with little doubt, create new treatments as soon as the food allergy problem is accurately identified (diagnosed).

New modes of treatment are already appearing, but "you ain't seen nothin' yet"!

Antimediators are already in the hoppers of research centers. Antihistamines 1 and 2, antiprostaglandins, anti-kinins, anti-lymphokines, anti-interleukins, plus anti-mediators yet to be discovered will make effective treatment easy once diagnosis is accurate, simple, and inexpensive.

Until that day, however, we must be thoroughly aware of the current state of the art. On behalf of all the authors, I hope this handbook fulfills that mission.

The gut wall is the site of food allergy generation. Temporary (usually) loss of sufficient barriers (immune integrity) permits antigens to cross the absorbing surface and contact underlying immune structures. The causes of defense barrier loss are as follows:

1. Immaturity
2. Inheritance
3. Injury:
   Infection (viral, bacterial)
   Infestation (*Giardia* and other agents)
   Irradiation
   Ischemia

Probably a macrophage is the first structure to respond immunologically. (1) It recognizes and processes the food antigen. (2) It then decides to eradicate the antigen itself, or (3) it calls in assistance to handle the invader. If so, the macrophage will assign specific antibody, complement, and/or specific T lymphocytes if they are available. If not, allogenic T cells (cytotoxic) will be recruited. (4) If specific immune structures are not available, the macrophage will either call in all the nonspecific immune structures it needs, and/or it will turn the specific antigen over to the immune system to create a specific immune defense against a possible future invasion by the same antigen. This process is inaugurated by a messenger material, interleukin-1 (Il-1) sent by the macrophage to the T lymphocytes. Figure 1 shows diagrammically how the defenses of the gut are breached using milk antigens as the example.

If the allogenic (nonspecific or cytotoxic) T cell cannot immediately control control the invasion, antigen-specific T lymphocytes are stimulated. Nonspecific T lymphocytes also respond to this interleukin-1 by sending orders via interleukin-2 (Il-2) to B lymphocytes to begin production of specific antibodies against the invading antigen. The result is that future invasion by this same antigen would be met by a much more vigorous immune response.

Not every breach in defense leads to sensitization. In normal situations, the "turn-on" and "turn-off" mechanisms of the immune system are balanced sufficiently to avoid development of food allergy sensitization. Abnormalities of either mechanism, however, can foster the production of allergy. Excessive turn-on lies in the overproduction of helper stimuli by T lymphocytes. Deficient turn-off stimulus by suppressor T lymphocytes may also allow excessive immune response to continue to produce excessive allergic antibodies. In either case, an allergic response is generated if these pathogenic factors make their contributions in this sequence.

STEPS IN THE DEVELOPMENT OF FOOD ALLERGY

I. Loss of gut defense barrier.

II. Food antigen contacts immune structure after breaching the gut defense barriers.

III. First immune structure contacted (macrophage) begins defense mobilization. The macrophage receptor site accepts the antigen. It may

A. By itself, control the invasion.

B. Perceive that the antigen has been previously encountered and generated specific immune structures. These structures (specific antibodies, antigen-specific T cells) are beckoned, probably by interleukin-1 messenger.

C. Perceive that this food antigen is new and that it (the macrophage) cannot control the invasion. It will set up the sensitization process.

IV. Sensitization process is begun. The macrophage via interleukin-1 stimulates the T lymphocyte to "organize and train" new defenses. Via interleukin-2, the T lymphocyte stimulates the B lymphocyte to form specific antibodies. Helper T lymphocytes sustain the stimulus for antibody production until adequate defenses are established. At this time, suppressor lymphocytes turn off the process.

V. Hypersensitization (allergy) may ensue. If this suppressor effect is inadequate, hypersensitization (allergy) is produced because the helper-cell effect is not curbed adequately.

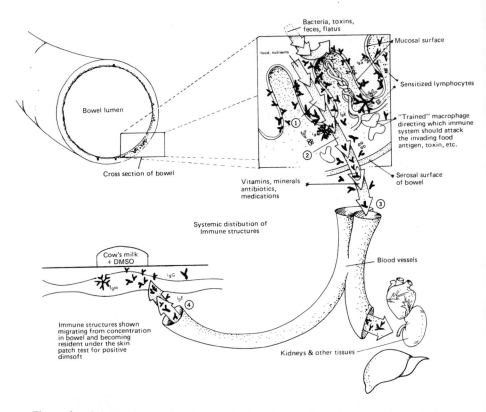

Figure 1a (1) Nutrients, vitamins, and minerals are allowed to pass through the mucosal barrier unimpeded; undesirable products, toxins, bacteria, and food allergens are normally repelled at the mucosal surface. Secretory IgA and mucus film are a significant factor in this impediment. (2) Food allergens, after absorption, contact the macrophage by occupying a receptor site on the macrophage cell membranes. A signal (interleukin-1) is generated and sent to T lymphocytes, which in turn respond either by (a) calling in nonspecific T lymphocytes (killer cells) via interleukin-2, or (b) calling in previously sensitized structures, that is, specific antibodies or specific T cells, or (c) summoning B lymphocytes to produce specific antibodies. (3) These immune structures inevitably wash free of the sensitizing arena and via blood and/or lymph stream are distributed into various body tissues, including skin. (4) Those immune structures that wash to the sub-q. areas affix to subcutaneous tissues. Surface food antigens, when mixed with DMSO, are able to penetrate to sufficient depth to contact these immune structures. This contact results in a controlled, localized immune reaction to a specific food antigen, resulting in a positive Dimsoft test.

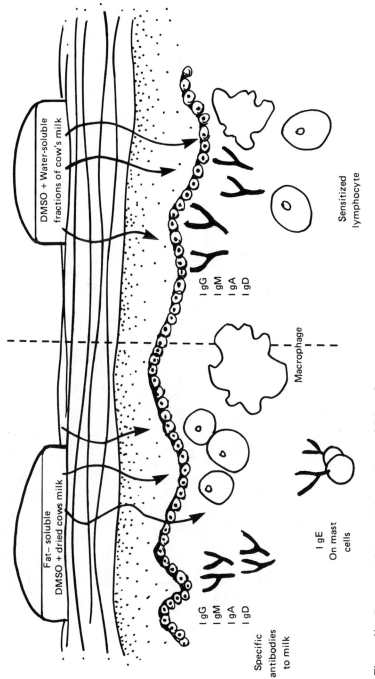

Figure 1b Diagram of dermal immunology of Dimsoft.

VI. The specific allergen again enters the now hypersensitized host and
the allergic reaction follows. In food allergy, this probably involves
all four Coombs immune reactions.
  A. Type I. If there is significant mast cell-IgE involvement, the main
     symptoms will be immediate or histaminelike. Rhinorrhea, broncho
     bronchospasm, eczema, and uriticaria are usual symptoms.
  B. Type II. If the food antigen has attached to host tissue cells,
     specific IgG or IgM will attach to the antigen. Complement is
     recruited, and the host cells are destroyed along with the antigen.

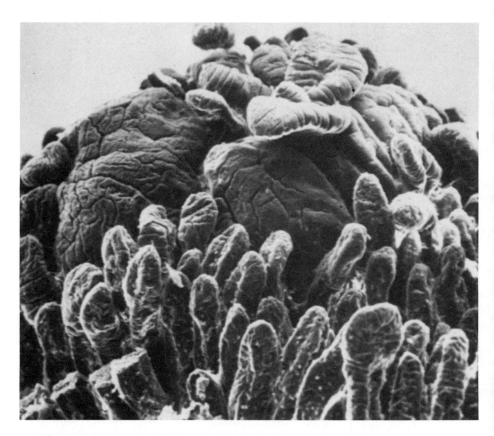

Figure 2 Surface of M cell in Peyer's patch. (Courtesy of Robert Owens,
Veterans Administration Medical Center, San Francisco, Calif.)

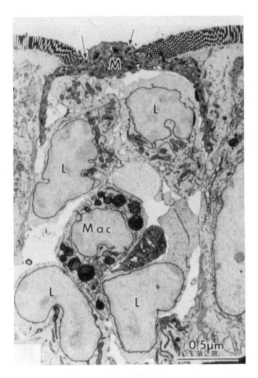

Figure 3 M cell cross section. (Courtesy of Robert Owens, Veterans Administration Medical Center, San Francisco, Calif.)

C. Type III. If the food antigen couples with the specific antibody (IgG or IgM) while in the fluid of the vascular system, it forms an immune complex. These complexes are trapped in tight vascular tufts (e.g., renal glomerulus), where they settle, receive complement, and destroy innocent bystander vascular structures.
D. Type IV. Specifically sensitized T lymphocytes are capable of recognizing the specific exogenous antigen. Nearby host cells are often injured during the process.

After food sensitization has taken place, the bowel monitors its content periodically. Through M cells in the Peyer's patches, soluble food products are sampled (see Figs. 2 and 3). If food antigens are detected, appropriate defenses, as recounted above, are summoned.

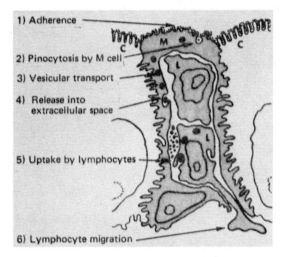

1) Adherence

2) Pinocytosis by M cell

3) Vesicular transport

4) Release into
   extracellular space

5) Uptake by lymphocytes

6) Lymphocyte migration

Figure 4   M cell diagramatic cross section.

Immune reactions in the skin parallel those in the bowel. Because of this, skin tests utilizing specific antigens can reflect allergic responses in the bowel. Since these immune structures migrate from the bowel wall to the skin, it is reasonable to assume they also are distributed to all body tissues. Therefore, the presence of these immune structures in the skin is reflective of the systemic distribution of these specific immune structures. Skin tests with appropriate food antigens, both fat and water soluble, delivered to sufficient depth to encounter these sensitized immune structures, ought then to predict food sensitivities. Breneman's Dimsoft, described by Dockhorn (Chap. 10), seems to fulfill these requirements. A positive Dimsoft patch test quite accurately diagnoses food sensitivity of immune etiology (See Fig. 1b).

In the skin, the macrophage is the intraepidermal Langerhans' cell. It performs the same immune functions as the bowel wall macrophage. It processes the the food antigen (provided by the Dimsoft patch). It stimulates allogenic (unrelated) T cells to help in general immediate defense. It induces food antigen specific T lymphocytes to assemble. It instructs nonspecific T cells to summon antibodies, complement, and so on.

The Langerhans' cell contacts all the T lymphocytes by means of food anti-antigens on the Langerhans' cell surface, the food antigen having been delivered to the Langerhans' cell by the Dimsoft test. This exogenous food antigen provides one signal for activation of T cells [2]. The second signal is interleukin-1, which is secreted by the Langerhans' cell and initiates the sequence of immune responses that set up the limited inflammatory response read as a positive Dimsoft patch test.*

REFERENCES

1. Breneman, J. C. (1984). *Basics of Food Allergy* (2nd ed.). Charles C Thomas Publishers, Springfield, Illinois, pp. 163–216.
2. Dahl, M. V. (1981). *Clinical Immunodermatology.* Year Book Medical Publishers, Chicago, Illinois.
3. Robert, L. K., Kruegor, G. G., and Daynes, R. A. (1984). Functional role for IA expression by keratinocytes. *J. Invest. Dermatol. 82*:418.
4. Sauder, D. N., and Katz, S. (1982). Immune Modulation by Epidermal Cell Products: Possible Role of ETAF in Inflammatory and Neoplastic Skin Disease. *J. Am. Acad. Dermatol. 7*:651–654.

*Corticosteroids will block the action of I-1; therefore, exogenous corticosteroids should be discontinued before and during Dimsoft patch testing.

2

Immunology of Food Antigens

MICHAEL J. SWEENEY and SOLOMON D. KLOTZ
Allergy/Immunology Research Laboratory of Central Florida and University of Central Florida, Orlando, Florida

FOODS AND THEIR POSSIBLE ROLE AS ANTIGENS AND ALLERGENS

We will define substances capable of eliciting an immune response as antigens. Whether the immune response initiated by these antigens are protective or lead to hypersensitivity states or to tolerance is the relevant information to be developed here.

General Properties of Antigens

Molecular Size

It has been known for many years that antigens have certain physical and chemical characteristics. The majority of antigens are proteins, polysaccharides, and glycoproteins. Other classes of macro-molecules have been implicated as having antigenic activity, such as nucleic acid and lipids, but overall they are not as strongly antigenic as the proteins and polysaccharides.

In general, antigens have molecular weights above 10,000 daltons (d), but some antigens fall below this weight range. Low-molecular-weight proteins that may be weakly antigenic may under certain circumstances become more strongly antigenic. This may occur if

1. Self-association of a low-molecular-weight compound leads to the formation of high-molecular-weight complexes.
2. In association with other proteins, macromolecules, or cell surfaces, either covalently or noncovalently, where these materials act as carriers for the low-molecular-weight substance.

3. The low-molecular-weight material is presented in association with adjuvant-like compounds.
4. A low-molecular-weight material is presented to the responder by a particular route of administration that is favorable for an immune response.

Antigenic Immunodeterminants

Antigens contain immunodeterminant groups. Immunodeterminants are defined as small areas of an antigenic surface that actually react — lock and key — with effectors of the immune response. The effectors can be antibody and/or cell surface receptors on immunocytes. The immunodeterminant sites are usually composed of between five and ten amino acids in proteins or approximately seven carbohydrate units in complex polysaccharides. These immunodeterminants may be in a linear sequence or act together to form a specific shape in space to which the effector binds with high affinity. To be effective, it is necessary for immunodeterminants to be expressed on the surface as a three-dimensional structure of the antigen, so that immunocompetent cells or antibodies may interact with them [1, 2].

Not all sequences of amino acids or carbohydrates, whether or not on the surface of an antigen, behave as immunodeterminants. Only specific groups within the molecules seem able to act in that capacity.

In a large complex protein or glycoprotein, many of the immunodeterminants are different. A particular macromolecule that is antigenic could have several hundred immunodeterminants. Each of those determinants could have a specific amino acid sequence, a characteristic charge, and a specific unique shape in space. Certain types of macromolecules, such as complex polysaccharides, may have repeating immunodeterminant groups. These immunodeterminants would have the same characteristics repeated over and over again within the molecule; however, this is the exception to the rule. It is not surprising, then, that an antibody response made to most complex antigens is heterogeneous in nature since each antibody would be reacting with various immunodeterminant groups present on that particular antigen.

Foreignness

The more foreign or chemically different an antigen is from the normal tissue of the responder, usually, the more antigenic the material would be. Proteins that are similar in nature to proteins already existing in the host quite often have little or no antigenicity in that host. Collagen, which is similar in most animal species, is therefore a poor antigen [3].

Adrenocorticotropic hormone (ACTH) consists of only 39 amino acid residues. Dayhoff and Eck studied this substance in various animal species. The animals studied shared some 24 of the 39 amino acid residues. The ACTH differed in these animal species in amino acid regions from 25 to 33. When antibodies were induced to the ACTH of the different species in these animals, it was found that the antibodies reacted with only the areas of variability, not with those areas that were common to the various species [4].

Thymus-Dependent and Thymus-Independent Antigens

Antigens can have varying degrees of antigenicity, depending upon the species into which they are injected. They usually induce a heterogeneous antibody population, not only in their idiotypes (specificity of the Fab binding site), but also in the class of antibody produced. Antigens, depending on their inherent nature, may predispose to induce mainly IgM and other antigens may initiate an IgG or any other antibody class response. These characteristics are observed with thymus-dependent and thymus-independent antigens. Thymus-dependent antigens need cooperation of functioning T and B cells for the production of antibody. Without the appropriate T-cell response, these antigens cannot initiate humoral responses. It is normally agreed that this type of antigen initiates the IgG, IgA, and IgE antibody classes. The thymus-independent antigens, on the other hand, initiate mainly an IgM response. Most thymus-independent antigens contain repeating immunodeterminant groups, are of very high molecular weight, and are slowly metabolized [5–8].

Complex antigens with many and varied immunodeterminant groups, which have highly complex tertiary structures, such as observed with proteins, lipoproteins, and glycoproteins, are usually T-cell dependent. T-cell-dependent antigens, with various types of treatments, can become T-independent antigens. This was shown with collagen, a thymus-dependent antigen [3]. It seems likely that the reverse of this may also occur.

Nature of the Response to Antigen

Antigens that initiate an antibody response may or may not induce a cellular immune response, and vice versa. There have been several reports in the literature in which antigenic material capable of inducing circulating antibody would, under various types of treatment, lose the ability to induce antibody but still be a potent inducer of a cellular immune response [9, 10].

Any one antigen can, under various circumstances, induce a range of immune responses. These responses may be strictly humoral or cellular or more likely a mixed response of both the humoral and cellular systems. The humoral response may be the production of one or more of the antibody classes, with one particular antibody class predominating, depending on the nature of the antigen presentation.

The general structure and chemical properties of an antigen alone cannot be used to predict the type of reaction one might observe in populations. Presentation of low concentrations of an antigen may lead to possible tolerance.

High concentrations of that same antigen may induce a very strong antibody or cellular response, but excessively high doses of that same antigen may abrogate the response and cause tolerance by a different mechanism from that observed in the low-dose presentation.

The concentration of an antigen reaching the immune system is somewhat influenced by the route of immunization. Intravenous injection causes antigens to concentrate in certain organs, especially the liver, with smaller amounts going to other tissues of the reticuloendothelial system (RES). The liver may degrade certain antigens in such a way that it may eliminate antibody production in other tissue organ systems, but that same antigen presented by another route may be a potent inducer of antibody [11, 12]. Antigens given subcutaneously are concentrated mainly in the regional lymph nodes; antigens that interact with mucosal membranes are presented to lymphoid tissues characteristic of that particular area of the mucosal membrane system [12].

The route of immunization not only affects the concentration of the antigen, but it determines the type of cells with which the antigens will interact. The type of cellular interactions that take place determines the ultimate immune response observed.

In regions where a specific immunoglobulin class precursor cell is found in high numbers, along with the appropriate T helper and accessory cells, the immunoglobulin produced will be of that class. It is not surprising, then, that subcutaneous injection of antigen usually favors IgG production but antigens presented by the mucous membranes are highly effective in inducing IgA and, in some individuals, a strong IgE response. In order for an immune response to be made to any antigen, the host must be capable of recognizing it and processing it.

The ability of inbred strains of mice to make humoral response to specific antigens was found to be controlled by Ir genes contained within the I region of the major histocompatability complex (MHC) [13]. These genes and their products are believed necessary for antigen recognition and response by specific T-helper cells and macrophages. Since these genes are linked closely to serologically defined transplantation antigens, they can sometimes be associated with a particular tissue type. Association of certain tissue types in humans with their ability to produce specific IgE antibody to certain allergens is reminiscent of the relationship that exists in the animal system [14]. These observations and the fact that allergy is strongly familial suggest a genetic component, not only in making a humoral response, but also in the class of antibody made.

Foods as Antigens

Antigenicity of Foods

Macromolecules contained in foods have all the necessary properties of antigens. Injection of foods or their extracts gives rise to antibody production. Ingestion of food has also been shown to elicit the production of antibody. The type and specificity of the antibodies produced in rabbits by ingestion versus injection have been shown to be similar in their specificities and isotypes [15, 16].

In our laboratory, we have demonstrated, in adults, that precipitating antibodies could be detected to many foodstuffs other than those that are most frequently reported. In addition to the usual precipitating antibodies found to milk, egg and fish, our studies have shown precipitating antibodies to corn, corn products, and various fruits and vegetables. None of these precipitating antibodies were associated with clinical hypersensitivity in our population group. The antibody classes detected to these foods were IgG and/or IgM.

Assays of cellular immunity to food antigens, such as migration inhibition and antigen-induced blast transformation, have proven to be positive against some food products [17, 18].

Foods Implicated as Allergens

Many foods have been shown to be antigenic, but there seems to be a rather limited number of foods that are considered strongly allergenic. The most notable in order of importance are cow's milk, eggs, and fish. Tomatoes, oranges, bananas, meats, nuts, chocolate, and cereals have also been reported to be allergenic.

General Properties of Food Allergens

Chemical characterizations of foods that induce IgE production have certain characteristics in common. The molecular weight of these materials is usually between 10,000 and 40,000 d. They are nearly always protein or glycoprotein in nature. It has been reported that most of the food allergens are heat resistant and fairly resistant to enzymatic breakdown [16]. Other investigators have found that enzymatic breakdown may give rise to new allergens from the food products [19-21].

Determination of Allergic Reactions to Food and Food Products

Allergenicity of foods has been demonstrated by skin testing, the elicitation of allergic symptoms using the appropriate food or fraction of the food in blind challenge testing, radioallergosorbent testing (RAST) showing specific IgE binding to a particular antigenic component of the food, and, most recently, by using crossed radioimmunoelectrophoresis techniques, which allow the detection of specific antigen fractions binding with the patient's IgE.

Clinical assays to detect food sensitivities have been fraught with inconsistency, and many reasons have been postulated to explain this. Important considerations to be taken into account when dealing with food allergies is the ability of the testing material to correctly reflect the material to which the patient is sensitive. Most testing material is composed of antigen mixtures or extracts from the raw food. The patient, however, ingests the food, usually after it is pretreated by washing and cooking in various ways. The prepared food is ingested to be further subjected to acid hydrolysis, enzymatic breakdown, association with other molecules, and absorption in the intestinal tract, where it finally interacts with cells of the immune system. Whether the antigens (allergens) at this time are significantly altered from the natural food before ingestion is a critical point. If the antigens have been changed significantly by digestion, the antibody or other immune effectors produced in the gastrointestinal tract may not react with the unaltered antigen used for testing.

Alteration of Antigenicity and Allergenicity of Foods

Immunodeterminants of antigens are expressed on the surface of the macromolecules. These macromolecules owe their three-dimensional shape in space to the primary structure of their amino acids, intramolecular associations by hydrogen bonding, and hydrophilic and hydrophobic interactions within the molecule and with the solvent, as well as other complex interactions. This tertiary structure is unique for particular proteins. Any alteration of the tertiary structure by chemical treatment, such as acid hydrolysis, heating, high salt concentrations, or large changes in ionic strength, can induce changes in the tertiary structure. The immunodeterminants, which were originally outside the molecule, may now be deep within the molecule, and new immunodeterminants can be exposed on the surface. These new immunodeterminants can give rise to antibodies and other effectors that have different specificities than those induced to the native antigen. The production of "new food antigens" (immunodeterminants) has been demonstrated using milk proteins or β-lactoglobulin. This digestive process was similar to that occuring during digestion [19-21].

The investigations of Haddad not only give evidence for the production of "new antigens" but strongly suggested that some of these new antigens produced are more allergenic than the native protein [19]. This differs from conclusions drawn by other investigators, who have also produced new antigen on enzymatic treatment. Their data give evidence that the undigested protein is still more allergenic than the new antigens produced. The individuals who react to the new antigens are therefore likely to react more strongly to the native allergens [20, 22].

Presentation of Antigen or Allergen to the Immune System

Evidence of Immune Reactions to Antigens Absorbed via the Intestinal Tract

For many years it was presumed that macromolecules did not enter the circulation via the intestinal pathway. It is now clear that antigen does pass through the intestinal tract, both intact and partially digested, directly interacting with cells of the immune system. This was initially thought to occur mainly in children. Investigators have shown that antibody to food was more common in young children than in adults. Antibody titers to food antigens usually decrease after the first year of age [23, 24].

Direct measurement of serum antigen after ingestion revealed that, in premature and newborn infants, antigenic material appeared in the serum. Older children and adults showed no detectable antigen in their serum on ingestion of the same concentration of antigen. It seems likely that more antigen is absorbed in the more immature gut [25, 26]. However, intraluminal injections of horse-radish peroxidase, a readily detectable macromolecule, has been used to show that high-molecular-weight substances can also be absorbed across the mature gut, where it can interact with cells of the immune system [27, 28].

Mechanisms of Absorption

The absorption of food antigens via the gut appears related to the concentration of ingested foods. One mechanism by which antigen transverses the gut into areas containing immunocompetent cells is essentially an invagination process, similar to phagocytosis. The antigens first are trapped by the microvillous membrane of the epithelium. After a certain concentration of antigen is reached within the membrane, invagination occurs, producing a phagosome that fuses with lysosomes to form phagolysosomes. Depending on the concentration of the antigen, all or some of the antigen may be digested in the phagolysosomes. Excess antigen may escape the process and become deposited in intercellular spaces by exocytosis. Antigen can also cross tight junctions between barrier cells of the gut and enter directly into the intercellular spaces [28, 29]. Both mechanisms of antigen transport apparently occur even in the mature gut, but to a much lesser extent. The amount of antigen that traverses the intestine by these mechanisms decreases with closure. At this time, the immunologic host defenses are more developed and the intestinal epithelial cells are more mature functionally and immunologically [28].

Specialized Mechanisms of Absorption Related to Immune Responsiveness

Antibody-Dependent Absorption. A facilitated uptake of antigens by the gut has been reported in animals. This uptake is dependent upon the presence of "opsonizing" antibodies and specific F_c receptors for these antibodies on epithelial surfaces of the microvilli. The specific receptors bind antibody, whether alone or in complexes. These antibodies induce phagosome formation and uptake. The antigen, if present, is thought to be protected from intracellular enzymes when complexed with antibodies, as is the antibody itself. The antibody class in animals, has been identified as IgG. This observation may have important clinical considerations if it is applicable to humans, in certain inflammatory conditions in which IgG is found intraluminally [30, 31].

Absorption via M Cells.   A specialized membranous epithelial cell, the M cell may be essential for antigenic assimilation by the gut with production of a protective local immune response by IgA. The M cell has specific characteristics that suggest this: (1) a congregation of these cells directly above gut-associated lymphoid tissues (Peyer's patches) so that direct interaction of antigen with lymphoid tissue can take place; (2) a concentration-dependent uptake of antigen, demonstrating preferential uptake of small amounts of antigen by the M cell; (3) a surface poor in microvilli; (4) poorly developed glycocalyx; (5) lack of lysosomal organelles, suggesting little or no digestion of antigen; and (6) release of the antigen directly to lymphoid cells circulating through Peyer's patches.

The concentration dependency of antigen uptake by the M cell may also have clinical implications. When large amounts of antigen are present within the lumen, there is uptake by other epithelial cells besides the M cells. This suggests the method of uptake and perhaps processing by the lymphoid tissue is dependent on concentration. The type of specific antigen processing could predetermine the type of effector to be produced [32-34].

All methods of antigen uptake by the gut appear to be dependent upon the ability of the antigen to interact strongly with the surface of the epithelial cells. Anything that would block this close contact of antigenic materials with the cell surface could interfere with uptake by the intestine. The gastric barrier, normal flora, mucous secretions, peristaltic movement, or other neutralization of antigen binding by intestinal secretory IgA can and does interfere with the uptake of antigen via the gut.

The concentration of antigen ingested may be extremely important in overcoming some of these protective mechanisms. Two considerations appear important in this respect. One is in areas of excess antigen, where an equilibrium condition exists for interaction at the microvillous surface; large amounts of antigen or foods may predispose to binding enough material so that the microvillous surfaces are induced to undergo endocytosis. This increased concentration could exceed the amount of material that could be handled effectively by the phagolysosomes of the cell. Antigens that are not completely digested because of the high concentration could then escape into the intercellular space by exocytosis, giving direct interactions with immunocompetent cells of the gut. The second consideration postulates that with high concentrations of material in the lumen, epithelial cells other than the M cells, are involved in the uptake of antigen. The uptake of antigen by cells other than the M cells could lead to the production of immune effectors other than secretory IgA.

Effects of Allergen or Antigen Presentation on the Immune Response

Influence on Induction of Immunity or Tolerance

It is clear that antigen is capable of entering the vascular compartment via the gastrointestinal and lymphoid systems. This route has been used intentionally to establish certain types of immunization. The Sabin polio vaccine is an example of the induction of immunity by this route. This vaccine, which is given orally, induces high concentrations of intestinal antibodies, particularly of the IgA type. The Salk polio vaccine, which is a killed vaccine and given parenterally, is not accompanied by significant concentration of antibody in the gastrointestinal secretions; therefore, the type of antigen and the route of immunization are important to the type of response obtained [35].

Not only is the type of antigen and its route of immunization important, but other considerations previously discussed must be taken into account to explain antigen effects on the host. Antigenic stimulation may induce, depending on its presentation, a state of tolerance, only a local initiation of immune reactive cells, or a general immune reactivity reflected systemically. In a beautifully conceived set of experiments by Pierce and Koster, some of the complexity and consideration of these interactions are pointed out. They showed that the priming of the cells of the jejunal lamina propria was achieved with intraperitoneal injection of antigen. After this initial priming, when the jejunal lamina propria cells were directly exposed to the antigen, a strong secondary antibody response was observed. Attempts at priming these same cells by the intravenous or subcutaneous route had no effect, and the cells were not primed. If the investigators first primed the cells of the jejunal lamina propria by direct exposure to the antigen and then attempted to induce a secondary response with the same antigen by intravenous, intraperitoneal, or subcutaneous routes, they saw no secondary response. On the contrary, they saw a suppression of the immune response. This antigen-specific suppression lasted for many weeks. Their work seems to suggest that the induction of priming and the induction of suppression are independent and depend on the cells with which the antigen initially interacts. In their experiments, the successful priming response suggests contact between the injected, intraperitoneal antigen and nonintestinal lymphoid cells that are precommitted to produce IgA; these committed cells then migrate to Peyer's patches to establish mucosal priming. Likewise, it appears that cells that mediated suppression of the mucosal response appear to be distributed throughout the systemic lymphoid tissue, and these were induced by intravenous and subcutaneous inoculations [36].

The results of the above studies, as well as investigations by others, could have important clinical correlations with both prevention of food allergy and its acquisition since they suggest that previous exposure by another route may influence the outcome of exposure via the gut. Therefore, previous exposure to airborne allergens or cross-reacting allergens via the respiratory tract could influence reactions seen at the mucous membranes of the gastrointestinal tract. Studies using cholera vaccine showed that mothers who had never been exposed to cholera made virtually no secretory antibody in breast milk when they received parenteral immunization to the cholera antigen. This is unlike a group of

Pakistani mothers who were previously exposed and who on parenteral immunization made a marked secretory IgA response [37].

ANTIBODIES INDUCED BY FOOD ANTIGENS

Antibody Class IgA

IgA production seems to be the most common response to mucous membrane stimulation by antigens. In the intestinal tract, secretory IgA is believed to function by neutralizing antigen uptake via mucosal barriers and thereby to limit and / or control the immunologic responses to antigen in the mucosal environs of the gastrointestinal tract. The IgA is thought to be produced by plasma cells in the region of antigenic stimulation. In the intestinal tract, the IgA is synthesized by lymphoid cells of the lamina propria. The molecule at this time is dimeric and contains a J piece. The dimeric IgA can then cross the intestinal epithelial cells by a specific transport system.

Transport of IgA to External Secretions

Transport via Epithelial Cells. The specialized transport system for IgA is initiated by glycoprotein synthesized by intestinal epithelial cells. This glycoprotein, termed the "secretory piece," is expressed on the surface of the intestinal epithelial cells, where it acts as a specific receptor for polymeric IgA and under certain circumstances for IgM. When dimeric IgA binds to this cell receptor, it stimulates endocytosis of the dimeric IgA now in close association with the secretory piece. This secretory IgA(sIgA) is transported in vesicles by the epithelial cells and released into the lumen by exocytosis [38].

Transport of IgA via the Liver. Another mechanism of transport for IgA to the bowel has been demonstrated. Large amounts of polymeric IgA can be transported from the plasma into the bile. This transport has been shown to be via the liver and is secretory piece dependent. It occurs only with polymeric IgA. Monomeric IgA transport has not been observed [39]. Investigation of this type of liver transport of IgA has shown that the secretory piece is expressed on the surface of hepatic parenchymal cells and the transport mechanism was apparently similar to that observed in intestinal epithelial cell transport [40].

Secretory IgA in Various Secretions. High concentrations of sIgA can appear in the bowel lumen from (1) locally induced and locally synthesized IgA secreted into the bowel by intestinal epithelial cells and (2) serum IgA synthesized in response to an antigen in the bowel or at distant sites not necessarily associated with mucous membranes and its recruitment via the liver pathway into the bowel.

Serum IgA. The IgA concentration within the serum can reflect IgA produced by antigens entering the mucous membranes of the gastrointestinal tract. If IgA is secreted by the lamina propria, it can go via the lymphatics through the thoracic duct and drain back into the bloodstream. This deposition of locally produced IgA in the serum would be dependent upon the amount of IgA secreted and the number of binding sites available locally on cell membranes to either facilitate secretion or binding of the IgA in situ.

Biologic Activity of IgA

The high concentration of secretory IgA in the bowel implies its importance as a deterrent to the intestinal uptake of antigenic material. Generally speaking, any type of antigen that must interact at cell surfaces can be neutralized or blocked by binding with sIgA. This blocking mechanism has been demonstrated with viruses, bacteria, toxins, and foods, preventing their attachment to cell surfaces.

Other important biologic characteristics of sIgA demonstrate the uniqueness and special attributes of this antibody in the protection of the mucous membranes. The ability to withstand enzymatic degradation is an extremely important feature, as it allows the antibody to remain biologically functional in areas where enzymes are especially active.

Since sIgA is not believed to activate the complement system by the classic or alternate pathway, its reaction with antigens on sensitive cell surfaces does not initiate a potentially harmful inflammatory response and may preclude secretory IgA from playing a direct role in hypersensitivity states.

Until recently, opsonization mediated by IgA was considered nonexistent. Recent work has demonstrated that IgA receptors on neutrophils facilitated binding of IgA-coated target cells. This IgA enhancement of phagocytosis was most effective when IgG was absent or in low concentrations. When IgG antibody increased, there was a marked decrease in IgA activity [41].

An enhancement of antibody-dependent cell-mediated cytotoxicity (ADCC) by human neutrophils, monocytes, and lymphocytes has been observed when sIgA has acted in conjunction with IgG [42].

Both opsonization and enhancement of ADCC activity are associated with F_c receptors for IgA on cell surfaces. These recent findings of $F_c \alpha$ receptors on T cells and non-T lymphocytes, as well as on monocytes and neutrophils, suggest biologic activities for IgA that have not been considered earlier, $F_c \alpha$-bearing T cells are apparently T-helper cells, and as such, they are probably important in regulatory responses associated with IgA [43].

Some of the newly described activities associated with IgA make it tempting to speculate that the molecule acts in other ways than the simple blocking of antigen interactions at cell surfaces. Antigens, if they did enter the systems, could be removed before they interacted with distant lymphoid tissues, initiating other types of antibody or cellular responses. It is also possible that some of these newly described activities could play some role in certain types of hypersensitivity states, perhaps mediated through a mechanism like ADCC.

Antibody Class IgM

The presence of IgM-containing B cells in the lamina propria of humans has recently been shown [44]. These cells seem capable of activation by antigen with the local production of antibody. In humans, IgM has a strong association with secretory piece, with which it binds with high affinity [45].

Transport of IgM to External Secretions

It appears that IgM can transport via the intestinal epithelium by binding to the secretory piece in a fashion similar to that of IgA. This secretion of IgM seems competitive with IgA, in that if IgA is present, little IgM is transported. In IgA deficiency states, IgM can be found in the intestine in fairly high concentrations, having been transported there via the secretory mechanism. It is possible, since transport occurs via the secretory piece, that IgM could be transported across hepatic cells, again in a fashion similar to that described for IgA.

Biologic Properties of IgM

IgM is an avid binder of antigen because of its multiple binding sites. It has been shown to be an efficient opsonizing antibody and activates complement by the classic pathway. It can act as a cytotoxic antibody in the presence of complement or in ADCC.

If IgM is present in secretions, it can theoretically bind with antigen, complex in such a way as to form an insoluble readily phagocytized complex, and remove it from the system. It could also be possible that it forms aggregates with antigen that inhibit intestinal absorption. If IgM was formed in the lamina propria in high concentrations, it could travel via the lymphatics through the thoracic duct back into the bloodstream. It could then act with specific antigens that induced its production to form either soluble or insoluble complexes in the serum compartment. The type of complex formed would be dependent upon the amount of specific IgM available, as well as the concentration and nature of the antigen to which it is reacting. IgM could also form complexes with antigen within the intercellular spaces and travel via the lymphatics through the thoracic duct back into the blood.

If reactions of food antigens with IgM take place in areas other than in external secretions, this reaction could lead to a more rapid clearance, depending again on the size and solubility of the complex or to a hypersensitivity state mediated through type III and possibly type II mechanisms.

allergic symptoms with the appropriate food or fraction of the food in blind challenge testing [18, 19]. In vitro testing has also shown specific IgE binding to particular antigenic components of food antigens [19-22].

Type II Hypersensitivities

Cytotoxic antibodies, most probably of the IgG and/or IgM class, appear to be theoretically possible. Food antigens, native or altered, capable of binding to cell surfaces could result in this type of hypersensitivity. Studies that have shown a decrease in platelets in milk-induced anaphylaxis strongly suggest this possibility [59].

Type III Hypersensitivities

The production of immune complexes to food antigens has been found by several investigators [60, 61]. This type of hypersensitivity is demonstrated most clearly when there is a selective IgA deficiency. In this condition, ingestion of food antigens is followed by occurrence of immune complexes and/or circulating food proteins [62].

Type IV Hypersensitivities

Activation of T cells by orally presented antigens has been reported to lead to hypersensitivity reactions of the delayed type [63]. There have also been reports of cytotoxic lymphocytes in Peyer's patches and the induction of cellular reactions of T lymphocytes to milk antigens [64]. In animal studies, the passive transfer of primed T lymphocytes from the thoracic duct of rats infected with *N. brasiliensis* to a nonsensitized recipient induces goblet cell hyperplasia in noninfected animals [65].

CONTROL OF IMMUNE REACTIONS TO FOOD ANTIGENS IN THE GASTROINTESTINAL TRACT

Lymphoid cells with specific immune functions appear to have a predilection to migrate to specified areas of the reticuloendothelial system. Immunocytes of the mucosal surfaces are particularly rich in IgA precursor B cells and T-helper cells, which are IgA specific. There is mounting evidence that precommitted cells found in mucous membranes of one area may migrate as needed to other mucous membranes. Experiments eliciting specific IgA in the gastrointestinal tract by feeding and the subsequent detection of IgA-secreting cells of that specificity in secretions of lactating females suggest that some of the specific migration patterns might be hormonally controlled. This pattern of specific migration of cooperating cell populations to specified areas of mucosal lymphoid tissue has been termed "the common mucosal immune system" [66, 67].

We will sketch the essence of the mucosal immune system, as others will describe it more fully in this book. Following antigenic stimulation, precommitted B cells within the Peyer's patches of the gut migrate via the mesenteric lymph nodes into the circulation and then to the thoracic duct into systemic circulation, from where they can home into the diffuse lymphoid tissues of the gastrointestinal tract, lung, breast, genitourinary tract, and so on. This elaborate network seems most important in limiting a limitless number of ubiquitous antigens from reaching cells of the immune system. It is, undoubtedly, an important controlling mechanism when considering reactions to food antigens [66, 67].

Many investigators have described the requirements for T-helper lymphocytes for the production of IgE antibody via appropriate B cells [68]. It follows that T-helper cells must be present in the area of IgE production.

Ishizaka and Adachi have described production of specific T-helper cells when normal splenic lymphocytes of syngenetic animals were exposed to macrophages of animals sensitized to ovalbumin. This interaction of sensitized macrophages with normal nonsensitized splenic lymphocytes induced the formation of T-helper cells specific for IgE formation in vitro. It was also observed that when soluble ovalbumin was presented in the absence of macrophages, T-suppressor cells specific for IgE were generated instead [69].

Feeding experiments with animals have demonstrated that a previously fed antigenic substance would upon a second exposure of the same antigen produce specific T-helper cells for that antigen within the Peyer's patches [70]. Other experimenters have shown that adoptively transferred Peyer's patches containing T lymphocytes from animals given ovalbumin orally would inhibit the in vitro production of IgG and IgE. They also showed the lymphocytes from Peyer's patches were more easily tolerized than spleen cells removed from the same animal and that fewer Peyer's patches lymphocytes were needed for inducing tolerance in normal mice compared with that of the spleen cells. These investigators concluded from their studies that the lymphocytes of the Peyer's patches may be the source for T-suppressor cells in immunologic reactions of the gut, especially those dealing with IgE [71].

FUTURE NEEDS OF FOOD IMMUNOLOGY

The material presented in this chapter points out the complexity of antigen-induced immunologic reactions in the gastrointestinal tract. Much work still has to be done to understand more clearly the mechanisms that induce and control these responses. The need to characterize antigens that are present or induced in foods before and after processing and digestion are obvious. The generation of "new antigens" and altered antigenic reactivity needs extensive investigation, as this could have significant clinical application.

The concept of precommitted migration patterns of effector and controlling cells in the mucosal system is in its infancy where IgE is concerned. There seems to be mounting evidence that much of this migration may be under hormonal control and specific antigenic stimulation. This concept might be relevant for controlling responses to food antigens, as it already has been suggested that certain pathologies observed in the gastrointestinal tract could be caused, not by the presence of a specific antigen per se, but by altered migration patterns, where appropriate cells might be in geographic areas of lymphoid tissues, resulting injury to the host.

The geography of cell populations within the intestinal tract deserves more attention. The ability to recognize where appropriate T-helper cells, T-suppressor cells, and others are located within the lymphoid tissues would give one a distinct advantage in delivering appropriate antigens to locations of a particular cell type. This type of approach would be most interesting, especially to the allergist who is specifically trying to induce a suppression to those allergens that produce clinical symptoms.

The presence and significance of soluble immune complexes induced by food antigens has yet to be explained fully. In order for a complete study of this type of phenomena, however, one will need more information about the affinity of antibodies produced in the gastrointestinal tract and the size and solubility of complexes formed. This will be dependent upon the amount of antigen that could bind with the appropriate antibody. Concentration effects seem to be an overriding concern.

New and accurate methods for measuring and characterizing immune complexes are, it is hoped, on their way and may shed some new light on this very important aspect of reactions to food antigens.

The hypersensitivity states induced by cellular effectors remain virtually untouched. The significance of ADCC and the formation of activated T cells with the production of lymphokines seems relevant in that the effector, or its product, may interact with cells of the gastrointestinal tract, inducing or amplifying inflammatorylike responses.

SUMMARY

In summary, then, it has been demonstrated that antibodies can be made to food antigens. The antibodies can be of any class, with IgA the predominant antibody class induced. It has also been shown that antigens can be altered in such a way that antibodies with new specificities are produced, reacting with only the "new antigenic determinants." Whether these new antigens are relevant to the clinician has yet to be determined, but there seems to be no reason to suspect that some of the new antigens produced would not be important clinical entities.

It appears that the body by its geographic distribution of effector and controlling cells of the immune system has set up a barrier to avoid large numbers of ubiquitous antigens from entering its system. This system seems to revolve around IgA, which selectively coats antigens blocking absorption on the intestinal barrier and other mucous membranes. This antibody is exquisitely suited to its task because of its stability to various enzyme systems and its ability to traverse the epithelial barrier into sections of high concentrations. It is also not surprising that the accessory cells for the production of IgA seem to be strategically located within the mucosal system so that IgA is formed to the near exclusion of the other antibody classes. This can be seen with the large number of specific IgA T-helper cells associated with the precommitted B cells. The areas that are rich in T-helper cells for IgA seem to have negligible T-suppressor activities for that antibody but have a large number of T-suppressor cells for IgG and IgM. It appears that the body has developed a system to specifically induce secretory IgA in areas where antigens are in constant contact with the host via the mucous membranes so that these ubiquitous antigens are kept from initiating an uncalled-for serum compartment protective response utilizing IgG and/or IgM unnecessarily. This would hold for the upper respiratory tract as well as the gastrointestinal tract. This similarity strongly suggests that a large, or at least a moderate, number of individuals would also produce high enough quantities of IgE so that type I reactions to foods may not be as rare as previously thought.

REFERENCES

1. M. Atassi, *Immunochemistry, 12*:423 (1975).
2. M. Crumpton, in *The Antigens* (M. Sela, ed.), Vol. 2. Academic Press, New York, 1974.
3. H. K. Beard, W. Page-Faulk, L. E. Glynn, and L. B. Conachie, in *Immunochemistry: An Advanced Textbook* (L. E. Glynn and M. W. Steward, eds.). John Wiley and Sons, New York, 1977.
4. M. O. Dayhoff and R. V. Eck, in *Atlas of Protein Sequence and Structure.* National Biomedical Research Foundation, Silver Spring, Maryland, 1969.
5. W. D. Armstrong, E. Diener, and G. R. Shellam, *J. Exp. Med., 129*:3951 (1969).
6. M. Feldmann and A. Basten, *J. Exp. Med., 134*:103 (1971).
7. J. G. Howard, G. H. Christie, B. H. Courtenay, E. Leuchars, and J. S. Davis, *Cell. Immunol., 2*:614 (1971).
8. M. Sela, E. Moses, and G. M. Shearer, *Proc. Natl. Acad. Sci. USA, 64*:2696 (1972).
9. A. T. Ichiki and C. R. Parish, *Cell Immunol., 4*:264 (1972).

10. C. R. Parish, *J. Exp. Med., 134*:1 (1971).
11. H. C. Thomas, R. N. McSween, and R. G. White, *Lancet, 1*:1288 (1973).
12. E. J. Miller, in *Immunologic Diseases,* 2d ed. (J. Samter et al., eds.). Little, Brown, Boston, 1971.
13. B. Benacerraf, *Science, 212*:1229 (1980).
14. D. G. Marsh, S. H. Physo, R. Hussain, et al., *J. Allergy & Clin. Immunol., 65*: 322 (1980).
15. R. M. Rothberg, S. C. Kraft, and R. S. Farr, *J. Immunol., 98*:386 (1967).
16. E. Bleumink, *World Rev. Nutr. Diet., 12*:505 (1970).
17. G. K. T. Holmes, P. Asquith, and W. T. Cooke, *Clin. Exp. Immunol., 24*:259 (1976).
18. N. Shibasaki, S. Suzuki, H. Nemoto, and T. Ckuroume, *J. Allergy & Clin. Immunol., 64*:259 (1979).
19. Z. H. Haddad, V. Kalra, and S. Verma, *Ann. Allergy, 42*:368 (1979).
20. H. R. Schwartz, L. S. Nerurkar, J. R. Spies, R. T. Scanlon, and J. A. Bellanti, *Ann. Allergy, 45*:242 (1980).
21. J. R. Spies, M. A. Stevan, W. I. Stein, and E. J. Coulson, *J. Allergy Clin. Immunol., 45*:208 (1970).
22. D. R. Hoffman, *J. Allergy Clin. Immunol., 71*:481 (1983).
23. T. Matsumura, T. Kuromi, A. Mitomo, and K. Kabasahi, *Int. Arch. Allergy Appl. Immunol., 30*:341 (1966).
24. E. Gold and G. Godek, *Am. J. Dis. Child., 102*:542 (1961).
25. R. M. Rothberg, *J. Pediatr., 75*:391 (1969).
26. E. J. Eastham, T. Lichauco, M. I. Grady, and W. A. Walker, *J. Pediatr., 93*: 561 (1978).
27. R. Cornell, R. W. Walker, and K. J. Isselbacher, *Lab. Invest., 25*:42 (1971).
28. W. A. Walker, *Clin. Immunol. Allergol., 2*:15 (1982).
29. W. A. Walker and K. J. Isselbacher, *Gastroenterology, 67*:531 (1974).
30. D. R. Abrahamson, A. Powers, and R. Rodewald, *Science, 206*:567 (1979).
31. P. Brandtzaeg, *Nature, 266*:262 (1977).
32. D. E. Bockman and M. D. Cooper, *Am. J. Anat., 136*:455 (1973).
33. R. L. Owen, *Gastroenterology, 72*:440 (1977).
34. W. A. Walker, *Arch. Dis. Child., 53*:527 (1978).
35. T. L. Ogra, D. T. Karzon, and N. MacGillivarey, *N. Engl. J. Med., 279*:893 (1968).
36. N. F. Pierce and F. T. Koster, *J. Immunol., 124*:307 (1980).
37. A. M. Svennerholm, J. Holmgren, L. A. Hansen, B. S. Lindblad, F. Quereshi, and R. J. Rahimtoola, *Scand. J. Immunol., 6*:1345 (1977).
38. R. J. Genco, R. Linzer, and R. T. Evans, *Ann. N.Y. Acad. Sci., 409*:650 (1983).
39. B. L. Delacroix and J. T. Vaerman, *Ann. N.Y. Acad. Sci., 409*:383 (1983).
40. D. J. Sacken, K. N. Jeejeebhoy, H. Bazin, and B. J. Underdown, *J. Exp. Med., 50*:1538 (1979).

41. M. W. Fanger, S. N. Goldstein, and L. Shen, *Ann. N. Y. Acad. Sci.*, *409*:552 (1983).
42. L. Shen and M. W. Fanger, *Cell Immunol.*, *59*:79 (1981).
43. M. H. Endoh, Y. Sakai, Y. Nomoto, and H. Kaneshige, *J. Immunol.*, *127*: 2612 (1981).
44. R. T. MacDermott, M. G. Beale, S. D. Alley, G. S. Nash, M. J. Bertovich, and M. J. Bragdon, *Ann. N. Y. Acad. Sci.*, *409*:498 (1983).
45. J. J. Socken and B. J. Underdown, *Immunochemistry*, *15*:499 (1978).
46. P. Brantzaege and K. Baklien, *Acta Histochem.*, *21*:105 (1980).
47. J. Yodoi and K. Ishizaka, *J. Immunol.*, *124*:1322 (1980).
48. K. S. Durkin and B. H. Man, *High concentrations of IgE and IgA bearing cells in Peyer's patches of germ-free rats, Proc. Natl. Acad. Sci. USA, 38*: 1081 (1979).
49. H. G. Durkin, H. Bazin, and B. H. Waksman, *J. Exp. Med.*, *154*:640 (1981).
50. T. A. E. Platt-Mills, *J. Immunol.*, *122*:2218 (1979).
51. K. G. Huggins and J. Brostoff, *Lancet*, *2*:148 (1975).
52. J. Bienenstock, A. D. Befus, F. Pearce, D. Denbeurg, and R. Goodacre, *J. Allergy Clin. Immunol.*, *70*:407.
53. J. J. Harris, V. Petts, and R. Penny, *Aust. Paediatr. J.*, *13*:276 (1977).
54. A. Capron, A. J. Dezzin, M. Capron, and H. Bazin, *Nature*, *253*:474 (1975).
55. A. Haque, A. Ouaîssi, M. Joseph, M. Capron, and A. Capron, *J. Immunol.*, *127*:716 (1981).
56. J. Ruitenberg and J. Steerenberg, *J. Parasitol.*, *60*:1056 (1974).
57. R. C. Welliver and T. L. Ogra, *Ann. N. Y. Acad. Sci.*, *409*:321 (1983).
58. F. Arnaud-Battandier, B. M. Bundy, M. O'Neill, J. Bienenstock, and D. L. Nelson, *J. Immunol.*, *12*:000 (1978).
59. A. Lambert, P. H. Falmon, and J. Falmon, *Acta Allergol. (Kbh.)*, *22*:209 (1967).
60. R. I. Carr, M. Andrist, and F. McDuffie, *Studies on the possibility of food induced immune complex disease, Proc. Natl. Acad. Sci. USA, 35*:574 (1976).
61. J. Penner, L. A. Katz, and F. Milgrom, *Lancet, 1*:669 (1978).
62. C. Cunningham-Rundles, W. E. Brandies, R. A. Good, and N. K. Day, *Mild precipitation, circulating immune complexes and IgA deficiency, Proc. Natl. Acad. Sci. USA, 75*:3387 (1978).
63. J. L. Parroto, L. M. Hangl, J. J. Isselbacher, and K. S. Warren, *J. Exp. Med.*, *140*:296 (1974).
64. M. F. Kagnoff, *J. Immunol.*, *130*:395 (1978).
65. H. R. T. Miller and Y. Nawa, *Nouv. Rev. Fr. Hematol.*, *21*:31 (1979).
66. J. Bienenstock and A. D. Befus, *Immunology*, *41*:249 (1980).
67. M. R. McDermott and J. Bienenstock, *J. Immunol.*, *124*:2536 (1980).
68. K. Ishizaka, in *Cellular Events in the IgE Antibody Response and Advances in Immunology*, (H. G. Kunkel and S. J. Dixon, eds.). Academic Press, New York, 1976, Vol. 23, p. 1.

69. K. Ishizaka and T. Adachi, *J. Immunol., 117*:40 (1976).
70. N. F. Kagnoff, *J. Exp. Med., 142*:1425 (1975).
71. L. S. Kind, *J. Immunol., 120*:861 (1978).

3

Gastroenterology of Food Hypersensitivity

AUBREY J. KATZ

Harvard Medical School and The Children's Hospital, Boston, Massachusetts

Adverse reaction to foods are a feature of many gastrointestinal diseases. Although food hypersensitivity may account for some of these reactions, other causes, such as malabsorption, toxic effects from contaminents, additives, and psychological factors, should always be considered.

The clinical symptoms and signs of gastrointestinal food hypersensitivity depend upon the site of the gastrointestinal tract involvement. Food sensitivity may result in inflammation from the esophagus to the rectum. These patients may present with signs and symptoms of esophagitis, gastritis, enteropathy, and/or colitis, singly or in combination.

DEVELOPMENT OF ENTEROPATHY

Involvement of the small intestine is the hallmark of food sensitivity and is most commonly involved in gastrointestinal food sensitivity. Thus the development of enteropathy is the cornerstone of this chapter.

The functional unit of the small intestine is the villus and the crypt. As shown in Figure 1, the ratio of the villus to crypt is 4:1. As these cells migrate up the crypt, they aquire their full complement of disaccharidases. The normal cycle of epithelial cell renewal takes about 4 days [1]. The surface intestinal lining consists of regular columnar epithelial cells with basal nuclei. There are normally very few intraepithelial lymphocytes. The lamina propria consists of many cell types, most notably plasma cells, eosinophils, lymphocytes, fibroblasts, and macrophages. The predominant cell, the plasma cell, produces secretory IgA, both, subtypes IgA_1 and IgA_2. By rule of thumb, the length of

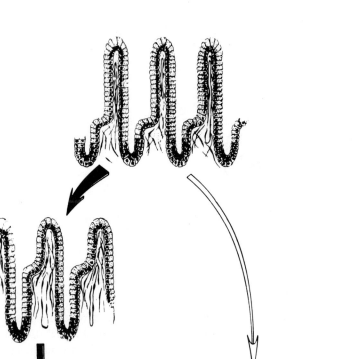

Figure 1   Evolution of the flat villus lesion.

the small intestine is about 2½–3 times the length of the body. The villi in the ileum are somewhat shorter than those in the jejunum, but any insult or resection that removes a large amount of jejunun will result in compensatory hypertrophy of the distal ileal villi.

The development of enteropathy or the flat gut syndrome is due to two basic mechanisms [2]. The prime one, which accounts for about 90% of enteropathies, occurs when the insult, be it a virus, parasite, allergy inflammation, or other event, results in epithelial cell damage. Compensatory crypt hypertrophy then ensues to compensate for this loss. If the insult continues, flattening of the villi occurs. The cells now lining the surface epithelium are immature crypt cells, which as we mentioned previously have a low complement of disaccharidases. This is the commonest mechanism for the development of a secondary disaccharidase deficiency, most notably lactase deficiency. This mechanism, as pointed out by Booth [3], is analogous to a hemolytic anemia, with the crypt cells akin to bone marrow cells and the villus cells to the peripheral blood cells. The rarer type of flat gut is characterized by short crypts; this is analogous to aplastic anemia. (See Figs. 1 and 2.) In addition to the villus and crypt changes, the lamina propria becomes infiltrated with specific types of cells, depending on the etiology of the inflammation, notably a large increase in the number of plasma cells. Etiologies of the flat gut are listed in Tables 1 and 2.

The development of diarrhea and/or malabsorption in patients with a flat gut syndrome, irrespective of etiology, depends on various factors. Primarily it is related to the extent of gut involvement and the degree of inflammation. Specific factors involved are as follows.

1. Secondary disaccharidase deficiency. Removal of lactose from the diet, for example, will alleviate diarrhea in any cause of the flat gut syndrome, since the osmotic effect of lactose will be removed.
2. Bile salt loss. Inflammation involving the distal ileum may prevent the reabsorption of bile salts. Increased bile acids in the colon lead to diarrhea; this form of diarrhea is ameliorated by the use of cholestyramine.
3. The hormones that influence pancreatic secretion and gallbladder contraction are located primarily in the surface epithelium of the small intestine. Thus, severe damage to the small intestinal mucosa results in decreased production of these hormones. In patients with the flat gut syndrome due to celiac disease, for example, pancreatic insufficiency and decreased contractility of the gallbladder contribute extensively to the malabsorption in this disease.

GLUTEN-SENSITIVE ENTEROPATHY (CELIAC DISEASE)

Gluten-sensitive enteropathy (GSE), or celiac disease, is a genetic disorder resulting in lifelong sensitivity to gluten, rye, oats, and barley. It is characterized clinically by malabsorption and pathologically by a flat villus lesion. Both are reversed by withdrawal of gluten from the diet and exacerbated on gluten challenge [4].

One of the earliest descriptions of this disease is attributed to Gee [5], who in 1888 thought that if the patient was to be cured at all, it must be by means of diet. Unfortunately, he chose bread and water. Gluten sensitivity remains the prime example of gastrointestinal food sensitivity. It was only in 1959 that Dicke in Holland described the role of gluten in this disease. He had noted that in Holland during World War II, the incidence of celiac disease decreased markedly

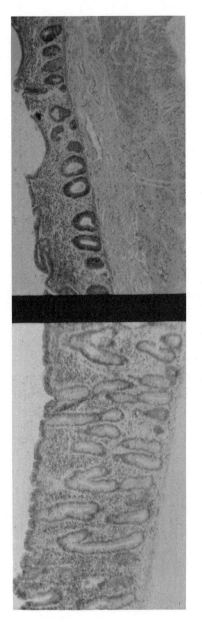

Figure 2 (left) Flat gut with crypt hypertrophy. (right) Flat gut, no crypt hypertrophy.

Table 1 Flat Gut Syndrome with No Crypt Hypertrophy

Chemotherapy: Methotrexate
Radiation therapy
Familial enteropathy

Table 2 Etiologies of the Flat Gut Syndrome (Enteropathy)

Infection
    Viral (rotovirus)
    Bacteria (*E. coli*)
    Parasitic (*Giardia*)
    Fungal (*Candida*)
Food hypersensitivity
    Gluten-sensitive enteropathy
    Milk-sensitive enteropathy
    Soy-sensitive enteropathy
    Eosinophilic gastroenteropathy
Tropical sprue
Immunodeficiency syndromes
    Transient hypogammaglobulinemia
    Acquired hypo- or disgammaglobulinemia
    Severe combined immunodeficiency
Protein calorie malnutrition
    (kwashiorkor, not marasmus)
Lymphoma
Crohn's disease
Whipple's disease
Zollinger-Ellison syndrome
Familial enteropathy

and that patients with celiac disease improved clinically, whereas after the war, the incidence of celiac disease returned to its prewar state and patients with the disease again developed symptoms. Looking for the link between food and this disease, he noted that wheat, which had been in plentiful supply before and after the war, was limited in supply to the Dutch people during the war. He therefore hypothesized that wheat was the cause of the syndrome, and this was subsequently borne out.

Pathology

Gluten sensitivity is limited to the small intestine. The esophagus, stomach, and colon are not involved. The hallmark of the small bowel biopsy in celiac disease is the flat gut. In any of the other conditions, except that in celiac disease the enteropathy is diffuse and not patchy. In other words, if one uses a capsule to obtain a small bowel biopsy of several fragments and there is a discrepancy between the samples, that is, some have evidence of flat gut and others are normal, this would virtually exclude the diagnosis of celiac disease and favor another etiology [6], provided the patient is on a regular (gluten-containing) diet.

Pathogenesis

The precise mechanism by which gluten produces the remarkable change in the intestinal mucosa of sensitive subjects is not known. The data regarding the pathogenesis of this disease have grown markedly over the last 30 years. Early theories favored gluten-sensitive enteropathy as a disease due to an inborn error of metabolism. However, evaluation only showed enzyme deficiencies in the presence of the flat gut, whereas studies of tissue from patients in remission never demonstrated any enzyme deficiency at all.

During the 1960s and the 1970s, when immunology was developing rapidly, features of celiac disease favored an immune mechanism for this disease. These factors included several observations that showed the presence of circulating anti-gluten antibodies in the bloodstream of patients with this disease. Plasma cells were increased in the lamina propria of the mucosa with increased local IgA synthesis; 50% of the increase in IgA was found to be specific anti-gluten antibody [7]. Intraepithelial lymphocytes were markedly increased in number. These have been recently shown to be T_8 cells (suppressor or cytotoxic cells). Wall et al. demonstrated that the patients with active gluten-sensitive enteropathy could be placed into remission by treatment with oral steroids [8], despite ingestion of gluten. This was corroborated in organ culture experiments [9].

To study the role of local immune responses and to determine whether gluten could be directly toxic to intestinal mucosal tissue, an in vitro model of gluten-sensitive enteropathy was developed by Falchuk et al. [10] using the organ culture techniques of Browning and Trier [11]. In the organ culture technique, intestinal biopsy specimens are cultured for periods of 24–48 hr. Tissue morphology and brush-border enzyme activity serve as markers of tissue condition. In organ culture of normal intestinal mucosa, brush-border alkaline phosphatase and other enzyme activities increase, indicating general maturation of immature crypt cells. Culture of gluten-sensitive enteropathy tissue in a gluten-free medium results in a similar maturation, with a dramatic increase in alkaline phosphatase activity. These changes are accompanied by the development of tall columnar epithelial cells with mature brush borders. This enzymatic and morphological change represents an in vitro remission of gluten-sensitive enteropathy. Cultures of tissue in the presence of gluten result in perpetuation of the abnormality with a minimal rise in alkaline phasphtase, and no improvement in morphology.

Culture of tissue in the presence and absence of gluten thus represents a model for gluten-sensitive enteropathy. Other foods, such as casein or β-lactoglobulin, do not result in perpetuation of the abnormality. When tissue from patients with gluten-sensitive enteropathy in remission is cultured in the presence of gluten, no difference is found. This suggests that gluten protein is not directly toxic to the epithelial cells of patients with gluten-sensitive enteropathy but that an endogenous effector mechanism must first be activated. When remission tissue is cultured with exacerbation tissue in the presence of gluten, the remission tissue appears susceptible to the toxic effect of gluten [12]. This experiment supports the concept that the active tissue produces either a lymphokine or sensitized cells, which can cross the medium and render the remission tissue sensitive to the effect of gluten. If cortisone is added to the gluten-containing medium, no inhibition by gluten occurs [9]. Steroids thus interfere with gluten toxicity. This mechanism remains unknown. It could be through either the steroid effect on the immune system or lysosomal stabilization. On the other hand, it may have nothing to do with the inhibition of gluten activity, since I have seen some patients with a flat gut syndrome not due to celiac disease in whom steroids have resulted in remission (unpublished observations).

Genetic Studies

In 1972, two separate investigative groups found that HLA-B_8 is found in 60–80% of patients with GSE, in contrast with 20–25% of this antigen in the normal population [13, 14]. Moreover, HLA-DW_3, a second HLA antigen, is present in 80% of patients with GSE. The HLA system is located on the sixth chromosome. Various markers on the sixth chromosome have also been found to be specifically increased in patients with gluten-sensitive enteropathy. The finding of these specific antigens, as well as the fact that celiac disease occurs to a much greater degree in populations with a high incidence of these genes, supports the concept that somehow these specific antigens are related to the development of the disease. However, 20% of patients with celiac disease have none of these antigens, and 20% of the normal population with these antigens do not have celiac disease. It should be mentioned, however, that 10% of the family members of patients with celiac disease may have the disease on biopsy but have no clinical symptoms. An acceptable control group, therefore, should have normal small bowel biopsies.

A higher frequency of HLA-B$_8$ is associated with other diseases in which generalized immune hyperresponsiveness occurs; these include myasthenia gravis, juvenile diabetes (type 2 diabetes), chronic active hepatitis, and Sjögren's syndrome. The mechanism, however, that results in the interaction between specific gene products governed by the sixth chromosome and gluten is still unknown. It is hypothesized that these genes govern specific receptors and their response to gluten on the surface epithelial cells [12].

Clinical Features

A classic description of a child with celiac disease is that of an irritable, anorectic child with chronic diarrhea, failure to thrive, a pot belly, and muscle wasting, particularly of the buttocks and proximal limbs [4]. The adult with this disease may in fact present in the same way, even with the pot belly and muscle wasting.

It should be noted that, in childhood, the common age for the onset and diagnosis of the disease is between 9 and 18 months. The disease occurs later in breast-fed babies, rather than bottle-fed babies, not because of any immune mechanism but solely because breast-fed babies tend to be fed gluten later than bottle-fed babies. It is much less common to diagnose the disease in adolescence for the first time, whereas in adulthood the incidence of diagnosis once again increases. Reasons for this age distribution at time of diagnosis are unclear and led investigators to surmise that gluten sensitivity was transient. Furthermore, "celiac children", despite cheating on their diets as they grew up, did not redevelop symptoms. Subsequent studies, however, demonstrated that so-called normal patients had abnormal biopsies despite a lack of clinical symptomatology [6]. Many theories evolved as to why these patients are asymptomatic, the most common that initially only proximal bowel involvement occurs, with sparing of the distal bowel; absorption therefore occurs distally and masks frank clinical malabsorption.

Many patients, not surprisingly, will not present with the classic form of diarrhea and malabsorption but with atypical features of celiac disease because of selective malabsorption [15]. These include growth failure alone, without gastrointestinal disease; anemia secondary to iron deficiency; folate deficiency or, rarely, B$_{12}$ deficiency; and osteoporosis or rickets. Many older women are classically diagnosed with postmenopausal osteoporosis, when in fact they may have osteoporosis on the basis of malabsorption. Bleeding disorders secondary to vitamin K deficiency or edema secondary to hypoalbuminemia have been described in several patients.

Of patients with dermatitis herpetiformis, an extremely pruritic, papulo-vesicular eruption of the skin, 80–90% have an associated gluten-sensitive entero-pathy [16]. Both the intestinal and eventually the skin lesions respond to gluten withdrawal [17]. This has not been described in childhood.

Diagnostic Evaluation

Diagnostic evaluation of a patient with gluten-sensitive enteropathy is that of malabsorption in general. In children, a sweat test should be performed in all patients. Cystic fibrosis is the commonest cause for malabsorption in childhood, and the coexistence of cystic fibrosis and gluten-sensitive enteropathy has been described [17]. Blood tests would indicate an anemia. Bleeding studies may indicate prolongation of prothrombin time. A 72-hr stool fat test will demon-strate the presence of steatorrhea. The xylose test and the lactose test may be abnormal, indicating intestinal mucosal damage. It must be emphasized, how-ever, that in some patients these tests may be normal because of the initial proxi-mal distribution of the disease. Intestinal biopsy has to be performed in all cases to make this diagnosis.

Treatment

The initial therapy includes omitting gluten, rye, oats, and barley, as well as lactose, from the diet. Lactose is withdrawn from the diet for a period of 6 weeks. The removal of lactose from the diet results in alleviation of some of the osmotic diarrhea. Lactose is then reintroduced after 6 weeks, provided the patient can tolerate it.

The most dramatic improvement initially is that of the central nervous system component. It is rather remarkable that patients with this disease have a marked tendency for irritability and easy frustration; after institution of a gluten-free diet, there is a complete change in personality. Diarrhea takes about 6 weeks to resolve.

It may take 6 months to 1 year for the biopsy to completely return to normal, provided the patient has remained on a strict gluten-free diet. Because there are other causes of the flat gut syndrome, some of which may in fact respond somewhat to withdrawal of gluten and lactose purely on the basis of symptoms, one has to be really sure that the patient indeed does have celiac disease.

When the patient is feeling well, 6 months to 1 year after the initial biopsy, and all blood tests are normal, the patient undergoes a second biopsy to assure that the small bowel mucosa is normal. The patient is then placed on a gluten challenge. It is important to emphasize that during the gluten challenge the majority of patients have no symptoms, and this should not dissuade one from performing the third biopsy. The patient is given gluten for 6 weeks. This can be administered in various forms. A minimum amount of two slices of bread per day or 10 gr of gluten powder should suffice. If the biopsy is abnormal and demonstrates a flat gut, the diagnosis is substantiated. If the biopsy is absolutely normal and the patient has been ingesting adequate amounts of gluten during this challenge, this probably rules out the diagnosis of celiac disease. Although some reports suggest a longer time of gluten challenge may be needed [18]. In this situation, the patient is kept on a gluten-containing diet for at least 1 year and then rebiopsied. If the mucosa is still normal, the disease is effectively ruled out. On the other hand, if the patient becomes symptomatic before the year is up, the patient is biopsied earlier.

Follow-up

The literature appears to suggest that patients with celiac disease are at a greater risk for the development of gastrointestinal malignancy than are other patients. This malignancy usually takes the form of lymphoma [19]. Initial studies could not differentiate between the flat gut due to lymphoma or celiac disease, since the development of lymphoma occurred so quickly after the original diagnosis. Subsequent data, however, tend to support the fact that lymphoreticular malignancies do in fact appear in patients with celiac disease. It should be emphasized, however, that the incidence appears to be low. There is no evidence of difference in incidence whether or not the patient adheres to the gluten-free diet.

COW'S MILK PROTEIN SENSITIVITY

Cow's milk protein sensitivity is a common food sensitivity in infants, with an incidence estimated at 0.5–5% of all infants less than 1 year old. It is rare in older children and adults.

Pathology

Unlike gluten-sensitive enteropathy, in which the sensitivity is limited to the small intestine, cow's milk sensitivity can affect the stomach with subsequent gastritis [20], the small intestine with an enteropathy [20], and the colon with colitis [21]. The symptoms and signs of this entity therefore depend on which organ system is more involved. Eosinophilic infiltration of tissues is the hallmark. Gastric involvement of this disease is usually limited to the antrum. Inflammation of the antrum with eosinophilic infiltration should always alert one to an allergic etiology (see Fig. 3). The small intestine reveals a patchy, flat villus lesion with varying degrees of eosinophilic infiltration. Colonic involvement is also patchy in nature; therefore, in many of these patients it is not unusual to perform a sigmoidoscopy and see evidence of colitis and yet obtain a normal

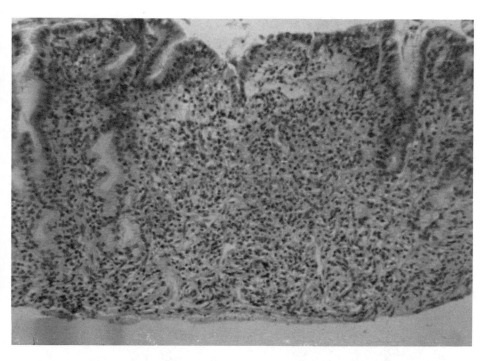

Figure 3 Gastric antral mucosal biopsy. Extensive necrosis of glands; inflammatory exudate with many eosinophils. (X54) (Reproduced with permission from A. J. Katz, H. Goldman, and R. J. Grand: Eosinophilic (allergic) gastroenteritis, *Gastroenterology*, 73:707, 1977.)

rectal biopsy. In the classic cases, however, rectal biopsy demonstrates focal area of colitis with eosinophilic infiltration (Fig. 4).

Clinical Features

Classic cow's milk protein sensitivity may result in both systemic and/or gastrointestinal disease. Systemic symptoms include anaphylaxis, rhinitis, urticaria, eczema, wheezing, and pulmonary hemosiderosis. The gastrointestinal manifestations, as mentioned previously, depend on the site(s) of gastrointestinal involvement [20]. Various manifestations include vomiting, diarrhea, or malabsorption; protein-losing enteropathy with low albumin and low immunologlobulins; edema secondary to hypoalbuminemia; anemia secondary to gastrointestinal bleeding; colic; and rectal bleeding (see Table 3).

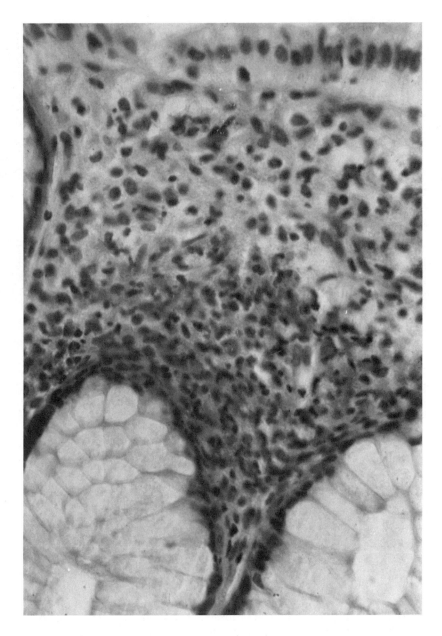

Figure 4   Rectal mucosal biopsy. Marked infiltration of eosinophils. (X135)

Table 3 Cow's Milk Protein Sensitivity

Gastritis	Enteropathy	Colitis
"Colic"	Diarrhea	Rectal bleeding
Vomiting	Malabsorption	
Guaiac-positive stools	Failure to thrive	
↓	Protein-losing enteropathy	
Anemia	↓	
	Edema	

Pathogenesis

The symptoms and the pathological changes of cow's milk-sensitive enteropathy, or gastroenteropathy, are reversed when the cow's milk protein is removed from the diet and is exacerbated on milk challenge. The mechanism of cow's milk protein sensitivity is unknown. However, unlike systemic allergic manifestations, IgE mediation does not appear to play a role in the gastrointestinal tract. Systemic manifestations are accompanied by elevation of serum IgE; the radioallergosorbent test (RAST) and skin tests are very positive to milk and milk products. In patients with gastrointestinal disease alone, serum IgE is normal and the RAST and skin tests to milk are negative [20]. Similar results are found in gluten-sensitive enteropathy, in which skin and RAST tests to gluten are negative and the IgE is normal. Many of these infants have associated transient hypogammaglobulinemia.

Treatment

It is estimated that up to about 30% of patients with cow's milk sensitivity are also sensitive to soy protein, and therefore, an initial milk- and soy-free formula is tried. Examples of these are Pregestimil, Portagen, and Nutramigen. Since these formulas are expensive, they are tried for 6-8 weeks initially, and if the patient responds dramatically, soy protein is then slowly introduced. If the patient's symptoms recur on soy protein, the patient is placed back on one of the casein hydrolysate formulas.

Follow-up Studies

Cow's milk sensitivity in the majority of cases is transient. It disappears by the age of 1-3 years. In patients with transient hypogammaglobulinemia, when the gammaglobulin levels rise to normal, the sensitivity disappears (unpublished observations). There appears to be no increased incidence of food sensitivity later in life, nor the development of any other allergies [20]. No specific HLA linkages have been found in these patients.

SOY PROTEIN SENSITIVITY

Gastrointestinal involvement due to soy protein sensitivity was first described by Ament and Rubin [22]. It occurs in 20–30% of infants with known milk sensitivity and may occur in patients without known milk sensitivity. Both enteropathy and colitis are described [23]; as yet gastritis has not been described. The pathophysiology appears to be the same as that for cow's milk sensitivity, in that IgE levels are normal, and RAST and skin tests to soy are negative. This disease also appears to be transient and disappears by the age of 1–3 years.

ALLERGIC DISEASE TRANSMITTED VIA BREAST FEEDING

It has now become apparent, as predicted by Gerrard in 1979 [24], that allergy in breast-fed babies due to ingredients in breast-milk would increase as breast-feeding became more popular. The first report of the development of eczema in a 3-week-old breast-fed baby after the mother had eaten a pound of chocolate was described in 1918 [23]. The eczema cleared when the mother avoided chocolate and returned when she ate it again.

The most common symptoms described with breast-feeding babies are colic [25] and colitis [26]. In the former group, a significant percentage of these patients developed classic cow's milk-sensitive enteropathy when they were weaned onto cow's milk. Lake et al. [26] described colitis in infants who are breast-fed. My experience with this entity has been that only 20% of these patients will improve if the mother goes on a milk-free diet, whereas 80% persist (unpublished observation). The colitis, however, is not severe enough to cause constitutional symptoms. The babies usually present with blood or mucus in the stool but are otherwise healthy, have no weight loss, and have no other signs of allergy. Interruption of breast-feeding results in complete amelioration of the colitis. However, the majority of the mothers do not wish to stop breast-feeding. It can be permitted only with continuing evaluation of the child. If the bleeding becomes very severe, the baby is placed on a casein hydrolysate formula. This is apparently a transient phenomenon; sufficient follow-up study is lacking on these patients to see whether they will develop any other sensitivities later in life.

EOSINOPHILIC (ALLERGIC) GASTROENTERITIS

Idiopathic eosinophilic infiltration of the gastrointestinal tract, both diffuse and circumscribed, was well reviewed initially by Ureless et al. in 1961 [27]. Klein et al. [28] subsequently proposed that eosinophilic gastroenteritis be divided into into three pathological entities:

1. Primary mucosal disease leading to malabsorption and gastrointestinal protein loss
2. Predominant muscle layer disease characterized usually by pyloric obstruction
3. Predominant serosal disease, a rare form presenting with eosinophilic ascites

It now appears that eosinophilic infiltration of the gastrointestinal tract may occur from the esophagus to the rectum. Different symptoms and signs will depend upon the site of inflammation. The mucosal form appears to be most common.

Clinical Features

Mucosal involvement can extend from the esophagus (personal observation) to the stomach, intestine, and the colon. Patients may therefore present with symptoms and signs of esophagitis, gastritis, enteropathy, ileitis, or colitis. Irrespective of the site of gastrointestinal involvement, these symptoms and signs are always accompanied by peripheral eosinophilia and systemic signs of allergy, most notably asthma, eczema, and rhinitis.

Patients with esophageal involvement may present with recurrent vomiting. Patients with gastritis present with gastrointestinal blood loss, that is, anemia, and recurrent abdominal pain [29]. Patients with enteropathy present with diarrhea, protein-losing enteropathy (hypoalbuminemia and hypogammaglobulinemia), and malabsorption. Patients with colitis present with rectal bleeding. The most common form of gastrointestinal involvement is gastritis and enteritis.

Pathophysiology

It would appear that a large majority of the patients presenting with the mucosal form of eosinophilic gastroenteritis have evidence for an allergic diathesis [29]. They all have markedly elevated serum IgE levels, usually in excess of 1000 IU/ml. RAST and skin tests are positive not only to all foods, but also to inhalant allergens. The only immunoglobulin changes are usually secondary to protein loss and are not primary. Studies of T- and B-cell functions by means of mitogen and antigen assays have demonstrated no abnormality. T-cell subsets have been normal. Many investigators in this field have wondered about the allergic etiology of this disease, but numerous attempts at dietary manipulation have failed to produce an absolute remission. Certain foods, however, may produce more severe symptoms and signs in some patients [30]. A recent study of one patient (personal observation) demonstrated that features of disease, includ- ing asthma, eosinophilia, and gastrointestinal disease, disappeared when the patient was placed on hyperalimentation. Subsequent attempts at refeeding, however, wer unsuccessful in preventing the recurrence of the disease. This would establish a role for food allergy in some of these patients; the specific allergic component(s) in the foods, however, still remain to be isolated. Certain patients have been described with specific allergies to specific substances, such as metabisulfite.

Treatment

The mainstay of treatment for eosinophilic or allergic gastroenteritis is corticos- teroids. Remission occurs on adequate steroid dosage. Some patients must be maintained on an alternate-day regimen of prednisone, and many other patients can be weaned off prednisone and placed back on accordingly when their symp- toms become severe. In all patients, dietary manipulation is usually of limited value, except in some patients with severe reactions to certain foods. Elimination of these foods can alleviate some of the symptomatology. Cromolyn has been unsuccessful as therapy in these patients. Hyperalimentation has been alluded to and should be reserved for those patients with severe steroid toxicity and/or persistence of symptoms preventing resumption of normal life activities.

Prognosis

This is a chronic lifelong condition; some patients have much more marked symptoms than others.

SUMMARY

In conclusion, food can adversely effect the whole of the gastrointestinal tract, extending from the esophagus to the colon. The symptoms and signs of these diseases depend upon which part of the gastrointestinal tract is affected.

REFERENCES

1. Trier, J. S., and Browning, T. H.: Epithelial cell renewal in cultured duo- denal biopsies in celiac sprue. *N. Engl. J. Med., 283*:1245, 1970.
2. Katz, A. J., and Grand, R. J.: All that flattens is not sprue. *Gastroenter- ology, 76*:375, 1979.
3. Booth, C. C.: The enterocyte in celiac disease. *Br. Med. J., 3*:725, 1970.

4. Katz, A. J., and Falchuk, Z. M.: Current concepts of gluten sensitive entero enteropathy (celiac sprue). *Pediatr. Clin. North Am., 22*:767, 1975.
5. Gee, S.: On the coeliac affliction. *St. Bartholomew's Hosp. Rep., 24*:17, 1888.
6. Rubin, C. E.: Malabsorption: Celiac sprue. *Annu. Rev. Med., 12*:39, 1961.
7. Falchuk, Z. M., and Strober, W.: Gluten sensitive enteropathy: Synthesis of antigliadin antibody in vitro. *Gut, 15*:947, 1974.
8. Wall, A. J., Douglass, A. P., and Booth, C. C.: Response of the jejunal mucosa in adult celiac disease to oral prednisone. *Gut, 11*:7, 1970.
9. Katz, A. J., Falchuk, Z. M., Strober, W., et al.: Gluten sensitive enteropathy: Inhibition by cortisol on the effect of gluten protein in vitro. *N. Engl. J. Med., 295*:131, 1976.
10. Falchuk, Z. M., Gebbard, R. C., Sessoms, C., et al.: An in vitro model of gluten sensitive enteropathy. *J. Clin. Invest., 53*:487, 1974.
11. Browning, T. H., and Trier, J. S.: Organ culture of mucosal biopsies of human small intestine. *J. Clin. Invest., 48*:1423, 1969.
12. Strober, W., Falchuk, Z. M., and Rogentine, G. N.: The pathogenesis of gluten sensitive enteropathy. *Ann. Intern. Med., 83*:242, 1975.
13. Falchuk, Z. M., Rogentine, G. N., and Strober, W.: Predominance of histocompatibility antigen HLA-8 in patients with gluten sensitive entero-pathy. *J. Clin. Invest., 51*:1601, 1972.
14. Stokes, P. L., Asquith, P., Holmes, GKT, et al.: Histocompatibility antigens associated with adult celiac disease. *Lancet, 2*:162, 1972.
15. Mann, J. G., Brown, W. R., and Kern, F.: The subtle and variable clinical expressions of gluten induced enteropathy. *Am. J. Med., 48*:357, 1970.
16. Katz, S. I., Hall, R. P., Lawley, T. J., et al.: Dermatitis herpetiformis: The skin and the gut. *Ann. Intern. Med., 93*:857, 1980.
17. Katz, A. J., Falchuk, Z. M., and Shwachman, H.: The co-existence of cystic fibrosis and celiac disease. *Pediatrics, 57*:715–721, 1976.
18. Visakorpi, J. K.: Definition of celiac disease in children. In *Celiac Disease.* Proceedings of Second International Symposium. PTO.
19. Harris, O. D., Cooke, W. T., Thompson, H., et al.: Malignancy in adult celiac disease and idiopathic steatorrhea. *Am. J. Med., 42*:899, 1967.
20. Katz, A. J., Twarog, F. J., Zieger, R., and Falchuk, Z. M.: Milk sensitive enteropathy: Similar clinical features with contrasting mechanisms and clinical course. *J. Allergy Clin. Immunol., 74*:72, 1984.
21. Grybowski, J. D.: Gastrointestinal milk allergy in infants. *Pediatrics, 40*: 354, 1967.
22. Ament, M. E., and Rubin, C. F.: Soy protein–another cause of the flat intestinal lesion. *Gastroenterology, 62*:227, 1972.
23. Powell, G. R.: Milk and soy induced enterocolitis of infancy. *J. Pediatr., 93*:553, 1978.
24. Gerrard, J. W.: Allergy in breastfed babies to ingredients in breast milk. *Ann. Allergy, 42*:69, 1979.
25. Jakobsson, I., and Lindberg, T.: Cow's milk as a cause of infantile colic in breast fed infants. *Lancet, 2*:437, 1978.

26.   Lake, A. M., Whitington, P. F., and Hamilton, S. R.: Dietary protein–
      induced colitis in breast-fed infants. *J. Pediatr., 101*:906, 1982.
27.   Uretes, A. L., Alshibaya, T., Lodico, D., et al.: Idiopathic eosinophilic
      infiltration of the gastrointestinal tract; diffuse and circumscribed. *Am. J.
      Med., 30*:899, 1961.
28.   Klein, M. C., Hargrove, R. L., Sliesenger, M. H., et al.: Eosinophilic gastro-
      enteritis. *Medicine (Baltimore), 49*:299, 1970.
29.   Katz, A. J., Goldman, H., and Grand, R. J.: Gastric mucosal biopsy in
      eosinophilic (allergic) gastroenteritis. *Gastroenterology, 73*:709, 1977.
30.   Leinbach, G. E., and Rubin, C. E.: Eosinophilic gastroenteritis. A simple
      reaction to food allergies. *Gastroenterology, 59*:876, 1970.

4

Pediatric Food Allergy

SAMI L. BAHNA and MOHAN D. GANDHI
Louisiana State University School of Medicine, New Orleans, Louisiana

Food allergy in the pediatric age group is distinct from that in adults in several features, including incidence, certain clinical manifestations, the causative food allergens, diagnostic procedures, management, and prognosis. This chapter is not intended to provide a comprehensive review of food allergy in children, but rather to shed light on those features that are of special importance during childhood. Even though a special effort has been directed toward avoiding duplication, certain areas may overlap to some degree with information in other chapters.

INCIDENCE

The incidence of food allergy, which has not been adequately addressed, varies because it depends on the investigator's attitude, the study population (age, mode of feeding, and associated illnesses), and the study design (symptoms included, food allergens looked for, diagnostic procedures, and duration of observation). It is our experience, as well as that of several others [1-3], that the most offending food allergen in children, and probably in persons of other ages, too, is cow's milk, with an estimated prevalence of 1-3% [4]. An incidence of 4-7% for food allergy in children is probably a reasonable estimate. Because the symptoms of food allergy resemble those of many other diseases and may persist for several months or years before being diagnosed or spontaneously "outgrown," the problem might have substantial impact (financial, social, physical, and emotional) on the patients as well as the family. The awareness on the part of physicians of food allergy and its diagnosis and management might obviate the need for subjecting the youngster to unnecessary diagnostic procedures, improper therapy, and prolonged suffering.

PREDISPOSING FACTORS

Development of allergy, in general, seems to be under the control of both genetic and environmental (intrinsic and/or extrinsic) factors. Certain such factors will be focused on here as they relate to the development of food allergy in children.

Heredity

Several studies have shown that, the stronger the family history of allergy, the higher is the incidence of allergy in the offspring [5-8], as well as the earlier the age at onset of symptoms [9-12]. Evidence also indicates that the IgE response is under genetic control [13]. Clinical observations suggest a role of heredity in the development of sensitivity to specific allergens. We, as well as others [14, 15], have seen examples of families with a high incidence of allergy to certain food allergens, particularly to cow's milk. Langeland observed an increased risk of intolerance to egg, milk, or fish among relatives of egg-sensitive patients [16]. Our studies on twins, however, did not provide any evidence that the sensitivity to specific allergens or the development of specific allergy manifestation is genetically determined [17, 18]. Probably both genetic and environmental factors influence the development of specific sensitivities.

Intrauterine Sensitization

Maternal IgE antibodies cannot cross the placenta, but the fetus can be sensitized to environmental antigens that reach the maternal circulation and cross the placenta. In 1928, Ratner demonstrated intrauterine sensitization to cow's milk proteins in the guinea pig [19]. Subsequently, several workers documented the same phenomenon in the human [6, 20-22]. Detection of specific IgE antibodies to foods in cord serum samples of newborns whose mothers had no such antibody supports a prenatal sensitization [23, 24]. The human fetus is capable of mounting an IgE response by 11 weeks' gestation [25].

Gastrointestinal Maturation

The increased permeability of intestinal mucosa and the poorly developed secretory IgA system during infancy enhance the chance of sensitization to ingested proteins during that period [26-28]. Such a phenomenon is most remarkable in the neonatal period, particularly in premature infants [29, 30]. Preterm neonates had significantly higher concentrations of circulating β-lactoglobulin than term neonates given similar amounts of cow's milk formula [28]. The clinical observation that most food-sensitive infants become able to tolerate the offending food by the age of 1-2 years further supports the protective role of gastrointestinal mucosal maturity against ingested antigens.

Mode of Feeding

Several studies showed that, at least in children, the most common food allergen is cow's milk. Cow's milk is the principal food for bottle-fed infants during the first year of life, and it contains more than 30 identifiable separate antigenic protein fractions. Evidence is sufficient that the incidence of allergy, as well as several other morbid conditions, is lower in breast-fed than in bottle-fed infants [31-35]. The beneficial effect of breast-feeding is much more obvious in protecting against allergy to ingestants than to inhalants and is more pronounced when it is for 6 months or more, particularly in the offspring of atopic families [31-33, 36, 37]. Also, mothers who breast-feed tend to avoid an early introduction of solid foods [38], which in turn should reduce the incidence of food allergy [39, 40].

In most instances, the development of sensitization is influenced by the degree of exposure. In general, the sensitizing dose is much greater than the provocative dose. Certain subjects, however, may become sensitized by quantities of allergens so minute that they may pass unnoticed. This phenomenon is obvious in those infants who are totally breast-fed yet in whom allergy symptoms develop from minute quantities of food antigens that reach the mammary gland from the maternal circulation [41-43].

Some studies suggested a lower allergenicity of soybean infant formula than of cow's milk formula [35, 44]. Like most other proteins, however, soy protein is antigenic in humans. In a study of circulating antibodies of the non-IgE class in young infants, soy protein and cow's milk protein were found to have equal antigenicity [26]. That study, however, did not address clinical allergenicity. Soybean formula has been a common milk substitute in infants sensitive to cow's milk. Clinical hypersensitivity to soy protein, although seemingly less common than to cow's milk, certainly exists [45-47]. An increased use of soybean formula may result in an increased incidence of hypersensitivity to its protein [7].

Other milk substitutes are available for infant feeding [4, 48]. Several are less allergenic than cow's milk formula, but their usefulness in preventing food allergy in infants has not been adequately studied.

Heat treatment of cow's milk results in denaturation of its heat-labile protein fractions, notably bovine serum albumin and immunoglobulin. Clinical reactions to these fractions, however, are much less common than to β-lactoglobulin or casein [4].

Enzymatically digested bovine casein (Nutramigen and Pregestemil by Mead-Johnson) is available for infant feeding. Such protein hydrolysates are more readily assimilated and less allergenic than cow's milk formulas. They are also, however, more costly.

Elemental diets, in which protein consists of synthetic amino acids (Vivonex by Norwich-Eaton), is a promising hypoallergenic formula, but expensive.

Goat's milk resembles cow's milk in composition, and certain protein fractions actually cross-react in both types of milk [49–51], which makes goat's milk an unsatisfactory substitute for cow's milk.

Immunodeficiency

Immunologic disorders may predispose to food allergy by enhancing the absorption of incompletely digested food proteins and/or disturbed T-cell–B-cell interaction. The most frequently encountered immunologic disorders are IgA deficiency and transient hypogammaglobulinemia of infancy [52–55]. Juto observed an increased risk of food allergy in infants with low T-cell numbers [56].

Associated Diseases

The development of food allergy could conceivably be enhanced by diseases that disturb either the local defense mechanisms of the gastrointestinal tract or the systemic immunologic balance. Increased intestinal mucosal permeability during and after diarrheal diseases may facilitate excessive absorption of macromolecules and subsequent sensitization [57, 58].

In infants of atopic families, Frick et al. noted a relationship between development of allergy, including food allergy, and precedent respiratory viral infections [22]. Such an effect is probably through a general enhancement of the humoral immune responses, particularly of the IgE system, by acute viral illnesses [59–61].

CLINICAL MANIFESTATIONS PECULIAR TO CHILDHOOD

The most common shock organ for food allergy is the gastrointestinal tract, followed by the respiratory tract and the skin. Other systems seem to be much less commonly involved. Multiple system involvement is not uncommon and may develop so acutely that it results in systemic anaphylaxis.

In this chapter, only certain clinical manifestations will be addressed and their peculiarities to childhood will be highlighted.

Gastrointestinal Tract

A wide variety of gastrointestinal manifestations has been ascribed to food allergy [4]. Abdominal pain, vomiting, and diarrhea are the most common and usually occur within a short time after the ingestion of the offending food. The length of the latent period depends on the quantity of the food allergen ingested, the degree of sensitivity of the patient, and the type of hypersensitivity reaction involved (immediate or late).

In infants, the abdominal pain seems to be more of the colic type (infantile colic), whereas in older children it is more of the vague, diffuse type, in the epigastric or periumbilical regions.

Less common gastrointestinal symptoms are steatorrhea, protein-losing enteropathy, enterocolitis, and bleeding.

Gastrointestinal bleeding has been reported in connection with cow's milk hypersensitivity; whether it can also be caused by other food allergens is unknown. The bleeding may be gross or, more commonly, occult. Gross bleeding occurs usually in very young infants and seems to originate from the large intestine. On proctoscopy, the mucosa may appear red, friable, and ulcerated [62]. Avoidance of cow's milk results in improvement usually within a few days, and most infants outgrow the problem within a few months of avoidance of milk. The occult form of bleeding usually occurs in older infants and young children and may persist for several months to a few years, resulting in a profound iron-deficiency anemia. Occult bleeding was noticed in 40% of infants with iron-deficiency anemia [63] and was associated with serum precipitating antibodies to multiple bovine milk protein fractions, mostly the heat-labile ones [64]. The fecal blood loss may reach 10 ml/day and varies with the quantity of milk intake [65]. Improvement follows avoidance of homogenized milk. These patients normally do well on heat-treated milk, and most of them will be able to ingest homogenized milk within 1-2 years.

Respiratory Tract

Food allergy seems to involve the respiratory tract in children more than in adults. The most common manifestations are rhinitis, chronic serous otitis media, and cough. Less common manifestations are asthma and bronchitis, and least common are chronic or recurrent pulmonary disease, and upper airway obstruction by pharyngeal lymphoid hyperplasia [4].

Chronic or recurrent pulmonary disease due to cow's milk hypersensitivity has been described by Heiner and coworkers in infants and young children [66-68]. In the Heiner syndrome, the chronic or recurrent pulmonary disease is often associated with upper respiratory symptoms, wheezing, failure to thrive, gastrointestinal symptoms, and eosinophilia. The chest x-ray shows persistent or changing patchy infiltrate, frequently associated with areas of atelectasis, reticular densities, hilar adenopathy, and pleural thickening [69]. The sera of such patients, when tested against cow's milk by double diffusion in agar (Ouchterlony technique), show multiple precipitin lines in high titers, indicating precipitating antibodies (IgG and IgM) to multiple protein fractions in cow's milk. The immunologic mechanism in this syndrome seems to be primarily an immune complex reaction, and in some patients cell-mediated and possibly IgE-mediated reactions may also be involved. Increased levels of IgG_4 antibodies to cow's milk have been noted in some patients [70]. Whether milk aspiration plays a role in the pathogenesis of this disease is not clear. Symptoms improve, usually within a few days of avoidance of milk, but the radiological findings may not completely disappear before several weeks. Although pulmonary disease has been described in relation to cow's milk, it might also be caused by other foods [70].

Pulmonary hemosiderosis should be suspected in infants who have the Heiner syndrome, hemoptysis, and iron-deficiency anemia [71, 72]. The disease should be verified by the demonstration of iron-laden macrophages in the tracheobronchial secretion or in the morning gastric lavage.

Dermatology

Skin involvement in food allergy is fairly common in children and may be in the form of urticaria, angioedema, atopic dermatitis, contact rash, and, less commonly, other manifestations [4].

The role of food allergy in atopic dermatitis has been documented by several studies [73-75]. Allergy to one or more foods is probably implicated in one-third to one-half of infantile eczema cases. Cow's milk, egg, and nuts are the most common offenders.

Miscellaneous

Hypersensitivity reactions to foods reportedly may occur in almost any system in the human body.

A wide variety of neurological and behavioral symptoms have been reported as possibly caused by ingestants (foods or chemicals) [76-79]. They include hyperkinesis, learning disorders, irritability, nervousness, headache, fatigue, musculoskeletal pains, and dizziness. Because of the subjectivity and nonspecificity of these symptoms, as well as lack of well-controlled studies, the role of hypersensitivity to foods, food additives, or food coloring has not been well documented. From a careful review of the literature and from our experience, hyperkinesis and other neurological symptoms apparently can occur from ingestant intolerance, although such occurrence is not as common as some clinicians believe. According to several studies, the offenders are more commonly chemicals than food proteins [80-83]. The problem is further compounded by the fact that, even in well-documented cases, the underlying immunologic mechanism is not understood. The reactions could possibly be idiosyncratically pharmacological in nature.

The urinary tract as a shock organ for food allergy in children has been suggested by a few workers. We have seen a few children with respiratory allergies whose coexisting enuresis disappeared after avoidance of certain foods and recurred after oral challenge. Enuretic children were noted to have associated allergic disorders more often than did nonenuretic controls [84]. In 1959, Breneman described 65 patients with nocturnal enuresis related to the intake of specific foods [85]. In a later study, the same author reported a rise in the improvement rate of nocturnal enuresis when an elimination diet was added to the pharmacological treatment [86]. When a series of enuretic children was put on an elimination diet, the nocturnal enuresis ceased, the frequency of micturition during daytime decreased, and the bladder capacity increased [87]. Histologically, the urinary bladder resembles the gastrointestinal and respiratory tracts in having a mucosal membrane, a submucosa rich in blood vessels, and a smooth muscle layer. That an allergic reaction can occur in the urinary bladder and result in "allergic cystitis" should not be surprising. In addition to enuresis, food allergy in some patients may cause other symptoms in the lower urinary tract [88-91]. Urinary eosinophilia in association with such symptoms has been noted by some authors [92] but not by others [89].

Albuminuria [93] or the nephrotic syndrome [94, 95] in certain patients may be aggravated or induced by the ingestion of specific foods, particularly cow's milk.

Various degrees of thrombocytopenia have been reported in many food-sensitive patients shortly after ingestion of the offending food. In a series of 35 children sensitive to milk and egg, an oral challenge with the offending food was followed by a drop in platelet count by more than 35% in 80% of cases. Significant thrombocytopenia related to food allergy, however, is estimated to occur in less than 1% of all thrombocytopenia patients [96]. A well-documented case of severe thrombocytopenia (3000-6000 platelets mm^3) caused by ingestion of cow's milk was reported in a newborn whose platelet count stayed normal on a milk-free diet. When that child was 1 year old, his mother tried on two occasions to reintroduce milk to his diet but on both attempts severe wheezing and easy bruising developed.

DIAGNOSIS

Diagnostic procedures of food allergy are mentioned in detail in other chapters of this volume. In most cases, whether in children or in adults, a detailed medical history is probably the most important procedure for diagnosing food allergy. Physical examination is essential to verify the nature of manifestations and their possible relation to nonallergic diseases. Selected laboratory procedures may be needed to exclude or verify suspected nonallergic diseases or to support the diagnosis of allergy. In children in particular, a wide variety of diseases should be considered in the differential diagnosis (Table 1). For determining the offending food(s), in addition to the medical history, skin testing (scratch or prick complemented with intradermal) and/or the radioallergosorbent test (RAST)

Table 1 Differential Diagnosis of Food Allergy in Children

Gastrointestinal tract
  Lactase deficiency
  Gastroesophageal reflux
  Celiac disease
  Cystic fibrosis
  Gastroenteritis
  Parasitic infestation
  Ulcerative colitis
  Crohn's disease
  Galactosemia

Respiratory tract
  Rhinitis or asthma not related to food
  Bronchopulmonary aspergillosis
  Foreign body
  Airway obstruction by vascular rings or other anomalies
  Hypersensitivity pneumonitis
  Aspiration pneumonia

Dermatology
  Urticaria, angioedema, or eczema not related to food
  Seborrheic dermatitis
  Acrodermatitis enteropathica
  Ichthyosis

Immunodeficiency
  Selective IgA deficiency
  Hypogammaglobulinemia
  Combined immunodeficiencies
  Complement deficiencies

may be useful. In case of cow's milk, we recommend testing with whole milk as well as with individual protein fractions, such as casein, whey, β-lactoglobulin, α-lactalbumin, bovine serum albumin, and bovine serum globulin. Both skin testing and RAST require experience in performance and interpretation. Several other in vitro tests can be used to detect the food allergen [4], but they are mostly research procedures and are not easily available in routine clinical laboratories.

To verify a cause-and-effect relationship, the elimination-challenge test should be done to document disappearance or significant improvement in the symptoms after elimination of the offending food and recurrence of symptoms after oral challenge. When the result is equivocal, the test should be repeated once or more, using the suspected food and a placebo. The use of semiblind or double-blind procedures are rarely necessary in infants or young children, whose reactions can be objectively evaluated. A discrepancy between the result of skin testing or in vitro testing and the result of the elimination-challenge test is common [97]. Unless the expected reaction is life threatening, the oral challenge test should be conducted to settle the diagnosis of food allergy.

PROGNOSIS

In general, the prognosis of food allergy is much better in children than in adults. Cow's milk allergy in infancy seems to have the best prognosis; it often subsides within a few months of avoidance of milk, and in most cases it disappears or is greatly reduced within 1-3 years [35, 62, 98-101]. The duration of clinical food sensitivity tends to be shorter in infants than in older children; in patients with single rather than multiple symptoms; when the shock organ is the gastrointestinal tract rather than other systems; when the offending food is cow's milk, soy, cereals, or fruits rather than nuts or fish; and when the level of total IgE or specific IgE antibodies is low [102, 103]. Histological and immunologic abnormalities in the intestinal mucosa [104, 105] and skin reactivity [102] may persist after the development of clinical tolerance. Whether such a state of subclinical hypersensitivity can be of clinical significance whenever a concurrent illness occurs or when the food allergen load is increased is not known. The child who once had food allergy may continue to be allergy prone for years, during which time the symptoms and/or the allergens may change.

ACKNOWLEDGMENTS

The editorial assistance of Miss Virginia Howard and the secretarial assistance of Mrs. Caroline Yarbrough are deeply appreciated.

REFERENCES

1. Gerrard, J. W. (1974). Allergy in infancy. *Pediatr. Ann. 3*:9-23.
2. Speer, F. (1976). Food allergy: The 10 common offenders. *AFP 13*:106-112.
3. Ogle, K. A., and Bullock, J. D. (1980). Children with allergic rhinitis and/or bronchial asthma treated with elimination diet: A five year follow-up. *Ann. Allergy 44*:273-278.
4. Bahna, S. L., and Heiner, D. C. (1980). *Allergies to Milk*. Grune & Stratton, New York.
5. Orgel, H. A., Hamburger, R. N., Bazaral, M., Gorin, H., Groshong, T., Lenoir, M., Miller, J. R., and Wallace, W. M., (1975). Development of IgE and allergy in infancy. *J. Allergy Clin. Immunol. 56*:296-307.
6. Dannaeus, A., Johansson, G., and Foucard, T. (1978). Clinical and immunological aspects of food allergy in childhood. II. Development of allergic

symptoms and humoral immune response to foods in infants of atopic mothers during the first 24 months of life. *Acta Pediatr. Scand. 67*:497–504.

7. Kjellman, N. I. M., and Johansson, S. G. O. (1979). Soy versus cow's milk in infants with a biparental history of atopic disease: Development of atopic disease and immunoglobulins from birth to four years of age. *Clin. Allergy 9*:347–358.

8. Croner, S., Kjellman, N. I. M., Eriksson, B., and Roth, A. (1982). IgE screening in 1701 newborn infants and the development of atopic disease during infancy. *Arch. Dis. Child. 57*:364–368.

9. Bahna, S. L. (1970). A statistical study of allergic disorders among school children. Thesis, Doctorate Degree in Public Health, University of Alexandria, Alexandria, Egypt.

10. Kaufman, H. S., and Frick, O. L. (1976). The development of allergy in infants of allergic parents: A prospective study concerning the role of heredity. *Ann. Allergy 37*:410–415.

11. Kjellman, N. I. M. (1976). Immunoglobulin E and atopic allergy in childhood. Linkoping University Medical Dissertations No. 36, Linkoping, Sweden.

12. Wittig, H. J., McLaughlin, E. T., Leifer, K. L., and Belloit, J. D. (1978). Risk factors for the development of allergic disease: Analysis of 2190 patient records. *Ann. Allergy 41*:84–88.

13. Meyers, D. A., and Marsh, D. G. (1981). Committee report: Report on a National Institute of Allergy and Infectious Diseases-sponsored workshop on the genetics of total immunoglobulin E levels in humans. *J. Allergy Clin. Immunol. 67*:167.

14. Gerrard, J. W. (1966). Familial recurrent rhinorrhea and bronchitis due to cow's milk. *JAMA 198*:605–607.

15. Deamer, W. C. (1973). Recurrent abdominal pain. A frequent manifestation of food allergy. *Curr. Md. Dialog 40*:130–154.

16. Langeland, T. (1983). A clinical and immunological study of allergy to hen's eggwhite. I. A clinical study of egg allergy. *Clin. Allergy 13*:371–382.

17. Prather, B., and Bahna, S. L. (1981). Does heredity determine the allergic manifestation or the sensitivity to a specific allergen? *J. Allergy Clin. Immunol. 67* (January Suppl.):61.

18. Bahna, S. L. (1983). Concordances in atopic twins. *J. Allergy Clin. Immunol. 71* (No. 1. part II):100.

19. Ratner, B. (1928). A possible causal-factor of food allergy in certain infants. *Am. J. Dis. Child. 36*:277–288.

20. Kaufman, H. S. (1971). Allergy in the newborn: Skin tests reactions confirmed by Prausnitz-Kustner test at birth. *Clin. Allergy 1*:363–367.

21. Kuroume, T., Oguri, M., Matsumara, T., Iwasaki, I., Kanbe, Y., Yamada, T., Kawabe, S., and Negishi, K. (1976). Milk sensitivity and soybean sensitivity in the production of eczematous manifestations in breast-fed infants

with particular reference to intra-uterine sensitization. *Ann. Allergy 37*: 41–46.

22. Frick, O. L., German, D. F., and Mills, J. (1979). Development of allergy in children. I. Association with viral infections. *J. Allergy Clin. Immunol. 63*:228–241.

23. Michel, F. B., Bousquet, J., Greillier, P., Robinet-Levy, M., and Coulomb, Y. (1980). Comparison of cord blood immunoglobulin E concentrations and maternal allergy for the prediction of atopic diseases in infancy. *J. Allergy Clin. Immunol. 65*:422–430.

24. Businco, L., Marchetti, F., Pellegrini, G., and Perlini, R. (1983). Predictive value of cord blood IgE levels in at risk newborn babies and influence of type of feeding. *Clin. Allergy 13*:503–508.

25. Miller, D. L., HirVonen, T., and Gitlin, D. (1973). Synthesis of IgE by the human conceptus. *J. Allergy Clin. Immunol. 52*:182–188.

26. Eastham, E. J., Lichauco, T., Grady, M. I., and Walker, W. A. (1978). Antigenicity of infant formulas: Role fo immature intestine in protein permeability. *J. Peadiatr. 93*:561–564.

27. Udall, J. N., Pang, K., Fritze, L., Kleinman, R. E., and Walker, W. A. (1981). Development of gastrointestinal mucosal barrier. I. The effect of age on intestinal permeability ot macromolecules. *Pediatr. Res. 15*:241–244.

28. Roberton, D. M., Paganelli, R., Dinwiddie, R., and Levinsky, R. J. (1982). Antigen absorption in the preterm and term neonate. *Arch. Dis. Child. 57*: 369–372.

29. Rothberg, R. M. (1969). Immunoglobulin and specific antibody synthesis during the first weeks of life of premature infants. *J. Pediatr. 75*:391–399.

30. Rieger, C. H. L., and Rothberg, R. M. (1975). Development of the capacity to produce specific antibody to an ingested food antigen in the premature infant. *J. Pediatr. 87*:515–518.

31. Kaufman, H. S., and Frick, O. L. (1979). The incidence of asthma in bottle and breast-fed infants. A prospective study. *Ann. Allergy 42*:128.

32. Saarinen, U. M., Kajosaari, M., Backman, A., and Siimes, M. A. (1979). Prolonged breast-feeding as prophylaxis of atopic disease. *Lancet 2*:163–168.

33. Chandra, R. K. (1979). Prospective studies of the effect of breast-feeding on incidence of infection and allergy. *Acta Pediatr. Scand. 68*:691–694.

34. Duchateau, J., and Casimir, G. (1983). Neonatal serum IgE concentration as predictor of atopy (letter). *Lancet 1*:413–414.

35. Businco, L., Marchetti, F., Pellegrini, G., Cantani, A., and Perlini, R. (1983). Prevention of atopic disease in "at-risk newborns" by prolonged breast-feeding. *Ann. Allergy 51*:296–299.

36. Soothill, J. F. (1976). Some intrinsic and extrinsic factors predisposing to allergy. *Proc. R. Soc. Med. 69*:439–442.

37. Hide, D. W., and Guyer, B. M. (1981). Clinical manifestations of allergy related to breast and cow's milk feeding. *Arch. Dis. Child. 56*:172–175.

38. Sleigh, G., and Ounsted, M. (1975). Present day practice in infant feeding. *Lancet 1*:753.
39. Saarinen U. M., and Kajosaari, M. (1980). Does dietary eleimination in infancy prevent or only postpone a food allergy?: A study of fish and citrus allergy in 375 children. *Lancet 1*:166–167.
40. Fergusson, D. M., Horwood, L. J., Beautrais, A. L., Shannon, F. T., and Taylor, B. (1981). Eczema and infant diet. *Clin. Allergy 11*:325–331.
41. Jakobsson, I., and Lindberg, T. (1978). Cow's milk as a cause of infantile colic in breast-fed infants. *Lancet 2*:437–439.
42. Gerrard, J. W. (1979). Allergy in breast-fed babies to ingredients in breast milk. *Ann. Allergy 42*:69–72.
43. Kaplan, M. S., and Solli, N. J. (1979). Immunoglobulin E to cow's-milk protein in breast-fed atopic children. *J. Allergy Clin. Immunol. 64*:122–126.
44. Johnstone, D. E., and Dutton, A. M. (1966). Dietary prophylaxis of allergic diseases in children. *N. Engl. J. Med. 274*:715–719.
45. Whitington, P. F., and Gibson, R. G. (1977). Soy protein intolerance: Four patients with concomitant cow's milk intolerance. *Pediatrics 59*: 730–732.
46. Ament, M. E., and Rubin, C. E. (1972). Soy protein – another cause of the flat intestinal lesion. *Gastroenterology 62*:227–234.
47. Powell, G. K. (1978). Milk and soy induced enterocolitis of infancy. Clinical features and standardization of challenge. *J. Pediatr. 93*:553–560.
48. Bahna, S. L., and Gandhi, M. D. (1983). Milk hypersensitivity. II. Practical aspects of diagnosis, treatment and prevention. *Ann. Allergy 50*:295–302.
49. Saperstein, S. (1960). Antigenicity of the whey proteins in evaporated cow's milk and whole goat's milk. *Ann. Allergy 18*:765–773.
50. Crawford, L. V., and Grogan, F. T. (1961). Allergenicity of cow's milk proteins. IV. Relationship to goat's milk proteins as studied by serum-agar precipitation. *J. Pediatr. 59*:347–350.
51. Jeness, R., Phillips, N. I., and Kalan, E. B. (1967). Immunological comparison of beta-lactoglobulins (abstract). *Fed. Proc. 26*:340.
52. Taylor, B., Norman, A. P., and Orgel, H. A., Stokes, C. R., Turner, M. W., and Soothill, J. F. (1973). Transient IgA deficiency and pathogenesis of infantile atopy. *Lancet 2*:111–113.
53. Cunningham-Rundles, C., Brandeis, W. E., Good, R. A., and Day, N. K. (1979). Bovine antigens and the formation of circulating immune complexes in selective immunoglobulin A deficiency. *J. Clin. Invest. 64*: 272.
54. Fineman, S. M., Rosen, F. S., and Geha, R. S. (1979). Transient hypogammaglobulinemia, elevated immunoglobulin E level, and food allergy. *J. Allergy Clin. Immunol. 64*:216–222, 1979.
55. Aiuti, F., and Paganelli, R. (1983). Food allergy and gastrointestinal disease. *Ann. Allergy 51*:275–280.

56. Juto, P. (1980). Elevated serum immunoglobulin E in T cell deficient infants fed cow's milk. *J. Allergy Clin. Immunol.* 66:402–407.
57. Gruskay, F. L., and Cooke, R. E. (1955). The gastrointestinal absorption of unaltered protein in normal infants, and in infants recovering from diarrhea. *Pediatrics* 16:763–769.
58. Walker, W. A. (1975). Antigen absorption from the small intestine and gastrointestinal disease. *Pediatr. Clin. North Am.* 22:731–746.
59. Bahna, S. L., Horwitz, C. A., Fiala, M., and Heiner, D. C. (1978). IgE response in heterophil-positive infectious mononucleosis. *J. Allergy Clin. Immunol.* 62:167–173.
60. Bahna, S. L., Horwitz, C. A., and Heiner, D. C. (1978). IgE response in cytomegalovirus mononucleosis. *J. Allergy Clin. Immunol.* 61:177.
61. Bahna, S. L., Heiner, D. C., and Horwitz, C. A. (1984). Sequential changes of the five immunoglobulin classes and other responses in infectious mononucleosis. *Int. Arch. Allergy Appl. Immunol.* 74:1–8.
62. Gryboski, J. D. (1967). Gastrointestinal milk allergy in infants. *Pediatrics* 40:354–362.
63. Wilson, J. F., Heiner, D. C., and Lahey, M. E. (1962). Studies on iron metabolism. *J. Pediatr.* 60:787–800.
64. Wilson, J. F., Heiner, D. C., and Lahey, M. E. (1964). Milk induced gastrointestinal bleeding in infants with hypochromic microcytic anemias. *JAMA* 189:122–126.
65. Wilson, J. F., Lahey, M. F., and Heiner, D. C. (1974). Studies on iron metabolism. V. Further observations on cow's milk-induced gastrointestinal bleeding in infants with iron-deficiency anemia. *J. Pediatr.* 84:335–344.
66. Heiner, D. C., and Sears, J. W. (1960). Chronic respiratory disease association with multiple circulating precipitins to cow's milk. *Am. J. Dis. Child.* 100:500–502.
67. Heiner, D. C., Sears, J. W., and Kniker, W. T. (1962). Multiple precipitins to cow's milk in chornic respiratory disease. *Am. J. Dis. Child.* 103:634–654.
68. Lee, S. K., Kniker, W. T., Cook, C. D., and Heiner, D. C. (1978). Cow's milk induced pulmonary disease in children. *Adv. Pediatr.* 25:39–57.
69. Diner, W. C., Kniker, W. T., and Heiner, D. C. (1961). Roentgenologic manifestations in the lungs in milk allergy. *Radiology* 77:564–572.
70. Heiner, D. C. (1983). Food allergy and respiratory disease. *Ann. Allergy* 51:273–274.
71. Boat, T. F., Polmar, S. H., Whitman, V., Kleinerman, J. I., Stern, R. C., and Doershuk, C. F. (1975). Hyper reactivity to cow's milk in young children with pulmonary hemosiderosis and corpulmonale secondary to nasopharyngeal obstruction. *J. Pediatr.* 87:23–29.
72. Stafford, H. A., Polmar, S. H., and Boat, T. F. (1977). Immunologic studies in cow's milk-induced pulmonary hemosiderosis. *Pediatr. Research* 11:898–903.
73. Hammar, H. (1977). Provocation with cow's milk and cereals in atopic dermatitis. *Acta Derm. Venereol.* (Stockh.) 57:159–163.

74. Atherton, D. J., Sewell, M., Soothill, J. F., and Wells, R. S. (1978). A double blind controlled cross over trial of an antigen avoidance diet in atopic eczema. *Lancet 1*:401–403.

75. Sampson, H. A. (1983). Role of immediate food hypersensitivity in the pathogenesis of atopic dermatitis. *J. Allergy Clin. Immunol. 71*:473–480.

76. Speer, F. (1970). *Allergy of the Nervous System.* Charles C. Thomas, Springfield, Illinois.

77. Campbell, M. B. (1973). Neurologic manifestation of allergic disease. *Ann. Allergy 31*:485–489.

78. Weinberg, E. G., and Tuchinda, M. (1973). Allergic tension-fatigue syndrome. *Ann. Allergy 31*:209–211.

79. Tryphonas, H., and Trites, R. (1979). Food allergy in children with hyperactivity, learning disabilities and/or minimal brain dysfunction. *Ann. Allergy 42*:22–27.

80. Amos, H. E., and Drake, J. J. P. (1976). Problems posed by food additives. *J. Hum. Nutr. 30*:165–178.

81. Werry, J. S. (1976). Food additives and hyperactivity. *Med. J. Aus. 2, 8*: 281.

82. Augustine, G. J., and Levitan, H. (1980). Neurotransmitter release from vertebrate neuromuscular synapse affected by a food dye. *Science 207*: 1489–1490.

83. Swanson, J. M., and Kinsbourne, M. (1980). Food dyes impair performances of hyperactive children on a laboratory learning test. *Science 207*: 1485–1488.

84. Zaleski, A., Shokier, M. K., and Gerrard, J. W. (1972). Enuresis: Familial incidence and relationship to allergic disorders. *Can. Med. Assoc. J. 106*:30–31.

85. Breneman, J. C. (1959). Allergic cystitis: The cause of nocturnal enuresis. *GP 20*:85–98.

86. Breneman, J. C. (1965). Nocturnal enuresis, a treatment regimen for general use. *Ann. Allergy 23*:185–191.

87. Esperanca, M., and Gerrard, J. W. (1969). Nocturnal enuresis: Comparison of the effect of imipramine and dietary restrictions on bladder capacity. *Can. Med. Assoc. J. 101*:721–724.

88. Powell, N. B., Boggs, P. B., and McGovern, J. P. (1970). Allergy of the lower urinary tract. *Ann. Allergy 28*:252–255.

89. Powell, N. B., Powell, E. B., Thomas, O. C., Queng, J. T., and Mcgovern, J. P. (1972). Allergy of the lower urinary tract. *J. Urol. 107*:631–634.

90. Horesh, A. J. (1976). Allergy and recurrent urinary tract infections in childhood. I. *Ann. Allergy 36*:16–22.

91. Horesh, A. J. (1976). Allergy and recurrent urinary tract infections in childhood. II. *Ann. Allergy 36*:174–179.

92. Pastinszky, I. (1959). The allergic diseases of the male genitourinary tract with special reference to allergic urethritis and cystitis. *Urol. Int. 9*:288–305.

93. Matsumara, T., Kuroume, T., and Fukushima, I. (1966). Significance of food allergy in the etiology of orthostatic albuminuria. *J. Asthma Res. 3*: 325–329.

94. Sandberg, D. H., McIntosh, R. M., Bernstein, C. W., Carr, R., and Strauss, J. (1977). Severe steroid-responsive nephrosis associated with hypersensitivity. *Lancet 1*:388–390.

95. Law-chin-Yung, L., and Freed, D. L. F. (1977). Nephrotic syndrome due to milk allergy. *Lancet 1*:1056.

96. Cohn, J. (1976): Thrombocytopenia in childhood. *Scand. J. Haematol. 16*:226–240.

97. Bjorksten, B., Ahlstedt, S., Bjorksten, F., Carlsson, B., Fallstrom, S. P., Juntunen, K., Kajosaari, M., and Kober, A. (1983). Immunoglobulin E and immunoglobulin G_4 antibodies to cow's milk in children with cow's milk allergy. *Allergy 38*:119–124.

98. Gerrard, J. W., Heiner, D. C., Ives, E. J., and Hardy, L. W. (1963). Milk allergy: Recognition, natural history and management. *Clin. Pediatr. 2*: 634–641.

99. Gerrard, J. W., MacKenzie, J. W. A., Goluboff, N., Garson, J. Z., and Maningas, C. S. (1973). Cow's milk allergy: Prevalence and manifestations in an unselected series of newborns. *Acta. Pediatr. Scand.* (Suppl.) *234*:1–21.

100. Hill, D. J., Davidson, G. P., Cameron, D. J. S., and Barnes, G. L. (1979). The spectrum of cow's milk allergy in childhood. Clinical, gastroenterological and immunological studies. *Acta Paediatr. Scand. 68*:847–852.

101. Jakobsson, I., and Lindberg, J. (1979). A prospective study of cow's milk protein intolerance in swedish infants. *Acta Paediatr. Scand. 68*:853–859.

102. Bock, A. S. (1982). The natural history of food sensitivity. *J. Allergy Clin. Immunol. 69*:173–177.

103. Ford, R. P. K., and Taylor, B. (1982). Natural history of egg hypersensitivity. *Arch. Dis. Child. 57*:649–652.

104. Shiner, M., Brook, C. G. D., Ballard, J., and Herman, S. (1975). Intestinal biopsy in the diagnosis of cow's milk protein intolerance without acute symptoms. *Lancet 1*:1060–1063.

105. Harris, M. J., Petts, V., and Penny, R. (1977). Cow's milk allergy as a cause of infantile colic: Immunofluorescent studies on jejunal mucosa. *Aust. Paediatr. J. 13*:276–281.

5

Food Allergy in Adults

VINAY K. JAIN and R. K. CHANDRA
Memorial University of Newfoundland, St. John's, Newfoundland, Canada

Food allergy is presumed by the general public to be responsible for a wide variety of physical and psychiatric symptoms. The true incidence of food allergy in adults has not been determined, but estimates vary from 1 in 1000, upward. Acute reactions to food can occur in adults who had previously tolerated the same food well. These reactions are easy to diagnose, and their relationship to food intake can be easily demonstrated. It is much more difficult to prove the association between food intake and chronic disease, like asthma, eczema, or psychiatric syndromes.

There is a lack of reliable diagnostic tests. Despite the plethora of tests available, the only test that conclusively proves food allergy is the double-blind food challenge. In patients with psychiatric or gastrointestinal disease, unpleasant symptoms can follow ingestion of a wide variety of foods, not all of which may be mediated through immunologic means; hence a critical approach must be maintained while diagnosing food allergy.

FOOD TOXICITY, IDIOSYNCRASY, AND ALLERGY

At the outset, it is important to distinguish between the above three distinct entities. In food toxicity, everything depends on the food, which contains some substance that, when ingested, is harmful to human beings. Many mushrooms, fish, and shellfish contain toxins that cause gastrointestinal and systemic illness. Bacterial toxins present in food can cause similar illnesses. Hexachlorobenzene used on wheat in Turkey caused acquired porphyria. Acetanilid used to denature rapeseed oil leads to pneumonopathy and respiratory failure.

In idiosyncrasy, a food causes symptoms only in certain individuals who have some anomaly. This includes an abnormal sensitivity to pharmacologically active substances present in the food or an enzyme deficiency. Galactosemia, favism, and hemolytic anemia due to glucose-6-phosphate dehydrogenase deficiency can cause symptoms simulating food allergy. Deficiency of disaccharidases in the intestinal tract border can cause intolerance to other disaccharides.

Tyramine, present in foods like French cheese, cheddar, yeast, herring, and Chianti, can cause migraine. This can be due to an excessive consumption of foods rich in tyramine, excessive endogenous decarboxylation of tyrosine to tyramine by intestinal flora, or a partial deficiency of tyramine-metabolizing enzyme, like monoamine oxidase or phenosulfatransferase, in the platelets. Other amines, like phenylethylamine and histamine, can cause such symptoms as erythema and headache and even a fall in blood pressure. Large amounts of histamine are found in cooked pork meats, sauerkraut, fermented cheeses, and tuna. Tomatoes and strawberries can cause a release of histamine. Nitrite and nitrite compounds used as preservatives in such foods as smoked fish, salami, bologna, pepperoni, bacon, frankfurters, and corned beef can cause migrainous headaches, urticaria or functional intestinal disorders. Monosodium glutamate, an ingredient used in Chinese cooking, can cause a syndrome of burning sensation, facial and chest pain, and migrainelike headaches about 15–25 min after ingestion. Caffeine can also cause headaches during ingestion of or withdrawal from excessive quantities.

True food allergy with evidence of immunologic hypersensitivity constitutes only an indefinite percentage of all clinical reactions to foods.

PATHOPHYSIOLOGY

Gastrointestinal mucosal immunity is quite complex and distinct from systemic immunity. There are distinct gut-associated lymphoid tissues composed of Peyer's patches in the small intestine and single lymphoid cells. Peyer's patches contain both B and T lymphocytes separated in distinct zones and covered by an epithelium of enterocytes and microfold membrane (M) cells. Intraepithelial lymphocytes are distributed all over the gastrointestinal tract, in epithelium and the lamina propria. The majority are T lymphocytes of the suppressor-cytotoxic subset. Plasma cells are densely packed around the crypts; 82% contain IgA, 16 and 2% contain IgM and IgG, respectively. There are very few IgE-bearing plasma cells in the mucosa of normal people. Their number increases in patients with type I food allergy. Antibodies against food antigens have been found in the feces and intestinal secretions of healthy and food-allergic patients. In addition to locally synthesized immunoglobulins, circulating immunoglobulins also contribute to the intestinal pool.

During normal digestion, most food is broken up into simpler subunits before being absorbed. But some intact macromolecules are absorbed from the intestine even in normal individuals. Macromolecular absorption occurs across the villous epithelium and the Peyer's patch epithelium where the M cells actively take up antigens. Macromolecular uptake also occurs by persorption, that is, the transport of solid food particles through or between intestinal cells. Pinocytosis may also have some role in absorption of intact proteins. This absorption of intact macromolecules increases when the digestion is disordered, as in achlorhydria and gastroenteritis. A deficiency of secretory IgA, which binds to food antigens and retards their absorption, also leads to enhanced uptake of whole macromolecules. Helminthic infestations of the gastrointestinal tract cause increased intestinal permeability directly or via the IgE-mast cell system.

The intact macromolecules absorbed by the intestines provoke both a systemic and a mucosal immune response. Antibodies against food antigens are present in the serum of a large percentage of the normal population and are not diagnostic of food allergy. The mucosal immune response consists primarily of secretory IgA against that particular antigen and retards the further absorption of that antigen. It is hypothesized that T-suppressor cells cause systemic tolerance to that antigen and also suppress deleterious cell-mediated immune response in the gut.

Type I Hypersensitivity

Most of the clinical manifestations of food allergy are due to type I hypersensitivity. This is the classic IgE-mediated mast cell-dependent immediate hypersensitivity reaction. The exposure of a sensitized individual to the appropriate antigens leads to mast cell degranulation in the gut and release of the chemical mediators of inflammation. This causes edema of the epithelium, subepithelial blebs and increased permeability of the mucosa. The histopathological picture may frequently be normal. Gastroscopic examination of food-allergic patients after ingestion of the offending antigen have demonstrated hyperemia, nodularity, edema and thickening of rugal folds, diminished peristalsis, and excessive production of mucus. The food-specific IgE can often be detected in the serum by radioimmunoassay or enzyme-linked immunoassay (ELISA).

Type III Hypersensitivity

Immune complexes with dietary antigens may be detected after food ingestion in both healthy and food-allergic subjects. In healthy subjects, these complexes consist predominantly of IgA; in food-allergic patients, IgG and IgE complexes may also be found. The IgA complexes are rapidly cleared, but the other complexes may be deposited in the bowel wall and other parts of the body and activate complement. Immune complex deposition in the gut leads to the accumulation of polymorphonuclear leukocytes, generation of anaphylotoxins, and enhanced bowel wall permeability. Activation of complement by IgG against food antigen has been shown in patients with egg-white and fish allergy and results in asthma and urticaria. The exact contribution of immune complex hypersensitivity to food allergy has not yet been delineated.

Type IV Hypersensitivity

Delayed hypersensitivity has been shown to be involved in only two situations. Ingestion of the inedible portion of gingko tree fruit causes stomatitis, pruritus ani, perirectal burning, and tenesmus. Oral hyposensitization agains *Rhus* dermatitis leads to stomatitis, pruritis, urticaria, dyshidrosis, and rashes. Cell-mediated immune reactions are implicated in both conditions. A few French as well as Israeli investigations have reported delayed hypersensitivity to edible foodstuff.

CLINICAL MANIFESTATIONS

Almost all organ systems have been claimed to be involved by the protean manifestations of food allergy. There is well-documented evidence for the involvement of the gastrointestinal and respiratory tracts and the skin. The evidence for the involvement of other organs, like the nervous, musculoskeletal, and renal systems, is anecdotal and not accepted by all physicians.

Gastrointestinal Tract

Gastrointestinal symptoms usually accompany systemic allergic reactions although they may also occur alone. Isolated gut symptoms are attributed to direct exposure of intestinal mucosa to allergens. IgE-secreting plasma cells have been demonstrated in the intestinal mucosa of food allergic patients.

Symptoms include edema and pruritus of the lips, tongue, and palate, vomiting, diarrhea, and abdominal pain. Anal pruritus may be seen in patients with diarrhea. Hemorrhagic proctitis can occur with cow's milk allergy. Abdominal distention and constipation are often seen. Other symptoms, like malabsorption, protein-losing enteropathy, intestinal bleeding, iron-deficiency anemia, hypoproteinemia, and eosinophilia, have been described mainly in children but can persist or even develop in adult life. Other rare and infrequent manifestations include hepatosplenomegaly, eosinophilic gastroenteritis, anorexia, colitis, and functional intestinal obstruction.

In eosinophilic gastroenteritis, there is diffuse eosinophilic infiltration of the gut, especially in the pyloric region. There is also associated eosinophilia. Almost one-half of the patients have a history of allergic disease, including urticaria, angioedema, allergic rhinitis, and asthma. Only a few of these cases have been associated with food allergy. In a very small group of patients, reactions to food have been serious and have caused edema of gastric and duodenal mucosa and even sudden death. The identification of food allergy is such patients is important, as withdrawal of the offending food can cause remission of symptoms.

In a small subgroup of patients with inflammatory bowel disease, allergic mechanisms may play an important role. In patients with isolated proctitis, without involvement proximal to the sigmoid colon, there was an increased number of IgE-bearing plasma cells in the lamina propria. These patients improved on oral disodium cromoglycate. No specific food allergy could be demonstrated.

Skin

Urticaria and angioedema are among the commonest symptoms of food allergy. They are the presenting features in 22-44% of patients. Almost all foods implicated in food allergy can cause urticaria. Yeast is a common culprit and is found in bread, sausages, alcoholic drinks, and other foods. *Candida* infestations of the gastrointestinal or genital tract can also lead to urticaria. Food additives are another frequent cause of urticaria, especially azo dyes and preservatives. Salicylates in amounts found in fruits and vegetables can also provoke urticaria. Angioedema involves deeper tissues, and if it involves the glottis, it can be life threatening.

It is easy to link acute urticarial attacks to an offending food and eliminate that particular foodstuff. It is much more difficult to associate recurrent or chronic urticaria with food allergy. Many other factors, including exercise, emotion, stress, and fatigue, can by themselves provoke urticaria or lower the threshold for urticaria due to food allergies.

Eczema has been linked to food allergies in children. Cow's milk and eggs were the foods most commonly implicated, and their withdrawal led to remission in many cases. In adults, elimination diets are not as successful even in patients who give a definite history of an exacerbation of their skin condition by food intake.

Respiratory Tract

Food-induced asthma is a well-recognized entity, although its frequency varies in different studies. Almost one of five asthmatic patients interviewed believes that food had some role to play in the precipitation of the asthma. Many of these may be due to inhalation of food antigens rather than their ingestion. Baker's asthma is due to inhalation of wheat flour. Similar sensitization can occur by exposure to rye, oat, corn, and barley flour, soybeans, green coffee, castor bean, cotton seed, flax seed, and potatoes. Those people can ingest the food involved without any side effects. The smell of fish can provoke asthma in fish-sensitive individuals.

The ingestion of offending food generally leads to asthma after 1–2 hr. Rarely, asthma has been observed to occur within minutes of food intake. This has been confirmed by blind food challenge through a nasogastric tube.

The same food can provoke asthma in different patients by different routes. Alcohol can provoke asthma when taken orally. This may be due to the alcohol itself or other substances in it, like histamine, yeasts, fungi, and flavoring agents. On the other hand, pure ethanol when inhaled or taken intravenously rarely causes asthma and may even increase the vital capacity of asthmatic subjects. Most patients with food-induced asthma have high IgE and a positive radioallergosorbent test (RAST) to the offending food. A small group has low IgE levels and may be RAST negative.

In children with cow's milk allergy, there may be chronic respiratory disease followed by pulmonary hemosiderosis. There is no similar syndrome in adults, although patients with gluten enteropathy are more prone to develop bird-fancier's disease.

The simplest way of documenting food-induced bronchospasm is to measure peak flow values regularly at home and to correlate these with food intake. A regular and predictable correlation between intake of a specific food and a drop in expiratory flow rate implicates food allergy as the causative factor in bronchospasm. Many environmental factors may modify food-induced bronchospasm. For example, no symptoms develop if one avoids shellfish and does not exercise vigorously. Other environmental factors, like weather and other allergens, may modify the subject's response to ingested foods. Some patients develop asthma only after repetitive challenge by a particular food. This is associated with joint pains and diarrhea, implicating an immune complex-mediated reaction.

Rhinorrhea occurs quite commonly on smelling certain foods. It also has been reported in studies in which food was introduced in the stomach via a nasogastric tube.

Central Nervous System

There are over 200 reported cases of epilepsy related to food allergy. These reports were anecdotal and are not taken seriously. Opinion is sharply divided on the role of food allergy in precipitating migraine. It has been shown that foods like chocolates, cheeses, and alcohol, containing vasoactive amines, can cause migraine by their direct pharmacological action. Other studies have tried to demonstrate that allergic mechanisms mediate some of the migrainous attacks by food. Double-blind oral food challenge tests are important confirmatory aids in implicating food allergy as a cause of migraine.

Hematological Disorders

A rare adult patient with severe thrombocytopenia has been reported to recover dramatically on withdrawal of milk. Previously, some patients with congenital absence of radius had been shown to develop thrombocytopenia on ingestion of cow's milk.

Musculoskeletal System

It is the conviction of innumerable patients with arthritis that their condition is exacerbated by food. Recently, a few detailed studies have been done to investigate the relationship between food allergy and arthritis. Although not a common occurrence, an occasional patient with joint disease may have a fully documented association with ingestion of certain foods.

Renal System

A rare patient with steroid-responsive nephrotic syndrome may benefit clinically from elimination of cow's milk and other common allergens from the diet, and this may even lead to a dramatic decrease in proteinuria and edema.

Psychiatric Disorders

The spectrum of psychological illnesses attributed to food allergy range from anxiety and depression to hyperactivity and "foggy brain" syndrome. Most of the evidence is the result of uncontrolled or poorly designed trials.

Anaphylaxis

Systemic anaphylaxis is a potential life-threatening manifestation of food allergy. It can occur from minutes to hours after food intake. There may have been milder symptoms previously on consumption of the same food. There is a sudden onset of dyspnea, cyanosis, angina, hypotension, and shock. Cutaneous manifestations, like urticaria and angioedema, are frequently present at the same time. Nausea, vomiting, and diarrhea may occur. If untreated, anaphylaxis can be fatal.

DIAGNOSIS

Complex investigations are not usually required for the diagnosis of food allergy. A commonsense approach as outlined below will lead to the diagnosis in most cases. History, elimination diets, diet diary, and cutaneous testing will identify many patients with food allergy. Single- or double-blind provocative tests are only needed in patients in whom no clear-cut diagnosis can be made by the above tests. Laboratory investigations are mainly useful for confirming a diagnosis. They are, by themselves, not enough to make a diagnosis of food allergy.

History

A detailed history is the most important initial procedure in the diagnosis of food allergy. The history should include a description of the symptoms, time between ingestion of food and the onset of symptoms, and the nature and amount of food required to provoke symptoms. When severe allergic symptoms follow soon after food intake, patients themselves make the association and avoid that specific food. In other cases there might not be a straightforward association between ingestion of a specific food item and the symptoms. This occurs when the offending food is eaten very frequently and is, therefore, disregarded as a causative agent. Other confounding factors can make diagnosis difficult. Symptoms usually depend on the quantity of food ingested and may occur intermittently, even though the food is ingested daily. Symptoms generally occur within 48 hr of the ingestion of food but may rarely be delayed. Other foods consumed in this time period make identification of the offending food difficult. In some patients, raw food may provoke symptoms but cooked food can be eaten with impunity. Symptoms can be due to food additives or contaminants. Milk or other dairy products may contain traces of antibiotics like penicillin, tetracycline, or bacitracin. One must also keep in mind the various nonallergic mechanisms of food intolerance that can mimic food allergy. The commonest foods causing symptoms is double-blind food challenge are shellfish, dairy products, egg, wheat, peanuts, and citrus fruit.

Diet Diary

This is especially useful in patients with occasional symptoms in whom it may be difficult to make an association on history alone. The patient maintains a record of all foods, beverages, and drugs consumed within 48 hr of each occurrence. Recurrence of the same food with exacerbation of symptoms suggests a causal relationship. Many times no such causal relationship may be apparent. The diet diary can also be used as a guide for skin tests. Testing is only done with antigens temporally associated with symptoms.

Elimination Diets

In patients with severe and recurrent symptoms, an elimination diet can be used for confirming the diagnosis and identifying the offending food. The objective is to establish a diet on which the patient remains asymptomatic, after which the omitted foods are reintroduced one by one until a satisfactory maintenance diet is achieved or until symptoms reappear. It is essential to ensure that the final diet is nutritionally adequate. The elimination diet may follow three setps.

1. Elimination of particular suspect foods, such as milk, eggs, or seafood,
2. Introduction of an empirical basic exclusion diet that excludes most common offending foods, like milk, eggs, fish, nuts, and artificial flavors and coloring.
3. In rare cases, a very simple elimination diet that eliminates virtually all known allergens is used so that a baseline can be established on

which to plan a more adequate dietary regimen. These are generally amino acids from the enzymatic hydrolysis of casein. This is mixed with sucrose, corn oil, vitamins, and minerals.

Some foods, like milk, eggs, and wheat, may be difficult to avoid because of their widespread use in different forms. Kosher cookbooks can provide recipies without milk products. Other specialized recipes can be found in dietetic cookbooks. Elimination diets should be used for 7 days. If marked improvement does not occur, food allergy is not likely and a general diet should be resumed. If there is some improvement, elimination diets can be continued for up to 14 days. If the patient is symptom free on an elimination diet, then regular foods should be reintroduced at 5-day intervals. If there is any exacerbation of symptoms after the reintroduction of a food, that food is eliminated from the diet. Many physicians withhold an important food for a prolonged time only if there are three or more consecutive exacerbations.

Some improvement during an elimination diet does not definitely establish food allergy. Many diseases, such as asthma, have spontaneous remissions and exacerbations and any benefit seen may be coincidental. The placebo effect should also keep in mind while attributing benefits in psychological symptoms to the elimination diet.

Skin Tests

Skin tests neither establish nor confirm a definitive diagnosis of clinically significant food allergy. They only demonstrate the presence of reaginic antibody in the the skin. There are a significant number of false-positive results. False negatives are quite infrequent, and a negative skin test usually excludes type I food allergy to that particular food. Reliability of the skin tests depends on the food in question. The foods correlating most reliably with skin tests include peanuts, eggs, milk, soy, fish, and shellfish. Skin tests are almost always positive with immediate hypersensitivity reactions but may be negative with reactions of delayed onset.

Skin testing is usually done by the prick or scratch methods. Commercially prepared food extracts are commonly used for skin testing. Generally the forearm is used as this allows a tourniquet to be applied in case of a systemic reaction. Intradermal tests advocated by some have a much higher incidence of false positives and have a greater tendency to cause systemic reactions. This may be due to the much higher volume of antigen that penetrates the epidermis in an intradermal injection ($50 \mu l$) compared with the skin prick method ($10^{-3} \mu l$).

The quality of the antigen used in the skin testing is also important. The antigen should, preferably, be standardized by testing it on patients with confirmed allergy to that food. Poor quality of food antigen for skin testing leads to erroneous and unreliable results.

Radioallergosorbent Test

This technique demonstrates the presence of serum IgE antibodies to a specific antigen. It is an in vitro technique and is of special use in the investigation of immediate hypersensitivity reactions. The patient is not exposed to the risk of direct cutaneous testing. It is also useful in patients with extensive eczema, in whom widespread skin lesions contraindicate cutaneous testing. RAST is generally less sensitive than skin tests. Except for foods like eggs, nuts, and fish, the correlation between RAST and skin test is not good. Also, it must be kept in mind that many food reactions are not mediated by IgE antibodies. In these patients, RAST will be negative.

Other techniques, like enzyme-linked immunosorbent assay (ELISA) and radioimmunoassay, also detect serum IgE antibodies and provide information similar to that from RAST.

Basophil Histamine Release

Peripheral blood basophils from patients with type I food allergy release histamine when stimulated in vitro by food antigens. Results from these studies correlate with skin test results. The procedure is time consuming and can be done in well equipped laboratories only.

Controversial Techniques

Many controversial techniques have been claimed to be effective for the diagnosis of food allergy. None has been proven conclusively to be reliable or significant. The following is a brief description of the more common of these techniques.

Cytoxicity Testing (Bryan's Test)

This is based on the premise that the addition of specific allergen in vitro to whole blood or serum leukocyte suspensions will result in the death of leukocytes. It has never been proved effective by controlled scientific studies, nor has a scientific basis for its use been demonstrated.

Subcutaneous Provocation and Neutralization Test

In this technique a subcutaneous injection of antigen of sufficient quantity is administered to elicit symptoms corresponding to the patient's complaints. This is followed by the immediate injection of a stronger or weaker dilution of the same antigen to "relieve" the provoked symptom.

Sublingual Provocative Test

It consists of placing 3 drops of a 1:100 aqueous or glycerinated extract under the tongue of the patient and waiting 10 min for the appearance of symptoms.

Then a "neutralizing" dose, which is usually a dilute solution (1:300,000) of the same extract, is administered.

The American Academy of Allergy in position statements have categorized above techniques as of unproved efficacy. It was recommended that they should at present be performed in controlled trials only.

Controlled Oral Food Challenge

Controlled oral food challenge involves giving the patient one of the suspect foods and observing the results. When both the patient and the doctor are aware of what food is being given, it is called an open food challenge. A single-blind food challenge is one in which only the doctor knows about the food being tested and the patient is kept unaware. In a double-blind food challenge, both the doctor and the patient are unaware of the nature of the food being tested and a neutral observer is present to record the findings. Both the single- and the double-blind food challenges are generally placebo controlled. A double-blind food challenge is the only objective test for food intolerance. A single unequivocal positive result may be taken as evidence for sensitivity to that food.

Before the food challenge, the patient is put on a restricted diet, one on which he or she is symptom free. The food to be tested is camouflaged either in other foods or in opaque gelatin capsules or is introduced via a nasogastric tube. The amount of food given depends on the degree of sensitivity of the patient; it may vary from 10 mg to 8 g. A small dose is used initially and may be increased up to a maximum of 8 g or until symptoms appear. It must be remembered that dried food (as in gelatin capsules) contains much more protein than an equal amount of wet food. Depending on the history, sometimes the challenge must be done with raw food, as cooking may result in the destruction of the relevant antigen.

After challenge with food, the patient is observed for symptoms for at least 2 hr. This time period may be increased depending on the history. Any physical signs, like urticaria, angioedema, asthma, vomiting, diarrhea, rhinitis, or pruritus, are unequivocal indicators of food intolerance. In cases of subjective complaints, however, a number of positive tests along with a totally negative placebo test are required before making the diagnosis.

Food challenge merely confirms a diagnosis of food intolerance. As said before, not all cases of food intolerance are due to true food allergy. Bernstein and colleagues have shown that the correlation of double-blind food challenge with various laboratory tests for determination of immediate hypersensitivity to food is quite poor. There was a 21% correlation with positive basophil histamine release test and only a 7.6% correlation with RAST.

ADDITIONAL READING

Chandra, R. K. (ed.), *Food Intolerance.* Elsevier, New York, 1984.
Chandra, R. K. (ed.), *Food Allergy.* Nutrition Research Education Foundation, St. John's, Newfoundland, 1986.
Chandra, R. K. (ed.), *Food Sensitivity.* Marabou, Sundyberg, Sweden, 1984.
Heiner, D. C. (ed.), Food allergy. *Clin. Rev. Allergy, 2*:1-93, 1984.
May, C. D. and Block, S. A., A modern clinical approach to food hypersensitivity. *Allergy, 33*:166-188, 1978.
Second International Symposium on Immunological and Clinical Problems of Food Allergy. *Ann. Allergy, 51*:218-328, 1983.

6

Diseases Produced or Affected by Food Intolerance

JEAN A. MONRO

The Nightingale Hospital, London, England

Diseases produced by food allergy or considered to be due to food allergy include eczema, asthma, rheumatoid arthritis, colitis, and multiple sclerosis. Some of these are dealt with in other chapters in this book, but here I will cover some aspects of each of these conditions, to give an overall picture.

ECZEMA

The terms "eczema" and "dermatitis" are often used synonymously; however, eczema can be classified as endogenous or exogenous. In the latter group are allergic contact eczema or irritant contact eczema, sometimes infective or photo-allergic. Endogenous eczema includes atopic, seborrhoeic, stasis eczema, diskoid eczema, pompholyx, and asteatotic eczema. In atopy there is a hereditary pre-disposition to develop allergic reactions. These patients have an excessive IgE antibody response to common antigens, and this can result in asthma, eczema, rhinitis, and conjunctivitis. Features of the disease are that it occurs in early childhood, there is usually a family history of atopy, a history of asthma or rhinitis in the patient, a flexural distribution of the eczema, and positive prick tests to common allergens, such as grass pollens, animal fur, house dust mite, and some common foods. Serum IgE concentrations can be greater than 180 IU/ml.

Clinically, eczema starts in childhood in atopic individuals. It affects about 5% of the population. It often starts on the face or in the flexures, particularly the antecubital and popliteal fossae and the ventral aspects of the wrists or the anterior aspect of the ankles.

Immunologic Abnormalities in Atopic Eczema

In a normal subject, IgE responses to antigens will occur, IgE being in the serum in low concentrations, but in atopic disease there is an increased tendency to produce IgE antibodies and raised serum IgE levels occur.

The cutaneous manifestation of IgE-mediated hypersensitivity is urticaria, not eczema, and the mechanisms are more complex and delayed. Initially on exposure to an antigen, itching will occur; scratching in response to the itch may induce part of the eczematous response. In atopic eczema, the number of circulating T lymphocytes is reduced in many patients [1]. This may explain the decrease in cutaneous delayed hypersensitivity [2]. However, mononuclear cell infiltrate in eczematous skin predominantly contains T lymphocytes. If house dust mite is applied by contact to the involved skin of patients with atopic eczema, a delayed eczematous reaction occurs in which basophils form a major component of the cells involved. Cutaneous hypersensitivity may therefore be a result of basophil and mast cell degranulation on parasitic invasion.

Some patients with recurrent staphlococcal infection of the skin and chronic eczema have very high levels of IgE [3]. These patients may show impairment of neutrophil chemotaxis. Lobfer et al., 1979 have described a specific IgE antibody against *Staphylococcus aureus.* Cutaneous staphylococcal infection is very common in atopic eczema and frequently the cause of sudden relapse.

Other forms of infection, such as Kaposi's varicelliform eruption with vaccinia, a widespread cutaneous viral infection, or *Herpes simplex* (eczema herpeticum) can occur. Active immunization with some egg-based protein in culture fluids can result in exacerbation of eczema.

Food Sensitivity and Eczema

As atopic eczema usually presents in infancy, its relationship to the changing diet of the infant has been closely scrutinized. It often occurs with cessation of breast-feeding [4]. Matthew et al. reported decreases in the expected incidence of atopic eczema in 20 children, in whom cow's milk was completely avoided. Atherton et al. [5] reported a double-blind controlled crossover trial of an antigen avoidance diet in atopic eczema. Of 36 children, aged from 2 to 8, 20 with atopic eczema completed a 12-week trial of an egg and cow's milk exclusion diet. For the first and third 4-week periods, the patients avoiding egg and cow's milk were fed soya-based milk substitute or an egg and cow's milk preparation. The response of the children was assessed in terms of the number of areas affected, pruritus, sleeplessness, the antihistamine usage, and eczema activity. Of the 20 patients who completed the trial, 14 responded more favorably to the antigen avoidance diet than to the control diet, whereas only one responded more favorably to the control diet than to the trial diet. Those children who dropped out withdrew usually after a control period, it was concluded perhaps because of the lack of benefit experienced. A total of 3 patients stopped all symptomatic treatments after the eczema virtually cleared during the antigen avoidance period. Other 3 patients had a severe exacerbation of eczema within a few days of starting their final diet period; in these cases this was the control diet.

Any patient who lapsed during the trial by not taking the required milk or milk substitute or eating an excluded food was excluded from the diet if more than five lapses occurred in any 4-week period.

Prick tests were performed in all patients at the start of the second period with 10 allergen solutions: *Dermatophagoides pteronyssinus,* Timothy grass pollen, cat fur *Aspergillus fumigatus,* whole egg, egg white, cereals, egg yolk, x lactalbumin, and whole cow's milk. There was no correlation between positive prick test to egg and cow's milk antigen and response to the diet.

I would like to suggest that the results of the study indicate that the value of dietary treatment in atopic eczema is greater than had been widely appreciated and that critical appraisal of avoidance of other dietary antigens in patients responding incompletely to cow's milk and egg avoidance alone is required.

In allergic contact eczema, allergic sensitization can follow skin contact with a variety of nonprotein substances, such as nickel, chrome, or rubber, which presumably act as haptens. Cutaneous Langerhans' cells are considered to play a role in antigen presentation. If the substance is subsequently applied to the skin, an area of eczema will develop at that site between 24 and 96 hr later. The timing of this reaction indicates that it is a delayed hypersensitivity reaction. Foods can aggravate eczema by direct contact, and this is particularly important in food handlers, and of course any patients with atopic eczema may equally be prone to this by handling food for their own consumption.

Dietary Management

It has been suggested that dietary management of eczema should be considered for infants, but many adults respond to dietary manipulation also. The first antigens to be considered are milk and egg, but there are many allergens related to milk. The other foods that should be excluded are beef products. A list of a suggested milk-free diet is appended (Appendix 1). In general, it can be assumed that for some patients the amount of milk taken is crucial. In fact, as had been stated by Atherton et al. [5], lapses made the trial invalid if more than five lapses occurred in a period of 4 weeks. However, some milk-sensitive patients can tolerate milk in a "denatured" way: evaporated milk or heat-treated milk may be more acceptable, especially if cooked into foods, than fresh milk. Some patients can tolerate goat's or sheep's milk instead of cow's milk, yet others find these intolerable.

Egg avoidance is more readily observed, as egg is distinctly utilized in egg dishes. A number of dietary books have been produced describing milk and egg avoidance.

If egg- and milk-free diets are not adequate in preventing eczema, a controlled regime of identifying foods responsible for the eczema can be applied. Avoidance of all common foods for a period of 5 days can be instituted and thereafter common foods introduced sequentially one at a time. As eczema can take a delayed period to develop, over a period of 5 days any food that causes itching of the skin should be avoided and the uncommon foods reinstituted before the introduction of another common food. However, if this regime proves too difficult to institute, and it may well be so in children, a different regime may be required. Initially, remove additives, especially tartrazine and monosodium glutamate, because they have been known to initiate adverse responses.

Detailed information about tartrazine and benzoic-free diets are in Appendix 2; as is also a note concerning the additive labeling regulations applied in the United Kingdom.

Having instituted a coloring- and additive-free diet and recommended the use of fresh foods only, one can then eliminate groups of foods according to the food families in which they occur. As has already been mentioned, there can be cross-reactions between milk and beef, and similarly there can be cross-reactions between chicken and egg. In a similar way, there are other food groups that are related; that is grains, including wheat, rye, barley, oats, maize, millet, rice, and derivatives of these. For example, derivatives of maize include corn syrup, corn oil, corn starch, and dextrose, and those related to barley include malt. Lists of some food-related products are attached (Appendix 3). Each diet should be introduced sequentially for a period of a fortnight as eczematous reactions may take 5 days to come on and subside. After identification of individual foods that cause reactions, these may be excluded from the diet and a rotation diet devised. An example of a rotation diet is given in (Appendix 3).

URTICARIA

Urticaria is classically a condition resulting from the sudden localized accumulation of fluid in the dermis or deeper tissues due to increased vascular permeability. Mast cells in the vicinity release the vasoactive mediators and they degranulate, having been triggered by IgE antibodies or complement fragments or by direct mast cell degranulation by drugs. Immediate hypersensitivity reactions trigger urticaria in some patients; the effects usually last about 24 hr but can be as long as 3 days. These responses can be suppressed by H_1 histamine antagonists. Recurrent urticarial reactions, however, may not be IgE mediated as histamine suppression does not reduce the weal formation or erythema and prostaglandin E_2 (PGE$_2$) mediation is involved.

There is evidence that dietetic factors are involved, and in particular avoidance of azo dyes and benzoates may prove beneficial (see Appendix 2).

RHEUMATOID ARTHRITIS

This condition is discussed elsewhere in this book, but mention of two studies is of importance. That by Park and Hughes [10], in which a patient's rheumatoid arthritis appeared to be exacerbated by dairy produce, showed that challenge with milk and cheese resulted in a marked increase in synovitis and changes in immune complex IgE antibodies and heat-damaged red cell clearance rates. Exclusion of dairy produce from the diet produced a considerable improvement in her previously aggressive disease. Recently, raised levels of 5-hydroxyindo-leacetic acid after food challenge have been reported in the serum of rheumatoid arthritis patients. Their symptoms increased following challenge with certain foodstuffs.

IRRITABLE BOWEL SYNDROME

Jones et al. found specific foods provoked symptoms of irritable bowel syndrome in 14 of 21 patients. They challenged patients double blind, and in 6 food intolerance was found. Although they found no difference in changes in plasma, glucose, histamine, immune complexes, hematocrit, eosinophil count, or breath hydrogen excretion produced after challenge by controlled foods, they did find that prostaglandin E_2 increased significantly.

The irritable bowel syndrome is one of the commonest bowel complaints seen by gastroenterologists. Patients suffer from abdominal pain, diarrhea or con constipation, and flatulence. Often there is no radiological or histological evidence of organic disease. The patients that Jones et al. studied [11] showed a classic symptom pattern with no abnormality detected by barium enema, rectal biopsy, or stool culture. The group of 25 patients were asked to limit their diets for 1 week to a single meat, a single fruit, and distilled or spring water. Those whose symptoms remitted on this regime were then asked to reintroduce single foods daily to ascertain whether certain foods provoked their symptoms and were asked to retest foods they believed upset them on three separate occasions. Following this, in a second study, 6 patients who were symptom free were admitted to the hospital; each patient was given a diet free of all foods that provoked symptoms, and the same menu was eaten each day. In these patients breakfast was given as a double-blind challenge, a nasogastric tube was passed, and fasting samples were taken; thereafter they were given a test food believed to provoke symptoms or a control food believed to have no such effect. A third study was undertaken in which five patients were admitted for two periods of 4 days, 4 weeks apart. They were tested with foods single blind during the first 4 days and then received twice-daily control food disguised in a flavored soup. In a second phase, test food was administered in the same way. All other meals were foods thought to be innocuous. In their first study, 4 of the 25 patients refused to try the diet, but of the remainder, 14 found that their symptoms cleared. A number of foods were found to provoke symptoms: wheat in 9, corn, 5, dairy products, 4, coffee, 4, tea, 3, and citrus fruit, 2. The patients who were found to be intolerant of wheat had a jejunal biopsy, and in all cases the sample was found to be histologically clear. In their second study, randomized double-blind food testing in the six patients showed that 10 of 12 test days and 11 of 12 control days were correctly identified by the patients (the t-test comparison; $t = 4.93C$ = less than 0.01). In their third study, five female patients all correctly identified the test period. Investigators found no evidence of food allergy in that serum IgE concentrations were normal and there was no evidence of raised eosinophil count. They postulated that the altered levels of prostaglandins that they found implicated these in the pathogenesis of the syndrome. The mechanisms by which food ingestion leads to prostaglandin production remain obscure.

It has been suggested that food allergy is an IgE immune complex disorder in which the mast cell in the duct plays the central role: if activated, it initiates a variety of inflammatory actions affecting smooth muscle contractions, small vessel permeability, chemotaxis, and cell activation. The release of mediator leads to an increase in gut permeability, permitting the entry of antigen and immune complexes. Patients with delayed-onset food allergy may well have a chronic form of serum sickness in which many of the organ systems may be involved, explaining the polysymptomatology of the condition. If the patient eats foods in large amounts, immune complexes may be formed in antigen excess and are therefore soluble. On dietary exclusion, antigen concentration falls and precipitates of immune complexes are formed as the complexes become insoluble, but again when the antigens clear the complexes formed will be in antibody excess and soluble again. It has been well documented that patients who are put on exclusion diets have withdrawal symptoms that would fit this pattern of response.

REFERENCES

1. Byrom, N. A., and Timlin, D. M., *Br. J. Dermatol.*, *100*:491, 1979.
2. Champion, R. H., and Parish, W. E., in *Textbook of Dermatology* (3rd ed.). A. J. Rook, D. S. Wilkinson, and F. J. G. Ebling (eds.). Blackwell Scientific, Oxford, 1979, p. 353.
3. Hanifin, J. M., and Lobitz, W. C., *Arch. Dermatol.*, *113*:663, 1977.
4. Matthew, D. J., Taylor, B., Norman, A. P., Turner, M. W., and Soothill, J. F., *Lancet, 1*:321, 1977.
5. Atherton, D. J., Sewell, M., Soothill, J. F., Wells, R. S., and Chilvers, C. E. D., *Lancet, 1*:401, 1978.
6. Sheffer, A. L., Urticaria and angiodema. In *Proceedings of the XI Inter-*

national Congress of Allergology and Clinical Immunology, J. W. Kerr and M. A. Ganderton (eds.). McMillan Press, London, 1983, pp. 119-124.

7. Kaplan, A. P., Horakova, Z., and Katz, S. L., Assessment of tissue fluid hi histamine levels in patients with urticaria. *J. Allergy Clin. Immunol., 61*: 350-354, 1978.

8. Misch, K. J., Greaves, M. W., and Kobza, Black, A. Histamine and the skin. *Br. J. Dermatol.* (Suppl.) *5*:10-13, 1983.

9. Phanuphak, P., Schoket, A., and Kohler, P. F., Treatment of chronic idiopathic urticaria with combined H_1 and H_2 blockers. *Clin. Allergy, 8*:49-43, 1978.

10. Parke, A. L., and Hughes, G. R. V., Rheumatoid arthritis and food: A case study. *Br. Med. J., 282*:2027-2029, 1981.

11. Alan Jones, V., Shorthouse, M., McLaughlan, P., Workman, E., and Hunter, J. O., Food intolerance: A major factor in the pathogenesis of irritable bowel syndrome. *Lancet, 2*:1115-1117, 1982.

ADDITIONAL READING

Atherton, D. J., Atopic eczema in food allergy. *Clin. Immunol. Allergy, 1*:000, 1983.

Atherton, D. J., Sewell, M., Soothill, J. F., Wells, R. S., and Chilers, C. E. D., A double blind controlled crossover trial of an antigen avoidance diet in atopic eczema. *Lancet, 1*:401-403, 1978.

Barnetson, R. S. C., Merrett, T. G., and Ferguson, A., Studies on hyperinnunoglobulinaemia E in atopic diseases with particular reference to food allergens. *Clin. Exp. Immunol., 46*:54-60, 1981.

Rajka, G., *Atopic Dermatitis.* W. B. Saunders, London, 1975.

APPENDIX 1: MILK–FREE DIET

Basic Allergy Diet.

Remember To Read All Labels Carefully.

Be Aware: Lactose, lactic acid, whey, casein, sodium caseinate, are all extracted from milk.

No Milk Means: No cream, fresh, dried, or skimmed milk, goat's or sheep's milk, butter, cheese, yoghurt, butter.

Most Commercially Made Food contains *Milk* in some form: Bread, biscuits, cakes, sweets, chocolates, salad creams and dressings, pickles, sauces, instant food (potato), soups, cereals, baby foods, instant drinks (Bournvita, Horlicks, dandelion coffee, Ovaltine, etc.), margarines, artificial sweeteners, food covered in breadcrumbs. *Instead*

Homemade is the best; you know what you have put in it.

However, Most large food manufacturers, e.g., Sainsburys, Marks and Spencer,
Waitrose, will supply you with lists of their milk-free products. Apply
directly to the firm.
A liquidizer is a good investment.

Milk Substitutes
Soya milks — Be-mil Pro Sorbee (powdered only)
Do not have soya milks containing beet (white) or cane (brown) sugar.
Nut milks — coconut cream, almond milk.
Magic milk — if you can tolerate eggs:
Recipe:
     3 lightly poached eggs or 3 egg yolks
     1 c water   ½ c oil
     1 c oil   3-4 c water
Liquidize eggs and oil, and add water gradually.
Pour into jug and make up to 2 pints with water.
Keeps the same time as milk in refrigerator, but whisk up before use.
Excellent for a milk substitute in cooking.

Evaporated milk *sometimes* can be tolerated, but please consult your doctor or
dietician before testing it.

Butter Substitutes
Margarines: Kosher (Tomor), Waitrose, and superfine low-fat spreads contain
corn and other oils, artificial flavoring, and coloring, and therefore do not suit
everyone.
Vitaquel is cold-pressed, unrefined, wheat, maize (corn), sunflower.
Cold-pressed unrefined oils for cooking, sunflower, safflower, and sesame,
grapenut, olive oil.
Coconut oil (M.C.T.-med. chain triglyceride).
Cashew nut, peanut, sesame seed, sunflower seed spreads.
Lamb, beef, and pork lard can be used.
Ghee available at Indian stores,
Clarified butter is usually tolerated:
Recipe:
Bring unsalted butter to the boil and skim off curds. Then strain hot fat through
cotton sieve. When nearly set, add a little sea salt to taste. Keep in refrigerator.

*All the Above Substitutes Must Be Used Sparingly and on a Strict 3 Day or 4
Day Off Rotation.*
Beef cannot be tolerated by some milk-allergic people.
Vitamin supplements:
     Calcium carbonate — 1 tsp/day.
     1 tsp cold-pressed oils or margarines per day.
     Halibut oil capsule — 2 per week.

Recipe Books:
Grain free, milk free – Cherry Hills
The Milk and Egg Free Cookbook – Isobel Sainbury, M.D.
See A.A.A. book list.

ALLERGY SUPPORT SERVICE
COMMON SOURCES OF YEAST

The following foods contain yeast as an additive ingredient in preparation, (often called leavening).

Breads	*Crackers*
Cake and Cake mixes	*Canned ice box biscuits:*
Cookies	Bordens, Pillsbury & General Mills

Flour. Enriched with vitamins from yeast: General Mills, Inc. Flour Corporation flour and enrichment products. Pfizer Laboratories enrichment products. Hungarian Flour Mills.

Hamburger buns	*Pastries*
Hot dog buns	*Pretzels*
Milk, fortified with vitamins	*Rolls,* homemade or canned
Meat, fish or fowl, fried in cracker crumbs	*Salt rising bread*

The following substances contain yeast or yeast-like substances because of their nature of their manufacture or preparation.

Black tea	*Soy sauce*
Buttermilk	*Truffles*
Mushrooms	*Yoghurt*
Sour cream	

Cheese of all kinds, including *cottage cheese*

Citric acid – almost always a yeast derivative.

Citrus fruit juices, of all types, whether frozen or canned. Only home-squeezed are yeast-free.

Dried fruits, of all types (prunes, raisins, dates, etc.)

Fermented beverages of all types. Beer, brandy, gin, rum, whiskey, wine, vodka, root beer, ginger ale.

Malted products of all types. Cereals, candy and milk drinks, which have been malted.

Monosodium glutamate, may be a yeast derivative.

Vinegars of all types: Apple, pear, grape and distilled. These may be used as such or they will be used in the following foods: All baby cereals, Bar-B-Q sauce, catsup, condiments, chili and peppers, etc. French dressing, horseradish, mayonnaise, mince pie, olives, pickles, salad dressing, sauerkraut, tomato sauce.

Yeast extracts, marmite, bovril, natex.

The following contain substances that are derived from yeast or have their source from yeast:

Antibiotics: B-12, Chloromycetin, Linocin, Mycin drugs, Penicillin, Tetracylines, and any others derived from mold cultures. Multiple vitamin capsules or tablets with Vitamin B made from yeast vitamin B Capsules or tablets if made from yeast.

U.S. vitamin products
Citric acid
Endo vitamin products
Laxo-Funk
Lilly vitamin products that
  contain vit. B-12
Lederle vitamin products
Manibee tablets, S.C.T.
Massengill vitamins
Zylax, Zymelose, Zymenol

Mead Johnson vitamins that contain
  vit. B-12
Merck Sharp & Dohme vitamin products
  that contain vit. B-12
Parke Davis vitamin products: VIBEX
Phoscaron-D
Squibb vitamin products if indicated
  on label
Vi-Litron Drops
Dormison rest capsules

Be sure to read labels. Additions may be found to this list.

From: Yeast: A Brief Description of Common Sources of Contacts of Yeast, compiles by Dr. Brown, Jr., M.D., with additions by Edward L. Brinkley, Jr., M.D.

Fructose is in all Fruit and Vegetables and Nuts

Very low

Avocado
Cranberries
Currants (white)
Gooseberries
Lemons
Loganberries
Melons
Rhubarb
Almonds
Brazil Nuts
Coconuts
Walnuts
Artichokes
Asparagus
Beans (French/runner)
Broccoli
Sprouts
Cabbage (all)

Carrots
Cauliflower
Celery
Chickory
Cucumber
Egg Plant
Lettuce
Marrow
Mushrooms (nil)
Pumpkin
Radishes
Salsify
Spinach
Swede
Tomatoes
Turnips
Water Cress

Low

Apricots	Passion Fruit
Blackberries	Quinces
Currants (black)	Raspberries
Damsons	Strawberries
Figs (green)	Cob Nuts
Tangerines	Peanuts
Greengages	Beans (broad)
Grapefruit	Leeks
Mandarines	Mustard & Cress
Medlars	Onions
Mulberries	Sweet Potatoes
Oranges	

Medium

Apples	Plums
Apricots (dried)	Pomegranates
Cherries	Chestnuts
Grapes (black)	Beetroot
Grapes (white)	Horseradish
Melons (yellow)	Parsnips
Nectarines	Peas
Peaches	Potatoes (all)
Pears	Yams
Pineapple	

High

(all canned in syrup)	Raisins
Bananas	Sultanas (dried)
Currants (dried)	Beans (butter)
Dates	Beans (haricot)
Figs (dried)	Lentils (dried)
Peaches (dried)	Peas (dried)
Prunes (dried)	

APPENDIX 2: TARTRAZINE, AZO DYES, AND BENZOIC ACID–FREE DIET

Some people have been found to get an urticaria reaction from tartrazine, azo dyes, and benzoic acid, which are present in many yellow colorings and preservatives used in food. The following diet will help in this situation.

Foods Allowed

Bread
Cereals, e.g., flour, porridge, rice
Potatoes
Sugar
Salad oil
Honey, marmite
Eggs, milk, meat, and fish
Cream
Fresh fruit and vegetables
Any other foods free of preservatives, e.g., cooking oil, lard, and cooking
    fats, e.g., Trex; pure chocolate

Proprietary Foods That Are Free of Tartrazine, Azo Dyes, and Benzoic Acid

Winston Smith sausages
Sainsbury's jams and marmalades
Heinz salad cream
Unigate, Farmers Wife, St. Ivel: butter, cheese (not cheese spread), plain
    yoghurt
Express Dairies: butter, cheese
Sainsbury's butter, cheese, plain yoghurt
Van den Burgs: margarines
Schweppes: American and Dry ginger ale, ginger beer, soda water, tonic
    water, Slimline ginger ale, and tonic water

Foods That Contain Tartrazine: Avoid These Foods

Penny candies, caramels and chews, fruit drops
Filled chocolate but not pure chocolate
Soft drinks, fruit drinks, fizzy lemonade (except plain lemonade)
Jellies
Jams, marmalades (unless homemade)
Stewed fruit sauces, fruit gelatins
Fruit yoghurt
Ice cream
Pie fillings
Vanilla, butterscotch, or chocolate puddings
Caramel custard (unless homemade)
Whips and dessert sauces, e.g., vanilla custard

Foods That Contain Azo Dyes: Avoid These Foods

Cream in powder form, e.g., Coffeemate
Bakery foods except plain rolls, crackers, cheese puffs, crisps
Cake and cookie/biscuit mixtures
Waffle and pancake mixes
Macaroni and spaghetti (certain brands)
Mayonnaise, salad dressing/cream; sauces, e.g., ketchup, mustard
Ready-made sauces, e.g., bearnaise, hollandaise, curry, fish, tomato, white
    onion, and parsley sauces
Packet and canned soups
Canned anchovies, herrings, sardines, caviar, cleaned shellfish
Colored toothpaste, yellow food coloring
Purees except pure tomato puree

Foods That Contain Benzoic Acid and Derivatives: Avoid These Foods

Soft drinks, fruit drinks, ciders
Jellies, jams, marmalades
Fruit gelatins, stewed fruit sauces
Some cheese, especially cream cheese
Low calorie margarine, e.g., Outline
Salad dressings, mustard
Ready-made sauces, e.g., see above
Salads with dressings, e.g., coleslaw
Refrigerated preserves of herrings, sardines, anchovies, shellfish
White fish treated with preservatives; can be washed off and then allowed
Drinking chocolate concentrates

Marmite may worsen urticaria because of its concentrated yeast content.
Please check all tablets and medicine with your doctor or druggist as some may
contain these substances.

APPENDIX 3: FOUR--DAY ROTATION DIETS

Day 1

Food Families:
Citrus: lemon, orange, grapefruit, lime, tangerine, kumquat, citron
Banana: banana, plantain, arrowroot (*Musa*)
Palm: coconut, date, date sugar
Parsley: carrots, parsnips, celery, celery seed, celeriac, anise, dill, fennel,
    cumin, parsley, coriander, caraway

Pepper: black and white pepper, peppercorn
Herbs: nutmeg, mace
Subucaya: brazil nut
Bird: all fowl and game birds, including chicken, turkey, duck, goose, guinea, pigeon, quail, pheasant, eggs
Tea: comfrey tea (borage family), fennel tea
Oil: coconut oil, fats from any bird listed above
Sweetener (use sparingly): date sugar, orange honey if honey not used on another day of rotation
Juices: juices may be made and used without adding sweeteners from the following. fruits: any listed above in any combination desired; vegetables: any listed above in any combination desired, including fresh comfrey

Day 2

Food Families:

Grape: all varieties of grapes, raisins
Pineapple: juice pack, water pack, or fresh
Rose: strawberry, raspberry, blackberry, dewberry, loganberry, youngberry, boysenberry, rose hips
Melon (gourd): watermelon, cucumber, cantaloupe, pumpkin, squash, other melons, zucchini, acorn, pumpkin, or squash seeds
Mallow: okra, cottonseed
Beet: beet, spinach, chard, lamb's quarters (greens)
Pea (legume): pea, black-eyed pea, dry beans, green beans, carob, soybeans, lentils, licorice, peanut, alfalfa
Cashew: cashew, pistachio, mango
Birch: filberts, hazelnuts
Flaxseed: flaxseed
Swine: all pork products
Molluscs: abalone, snail, squid, clam, mussel, oyster, scallop
Crustaceans: crab, crayfish, lobster, prawn, shrimp
Tea: alfalfa tea, fenugreek
Oil: soybean oil, peanut oil, cottonseed oil
Sweeteners (use sparingly): carob syrup or beet sugar
Clover honey: if honey not used on another day
Juices: Juices may be made and used without added sweeteners from the following: fruits or berries: any listed above in any combinations desired; vegetables: any listed above in any combination desired including fresh alfalfa and some legumes

Day 3

Food Families:

Apple: apple, pear, quince
Mulberry: mulberry, figs, breadfruit
Honeysuckle: elderberry
Olive: black or green or stuffed with pimento
Gooseberry: currant, gooseberry
Buckwheat: buckwheat, rhubarb
Aster: lettuce, chicory, endive, escarole, artichoke, dandelion, sunflower, seeds, tarragon
Potato: potato, tomato, eggplant, peppers (red and green), chili pepper, paprika, cayenne, ground cherries
Lily (onion): onion, garlic, asparagus, chives, leeks
Spurge: tapioca
Herb: basil, savory, sage, oregano, horehound, catnip, spearmint, peppermint, thyme, majoram, lemon balm
Walnut: English walnut, black walnut, pecan, hickory nut, butternut
Pendalium: sesame
Beech: chestnut
Saltwater fish: sea herring, anchovy, cod, sea bass, sea trout, mackerel, tuna, swordfish, flounder, sole
Freshwater fish: sturgeon, herring, salmon, whitefish, bass, perch
Tea: Kaffir tea
Oil: safflower oil
Honey (use sparingly): buckwheat, safflower, or sage honey if not used on another day
Juices: juices may be made and used without added sweeteners from the following: fruits: any listed above in any combinations desired; vegetables and herbs: any listed above in any combination desired

Day 4

Food Families:

Plum: plum, cherry, peach, apricot, nectarine, almond, wild cherry
Blueberry: blueberry, huckleberry, cranberry, wintergreen
Pawpaws: pawpaw, papaya, papain
Mustard: mustard, turnip, radish, horseradish, watercress, cabbage, kraut, Chinese cabbage, broccoli, cauliflower, brussels sprouts, collards, kale, kohlrabi, rutabaga
Laurel: avocado, cinnamon, bay leaf, sassafras, cassia buds or bark
Sweet potato or yam

Grass: wheat, corn, rice, oats, barley, rye, wild rice, cane, millet, sorghum, bamboo shoots

Orchid: vanilla

Protea: Macadamia nut

Conifer: pine nut

Fungus: mushrooms and yeast (brewer's yeast, etc.)

Bovid: milk products — butter, cheese, yoghurt, beef and milk products, oleomargarine, lamb

Tea: sassafras tea or papaya leaf tea, maté tea, lemon verbena tea

Oil: corn oil, butter

Sweetener (use sparingly): cane sugar, sorghum, corn syrup, glucose, dextrose, avocado honey if honey is not used on another day

Juices: juices may be made and used without added sweeteners from the following: fruits: any listed above in any combination desired; vegetables: any listed above in any combination desired, including any of the tea herbs obtained fresh

7
Migraine and Allergy

JEAN A. MONRO

The Nightingale Hospital, London, England

DIAGNOSTIC CLASSIFICATION

The diagnosis of migraine is clinical and should not depend on mechanism or etiology [1]. The Ad Hoc Committee on classification of headache defines migraine as "Recurrent attacks of headache widely varied in intensity, frequency and duration" [2]. The distinction between clinical groups of migraine is rightly blurred in this definition, as susceptibility to one type of headache may change and another may predominate in the same individual at different times in the natural history of the disease. The groups are nevertheless classified for descriptive diagnostic purposes although their etiology may be the same. The classification is into common classic hemiplegic, ophthalmoplegic, and basilar migraine; migrainous neuralgia is regarded as a separate entity.

CLINICAL FEATURES

In common migraine, periodic headaches occur in association with nausea and dizziness. Classic migraine is characterized by severe unilateral headache preceded by teichopsia or scotomata. Following the onset of headache, nausea and vomiting, constipation or diarrhea, diuresis or urinary retention, alterations in temperature control with associated pallor, or sometimes hyperemia and some sensory phenomena, such as heightened perception of sound and photophobia, may occur.

Hemiplegic migraine is again unilateral, with sensory disturbances of paraesthesias and·motor associations of hemiplegic limb weakness or disturbances of speech that are generally fleeting but may occasionally become permanent.

Ocular palsies may be similarly temporary or permanent in ophthalmoplegic migraine. The third cranial nerve is the most commonly affected.

Basilar migraine is heralded by paraesthesias around the mouth and lips, bilateral paraesthesias of the hands and feet, and sometimes a sensation in the epigastrium and chest of a "rushing sensation." The ensuing headache is bilateral. Often with this form of headache there may be an associated feeling of fear, panic, and doom and strong emotional sensations that are difficult to dispel, though short-lived.

In migraine, the quality of the pain is described often as throbbing [3] and can be very intense. This accords with a vascular hypothesis of the etiology of migraine. The frequency of the attacks varies; in some patients it may occur as frequently as daily, in others as sporadically as once every few years. Each attack may last from a few hours to several days. The severity of attacks may also vary from simply the teichopsia or scotoma, perhaps with a slight awareness of pain, to intense severe headache that, with the accompanying other features, renders the patient helpless.

Horton's neuralgia, histamine headache, and cluster headache are all synonyms for a distinct form of migrainous neuralgia in which the headache occurs in clusters with long periods of remission. The headache is often extremely severe and associated with unilateral lacrimation and conjunctivitis.

The time of onset of attacks is often characteristic. Many patients wake with the migrainous attack. Sometimes there may be frequent attacks in paroxysms and then a remission with a period of relatively few attacks.

The association of headaches with the premenstrual phase of the menstrual cycle is common. Other hormonal factors play a part, such as the onset of migraine with the menarche, abatement with the menopause on occasion, aggravation with the contraceptive pill, and cessation during pregnancy.

Missed meals are almost certainly a trigger. Changes in temperature or visual, auditory, or olfactory stimuli will provoke attacks. In particular, zigzag patterns and flickering lights or stroboscopic effects will trigger migraine. Sometimes weather changes, such as impending storms, act as triggers. Fatigue, excitement, or stress may also provoke attacks. Food triggers are discussed later.

FAMILY HISTORY

There is often a strong family history of migraine in some cases. In others there is an association between migraine and epilepsy. The two disorders are reported to coexist in a greater number of patients than expected by chance [3]. An excess of migraine is reported in families of epileptics. Epilepsy occurs in 2-11% of migraine patients.

PATHOLOGICAL CHANGES

There are no gross anatomic changes seen after a migrainous attack, except in those subjects in whom residual neurological sequelae occur, when cerebral infarcts have been shown by computer axial tomography [4] or at necropsy [5].

Goltman [6] reported the case of a woman who was operated on during a migrainous attack and was found to have an edematous brain. She had a skull flap lifted. On a later occasion when she had a migrainous headache after eating wheat, edematous swelling was palpable through the skull opening.

Reduced cerebral blood flow has been demonstrated during the aura in particular. The ischemia may outlast the clinical manifestations of the aura [7, 8]. There is hyperemia in the headache phase. It has been suggested that this may be a compensatory effect from the hypoxia, or it could be that pain itself augments metabolism causing the blood flow to increase [9]. On occasion, although the headache is unilateral, the oligemia is bilateral. Olesen et al. [7, 8] have shown that intense oligemia starts in one occipital lobe in patients with classic migraine. The oligemia spreads slowly forward but is not confined to the major territories of the posterior or middle cerebral arteries.

Electroencephalographic (EEG) changes in migraine include both focal and generalized slow θ and δ activity that may precede the symptoms of the aura.

BIOCHEMICAL OBSERVATIONS

Histamine headache is associated with generalized vasodilatation, but this is not common in all forms of migraine.

Changes in serotonin metabolism during migrainous attacks have been demonstrated [10]. Plasma 5-HT has been found to rise just prior to the onset of headache in classic migraine and to fall during the headache phase [11, 12]. 5-Hydroxyindoleacetic acid (5-HIAA) excretion increases during attacks [11], indicating, as it is a metabolite of 5-HT, that more is being released and utilized. Of the 5-HT in blood, 98% is contained in platelets. Hence, release of 5-HT is likely to be from platelets when they aggregate. An increase in platelet aggregation has been described by Hilton and Cumings [13]. A serotonin-releasing factor has been demonstrated by Anthony and Lance [14] and colleagues to be active during the vasoconstrictor phase of migraine. This releases 5-HT from platelets. In the subsequent painful vasodilator phase, low levels of 5-HT are found. Increased platelet aggregability has been shown in patients with migraine [13], with a fall in platelet 5-HT and monoamine oxidase levels in migrainous attacks [15].

An increase in β-thromboglobulin during migrainous attack was reported by Gawel et al. [16]. This is regarded as an index of the platelet release reaction

[17]. Other aggregating agents have also been considered, including epinephrine, norepinephrine, and adenosine diphosphate [18-21].

Hanington has hypothesized that migraine is a blood disorder due to abnormal platelet function [00].

When platelets aggregate, arachidonic acid is released by the action of platelet phosphorylase A_2 via the cyclo-oxygenase pathway [22-24]. Prostaglandins and thromboxane A_2 are synthesized. Thromboxane A_2 is a potent vasoconstrictor and may be involved in the etiology of migraine.

IMMUNOLOGIC CONSIDERATIONS

Platelet hyperaggregability can be provoked by immune mechanisms. Soluble immune complexes do lead to platelet aggregation [25] and 5-HT release from platelets [26].

Little et al. [27] have shown that 5-HT fell and 5-HIAA levels rose in patients with rheumatoid arthritis known to be intolerant of various foods with which they were challenged. This indicates that 5-HT is released from platelets during food challenge in food-sensitive patients. The same phenomenon may be responsible for migraine.

The normal clearance mechanisms for food antigens entails complexes with IgG and IgA [28]. In food-allergic subjects, however, it has been shown that IgE complexes are also formed [29]. Platelets contain receptors for both IgG [30] and IgE [31].

Sodium cromoglycate blocks the immediate hypersensitivity reaction in patients with food allergy and prevents the formation of IgE complexes [32]. We have shown that the effects of food challenges can be blocked in patients with migraine by prior treatment with oral sodium cromoglycate [33].

HISTORICAL ASSOCIATION OF FOOD ALLERGY WITH MIGRAINE

Migraine has been known to be provoked by food for centuries, and there have been reports that the basis of this is food allergy. A consideration of the evolution of the human diet would be appropriate.

People differ in their dietary requirements, but the basis of the variations has not been elucidated. The aphorism "one man's meat is another man's poison" indicates that some foods do not suit everyone because of intolerance from pharmacological or immunologic effects.

Humans have chosen their food by trial and error over thousands of years. If the substance caused illness, it would not be used again. For example, the death cap fungus (*Amanita phalloides*) is poisonous, causing abdominal pain, diarrhea and vomiting, prostration, coma, and death within a day. Yet it looks similar to the field mushroom (*Agarious campestris*), which is a good food source rich in vitamins. The distinction between these two has been carefully noted; the edible variety has brown gills, the poisonous, pink, and the death cap has a volva, a cuplike socket supporting the bottom of the stem. There is obviously a pharmacological intolerance that affects everybody equally.

In other cases the effects can be mediated immunologically and can be just as dramatic due to anaphylaxis. The food may be one in customary use yet affects only certain individuals rather than everyone.

In other cases the "toxicity" of the food has not been identified as the effects are insidious, and again the effects can be either pharmacological or immunologic.

The bulk of knowledge about food has been accumulated painstakingly, and most vegetable intake is limited to very few plant families, and in these only some genera are edible.

The dividing line between edible and toxic foods is narrow, and the method of preparation of food also plays a part in tolerance or antigenicity.

In the development of humans through the millenia to our present omnivorous state, the sequence of dietary changes is important. Humans were thought to be herbivorous 2,000,000 years ago, eating mainly fruit and nuts. Then they became hunters. Only recently have they been cultivators, 8000 years ago, about one-half of 1% of the time of human existence. This is not a long time in biologic terms for adaptation to occur. That 1 in 305 people in the west of Ireland has been shown to have celiac disease is an indication of the lack of adaptation to gluten-containing cereals. This prevalence has also been shown in the west of England.

Furthermore, a technological revolution is now occurring in which humans are able to manufacture their own foods and preserve, refine, and adulterate foods with artificial sweeteners, preservatives, antioxidants, emulsifiers, colorings, and flavorings. These may not be overtly harmful, yet there is accumulating evidence that some of them are. Tartrazines are now to be banned from foods, for example. As this period is only 200 years, we are unable to evaluate the degree of adaptation required as yet. Certainly there is evidence of increasing frequency of many diseases of Western European civilization as opposed to those in the Asian and New World civilizations. Some of the diseases caused by foods are caused by pharmacological effects, some may be due to intolerance due to deficiency of enzymes, but others are definitely due to immunologic mechanisms. Strictly proven allergic reactions may be directly caused by the food or, in effect, indirectly caused through a hapten reaction, as may occur with some of the chemicals included in present-day diets.

That diet is involved in migraine has been recorded in the medical literature, and particular pointers to food allergy are recorded.

In his renowned treatise, "On Megrim, Sick Headaches and Some Allied Disorders," Liveling [34], in 1873, described the migrainous syndrome well —

its periodic recurrence, unilateral and bilateral attacks of headache, disturbance in sight, tactile sensations, speech, psychic functions, giddiness, nausea and vomiting, familial nature, and associations with other conditions. He states that "certain articles of diet occasionally act as exciting causes of the seizures." He reported a case in which headaches had occurred for 30 years from the smallest amount of wine or from burnt pastry.

Laroche et al. [35] stated their conviction that food allergy might cause migraine in 1919. In 1920, Brown [36] reported that cyclic headaches were caused by "a protein poisoning" after the injection of cow's milk, meat, eggs, fruit, tomatoes, mushrooms, rhubarb, coffee, tea, and chocolate (especially effective were tomatoes, mushrooms, and chocolate). He found that skin tests were of no value, and diet trial was suggested with rice, butter and toast, and a few green vegetables and water.

T. F. Brown, in 1921 [37], treated migraine subjects with a dietary regimen, believing that carbohydrate metabolism was at fault. A diet of vegetable and fats was recommended, or a vegetarian diet, and on this regimen he reported alleviation of headache in some cases.

Minot, in 1923 [38], also recommended limitation of starch, which proved beneficial in some cases of migraine. In others, elimination of a specific meat or meats as a whole was an effective remedy. In particular, cereals were eliminated in these regimens as they were a source of starch. Case reports corroborated the observations made.

In 1923, Miller and Raulston [39], believing allergy to be the basis of migraine, used peptone injections and reported alleviation of migraine in 21 of 25 patients.

In 1924, Ball [40 reported a further 20 cases, 10 of whom benefited from this treatment.

Of 1000 random cases, migraine occurred in 26.1% of the families; asthma in 16.2%; hay fever in 9.1%; urticaria in 19.9%; epilepsy in 2.7%; and eczema in 6.1%.

Vaughan, in 1922 [41], reported the control of migraine by the elimination of allergenic foods, followed by case reports published in 1922 and 1927 with analysis of his results in 1933. Good results were reported in 50.8% of his patients; 62 different foods were provocants in different combinations: wheat, milk, peanuts, chocolate, pork pie, bean, onion, egg, and bananas were the chief provocants, in this order.

Van Leeuwin [42], in 1925, reported that egg and chocolate at times provoked headache, which he attributed to allergy.

In 1927, Diamond [43] gave reports of food idiosyncrasies in migrainous subjects but accorded the condition to liver dysfunction.

McClure and Huntsinger, in 1927 [44], reported on eight patients with migraine, four of whom had positive skin scratch tests to food. These items (milk, meat, and eggs in particular) were eliminated and the patients improved.

Table 1 Association of Allergic Conditions with Migraine from Family History

	Migraine as a major complaint	Migraine as a minor complaint	Total
Number of cases	46	40	86
Male	16	7	23 (27%)
Female	30	33	63 (73%)
Age	38.4	41	39.6 (average)
Positive family history	39	25	64 (74%)
Associated allergic conditions			
Asthma	3	7	10 (12%)
Hay fever	4	11	15 (17%)
Cutaneous allergy	18	19	37 (43%)
Abdominal allergy	22	33	55 (64%)

Rowe, in 1928 [45], first reported 48 patients with migraine, all of whom had complete or almost complete relief from migraine with elimination diets. A further report (1931) [46] of 86 cases similarly managed and 139 cases were analyzed. Good results were obtained in 73.1%, fair in 6.9%, and poor in 20%. However, 21% did not cooperate well, and 14% of the patients who had cooperated well did not benefit.

Skin reactions were absent in 58% of the patients. He reported associations with migraine from family history (see Table 1).

Rowe further reported in *Food Allergy; Its Manifestations Diagnosis and Treatment* [47] statistics on 247 patients with headache as a major complaint, summarized in Table 2. Results of elimination diet treatment are shown in Table 3.

Rowe used a hypoallergenic diet for 2–3 weeks, subsequently adding one food at a time to observe symptoms. Thus two points were taken into consideration: the effect of withdrawal and the effect of challenge.

Balyeat and Rinkle, in 1931 [48], reported 202 cases of migraine in whom skin tests were used to detect allergy. Milk was the most prevalent allergenic food found; 22% of the patients reported excellent improvement and 38%, good.

Meyer [49] reported the detection of reactions to food by noting a relative tachycardia after its ingestion. He successfully treated 13 patients with migraine after this means of detection of allergens was used.

Unger and Unger [50] also used elimination diets in 55 patients with migraine; complete relief in 64% and marked improvement in 16% were reported.

Table 2 Summary of 247 Patients with Headache

	No. of cases		No. of cases		No. of cases
Age (years)		Personal history		Family history	
1–15	3	Nasal congestion	89	Headaches	113
15–35	72	Hay fever	35	Asthma	50
35–55	135	Asthma	25	Hay fever	39
>55	37	Chronic indigestion	98	Eczema	8
		Nausea	130	Urticaria	12
Sex		Vomiting	91	Chronic indigestion	42
Male	66	Abdominal pain	47		
Female	181	Constipation	142	Skin reactions	
		Diarrhea	24	Foods	65
Duration of symptoms		Eczema	40	Inhalants	45
(years)		Urticaria	68	Miscellaneous	26
½–1	23				
1–5	40				
>5	184				

Table 3   Results of Elimination
Diet Treatment

	No. of cases (%)
Results	
Failure	43(17.0)
Fair	49(19.5)
Good	155(63.5)
Cooperation	
None	6
Poor	15(19)
Fair	26
Good	200(81)

They used elimination diets, and following 14 days' avoidance of the food challenged the patients with individual foods, noting their response. The allergens were milk in 33%, chocolate in 31%, wheat in 22%, and pork in 18%. They reported that in those patients whose attacks occur more frequently than once in 6 weeks, the patients were usually sensitive to foods eaten in some form almost daily.

Shapiro and Eisenberg in 1965 [51], reported the results of skin testing 100 patients with migraine and headache. Of these, 13 had migrainous symptoms, such as teichopsia, and 88 had nausea, vomiting, vertigo, nasal disturbance, photophobia, or other symptoms. These patients showed positive skin tests for foods. With elimination diets and desensitization treatment, 36 became headache free and 40 improved greatly.

Speer, in 1977 [52], published results of identification of allergens in migrainous patients with elimination diets used for diagnostic purposes as well as skin tests. Milk, chocolate and cola, and corn were responsible for causing symptoms on challenge in 31, 24, and 17%, respectively.

A further report of migraine diagnosis by a combination of elimination diets and relative tachycardia was published by Grant [53]. In 60 patients, 10 common foods provoked reactions: wheat, 78%; orange, 65%; egg, 45%; tea, 40%; coffee, 40%; chocolate, 37%; and milk, 37%.

One group was placed on a diet free of cheese, chocolate, citrus fruit, and alcohol. Only 13% of these patients became headache free. Of the other group, 85% became headache free for 3 months with avoidance of the specific foods that by challenge produced their headache. Furthermore, the monthly incidence of migraine was reduced from 402 to 6, and the headache incidence from 533 to 22. IgE levels to specific foods were raised in some patients.

In our paper on food allergy in migraine [54], we showed that a proportion of severe migraine sufferers were shown by dietary exclusion and challenge to be

Table 4   Foods Considered Migraine
Precipitants and Excluded from the
Diet of 500 Patients

Food	Patients (%)
Chocolate	74
Dairy products (cheese)	46
Fruits (citrus)	30
Alcohol	25
Fatty fried foods	18
Vegetables (onion)	17
Meat (pork)	14
Tea and coffee	14
Seafood	10

allergic to various foods. The radioallergosorbent test (RAST) confirmed the relevance of these foods.

There have been sporadic reports about other food associations with headache. One example is "ice cream headache"; another is Kwok's disease, in which pressor reactions to the monosodium glutamate in Chinese food result in headache, among other symptoms.

This review of literature connecting migraine with allergy is not, of course, the only literature concerning food connected with migraine. There are many publications suggesting other etiological relationships, and it is appropriate to mention them here.

Hanington et al. [55] reported that approximately one-third of the patients attending a migraine clinic stated that some of their headaches are related to articles of food; Table 4 lists those cited most frequently.

A group of 11 migrainous patients, difficult to manage on a complex elimination diet, have been treated with immunotherapy using the provocation-neutralization method described by Lee and modified by Miller. The efficacy of their treatment was tested by double-blind assessment of immunotherapy versus placebo. The results indicate a marked preference for immunotherapy in protecting them from challenge with relevant food and inhalant allergens and chemicals they met during the course of the month of the study [56].

Eggear et al. [57] have shown by a double-blind trial of oligoantigenic treatment that migraine is likely to be due to food allergy. Of 88 children with severe frequent migraine, 93% recovered on oligoantigenic diets. The diet consisted of one meat (lamb or chicken), one carbohydrate (rice or potato), one fruit (banana or apple), one vegetable (*Brassica*), water, and vitamin supplements for 3-4 weeks. Those who did not improve were offered a different combination of foods. Thereafter, one food was reintroduced at a time. If no reaction occurred, the patient was advised to eat the food regularly. Foods that provoked symptoms were withdrawn at the end of the week. Commercial orange squash was given as a source of artificial color and preservative. If symptoms were provoked, they were investigated further by giving 150 mg tartrazine per day during the second week and 150 mg benzoic acid per day during a third week.

A double-blind, placebo-controled crossover trial that tested the response to one of the foods that provoked symptoms in the reintroduction phase was then instituted using a savory base and a sweet base in turn. The "active" base contained the suspected food. Tartrazine and benzoic acid were tested as capsules versus placebo capsules.

Many foods were found to be provocants, and the researchers conclude that it is therefore more likely to be an allergic rather than an idiosyncratic metabolic process. Other associated symptoms also improved; these included abdominal pain, behavior disorder, fits, asthma, and eczema. They also found that in those patients in whom migraine was provoked by nonspecific factors such as blows to the head, exercise, and flashing lights; these factors no longer provoked migraine while they were on the diet.

We showed that migraine in some patients can be relieved by dietary exclusion. Formal food challenge provoked migraine; pretreatment with oral sodium cromoglycate (SCG) exerted a protective effect. Challenging with the relevant food led to the appearance of immune complexes containing IgE. These were absent when the patient was pretreated with SCG. This drug acts locally on the gut mucosa, as it is poorly absorbed, and it is suggested that it blocks an immunologic trigger for the absorption of antigen immune complexes and possibly mediators [33].

DIAGNOSIS OF FOOD ALLERGY IN MIGRAINOUS SUBJECTS AND SUBSEQUENT MANAGEMENT

Elimination and challenge must be the cornerstone of diagnosis. A diet diary must be kept initially and definite provocants noted. Frequency, severity, and duration of migrainous attacks are recorded. Then a rare food diet is instituted for 4 days followed by single-food challenge sequentially. Those foods known to produce symptoms can be charted and avoided altogether. Then foods that are innocuous may be eaten freely but preferably on a rotation diet so that they are not taken too frequently. This is because food allergies are not immutable but are variable. New sensitivities may develop and others decline depending upon frequency of exposure. Then foods that are "suspect" but not definitely confirmed may be taken less frequently, perhaps once a week.

After a period of 4 or 5 months, some of the "forbidden" foods may be reintroduced only once a week to see if they can be tolerated. If there is any increase in the frequency, severity, or duration of the migrainous attacks, the allergenic food is discontinued once more.

Immunotherapy based on the Miller technique has been found helpful [56].

PHARMACOLOGICAL TREATMENT AND ITS RELEVANCE TO FOOD ALLERGY

Pretreatment with sodium cromoglycate has been found to be beneficial. The dose we have reported to be effective has been 1600 mg individual doses before meals [58].

Ketotifen has also proved beneficial; 1 mg twice daily has reduced the frequency, severity, and duration of migrainous attacks by 72% [58]. Like sodium cromoglycate, Ketotifen has been stated to have an inhibitory effect on the release of mast cell mediators by allergens. It is also reputed to act on neutrophils by inhibiting the release of slow-reactive substance of anaphylaxis (SRS-A).

Aspirin has a prophylactic effect in reducing the frequency of migraine attacks. Aspirin blocks the production of thromboxane A_2 by the cyclo-oxygenase pathway [20, 59].

The relief of pain by simple analgesics may be appropriate and symptomatic treatment for the nausea and vomiting.

α-Adrenergic drugs (e.g., ergot) may be employed in the most severe cases.

CONCLUSION

There is accumulating evidence to show that migraine is due to food allergy in many patients. The foods produce antibody-antigen complexes containing IgE. IgE-mediated allergy depends on the production of IgE antibodies to normally harmless substances. The levels of total IgE in migraine are not raised generally. The likely aberration is possibly an IgE-suppressive immunodeficiency due to defects in the T-lymphocyte system. There is evidence to show that cumulative exposure to antigens results in T-cell depletion [61] and that withdrawal from these antigens can lead to a restoration of immunocompetence. Hence the ideal management of migraine sufferers must be the withdrawal of the antigens and, if necessary, immunotherapy and drugs that protect against the effects of food allergy.

REFERENCES

1. Blau, J. N. Towards a definition of migraine headache. *Lancet, 1*:444–445, 1984.
2. Friedman, A. P. Ad hoc committee on classification of headache. *JAMA, 179*:717–718, 1962.

3. Pearce, J. M. S. Charles C. Thomas, *Migraine, Mechanisms and Management.* Springfield, Illinois, pp. 1–9, 1969.
4. Hungerford, G. D., du Boulay, G. H., and Zilkha, K. J. Computerized tomography in patients with severe migraine. *J. Neurol. Neurosurg. Psychiatry, 39*:990–994, 1976.
5. Neligan, P., Harriman, D. G. F., and Pearce, J. M. S. Respiratory arrest in familial hemiplegic migraine: A clinical and neuropathological study. *Br. Med. J., 2*:732–734, 1977.
6. Goltman, M. A. *J. Allergy, 7*:351, 1936.
7. Olesan, J., Tfelt-Hansen, P., Henriksen, L., and Larsen, B. The common migraine attack may not be initiated by cerebral ischaemia. *Lancet, 2*:438–440, 1981.
8. Olesan, J., Larsen, B., and Lauritzen, M. Focal hyperaemia followed by spreading oligaemia and impaired activation in CBF in classic migraine. *Ann. Neurol., 9*:344–352, 1981.
9. Edmeads, J. *Headache, 17*:48, 1977.
10. Sicuteri, F., Testi, A., and Anselmi, B. Biochemical investigations in headache: Increase in hydroxyindolacetic acid excretion during migraine attacks. *Int. Arch. Allergy Appl. Immunol., 19*:55–58, 1961.
11. Anthony, M., Hinterberger, H., and Lance, J. W. Total plasma serotonin migraine and stress. *Arch. Neurol., 16*:544–552, 1967.
12. Curran, D. A., Hinterberger, H., and Lance, J. W. Total plasma serotonin, 5-hydroxyindolacetic acid and p-hydroxy-m-methoxymandelic acid excretion in normal and migrainous subjects. *Brain, 88*:997–1010, 1965.
13. Hilton, B. P., and Cummings, J. N. An assessment of platelet aggregation induced by 5-hydroxytryptamine. *J. Clin. Pathol., 24*:250–258, 1971.
14. Anthony, M., and Lance, J. W. Serotonin in migraine. J. M. S. Pearce, ed., In *Topics in Migraine,* Heinemann, London, 1975.
15. Hanington, E. Further observations on platelet behavior in migraine. F. C. Rose and J. Zilkha, eds., In *Progress in Migraine Research, Vol. I,* Pitman, London, pp. 80–84, 1981.
16. Gawel, M. J., Burkitt, M., and Rose, F. C. The platelet release reaction during migraine attacks. *Headache, 19*:323–327, 1979.
17. Moore, S., Pepper, D. S., and Cash, J. D. The isolation and characterization of platelet specific globulin. *Biochem. Biophys. Acta, 379*:360–369, 1975.
18. Holmsen, H. Biochemistry of the platelet release action. K. Elliott and J. Knight, eds., In *Biochemistry and Pharmacology of Platelets,* Ciba Foundation Symposium No. 35; Elsevier, Amsterdam, pp. 175–205, 1975.
19. Couch, J. R., and Hassanein, R. S. Platelet aggregability in migraine. *Neurology, 27*:843–848, 1977.
20. Deshmukh, S. V., and Meyer, J. S. Cyclic changes in platelet dynamics and the pathogenesis and prophylaxis of migraine. *Headache, 17*:101–108, 1977.
21. Hanington, E., Jones, R. J., Amess, J. A. L., and Wachowicz, B. Migraine: A platelet disorder. *Lancet, 2*:720–723, 1981.
22. Bills, T. K., Smith, J. B., and Silver, M. J. Metabolism of [^{14}C] arachidonic acid by human platelets. *Biochem. Biophys. Acta, 424*:303–314, 1976.

23. Smith, J. B., Ingerman, C., Kocik, J. J., and Silver, M. J. Formation of prostaglandins during aggregation of human blood platelets. *J. Clin. Invest.*, *52*:965–969, 1973.

24. Hamberg, M., Svensson, J., and Samuelson, B. Thromboxane, a new group of biologically active compounds derived from prostaglandin endoperoxides. *Proc. Natl. Acad. Sci., USA, 72*:2994–2998, 1975.

25. Penttinen, K., Myila, G., Makela, O., and Vaheri, A. Soluble antigen-antibody complexes and platelet aggregation. *Acta Pathol. Microbiol. Scand.*, *77*:309–317, 1969.

26. Humphrey, J., and Jacques, R. The release of histamine and 5-hydroxytryptamine (serotonin) from platelets by antigen-antibody reactions (in vitro). *J. Physiol., 128*:9–27, 1955.

27. Little, C. H., Stewart, A. G., and Fennessy, M. R. *Lancet, 2*:297–299, 1983.

28. Brostoff, J., Carini, C., Wraith, D. G., Paganelli, R., and Levinsky, R. J. Immune complexes in atopy. J. Pepys, and A. M. Edwards, eds., In *The Mast Cell*. Pitman Medical, London, pp. 380–393, 1979.

29. Brostoff, J., Carini, C., Wraith, D. G., and Johns, P. Production of IgE complexes by allergen challenge in atopic patients and the effect of sodium cromoglycate. *Lancet, 1*:1268–1270, 1979.

30. Enderssen, G., and Farre, O. Studies on the binding of immunoglobulins and immune complexes to the surface of human platelets: IgG molecules react with platelet Fc receptors with cH3 domain. *Int. Arch. Allergy Appl. Immunol., 67*:33–39, 1982.

31. Joseph, M., Auriault, C., Capron, A., Vorng, H., and Viens. P. A new function for platelets: IgE-dependent killing of schistosomes. *Nature, 303*: 810–812, 1983.

32. Brostoff, J., Carini, C., and Wraith, D. G. Food allergy; An IgE immune complex disorder. In *Theoretical and Clinical Aspects of Allergic Diseases*. Almquist & Wiksell International, Stockholm, 1983.

33. Monro, J., Carinci, C., and Brostoff, J. Migraine is a food-allergic disease. *Lancet, 2*:719–721, 1979.

34. Liveling, E. J. and A. Churchill, *On Megrim, Sick Headaches and Some Allied Disorders*. London, 1873.

35. Laroche, G., Richet, C., and Saint Girons, E. *Alimentary Anaphylaxis*, Paris, 1919 (translated by Rowe, University of California Press, 1930).

36. Brown, R. C. The protein of foodstuffs as a factor in the cause of headache. *Wisc. Med. J., 19*:337, 1920.

37. Brown, T. R. Role of diet in etiology and treatment of migraine and other types of headache. *JAMA, 77*:1396, 1921.

38. Minot, G. R. The role of a low carbohydrate diet in the treatment of migraine and headache. *Med. Clin. North Am., 7*:715, 1923.

39. Miller, J. L., and Raulston, B. O. Treatment of migraine with peptone. *JAMA, 80*:1894, 1923.

40. Ball, F. E. Migraine, its treatment with peptone and its familial relation to sensitization diseases. *Am. J. Med. Sci., 173*:781, 1927.

41. Vaughan, W. T. Disease associated with protein sensitisation. *Virginia Medical Monthly* (September), 1922.
42. Van Leeuwen, W. S. *Allergic Diseases.* J. B. Lippincott, Philadelphia, 1925.
43. Diamond, J. S. Liver function in migraine, with report of 35 cases. *Am. J. Med. Sci., 174*:695, 1927.
44. McClure, C. W., and Huntsinger, M. E. Observations on migraine. *Boston Med. Surg. J., 196*:270, 1900.
45. Rowe, A. H. Food allergy: Its control by elimination diets. Westminster Hospital Nurses' Rev. 13 (1 and 2).
46. Rowe, A. H. Abdominal Food Allergy. Its treatment with elimination diets. *California Western Med., 29*:5, 1928.
47. Rowe, A. H. *Food Allergy, Its Manifestations, Diagnosis and Treatment.* Lea and Febiger, Philadelphia, 1931.
48. Balyeat, R. M., and Rinkel, H. J. Further studies in allergic migraine. *Int. Med., 5*:713-728, 1931.
49. Meyer, M. G. Non-reaginic allergy. *Ann. Allergy, 6*:417-427, 1948.
50. Unger, A. H., and Unger, L. Migraine is an allergic disease. *J. Allergy, 23*: 429-440, 1952.
51. Shapiro, R. S., and Eisenberg, B. C. Allergic headache. *Ann. Allergy, 23*: 123-126.
52. Speer, F. *Migraine.* Nelson-Hall, Chicago, 1977.
53. Grant, E. E. C. Food allergies and migraine. *Lancet, 1*:966-969, 1979.
54. Monro, J. A., Brostoff, J., Carini, C., and Zilkha, K. J. Food allergy in migraine. *Lancet, 2*:1-4, 1980.
55. Hanington, E., Horn, M., and Wilkinson, M. A. L. Cochrane, ed., Proceedings of the Third Migraine Symposium, Chap. 2. Heinemann, London, 1969.
56. Monro, J. A. Food allergy in migraine. *Proc. Nutr. Soc., 42*:241, 1983.
57. Egger, J., Carter, C. M., Wilson, J., Turner, M. W., and Soothill, J. F. Is migraine food allergy? A double blind trial of oligoantigenic diet treatment. *Lancet, 2*:865, 1983.
58. Monro, J. A. Food allergy and migraine. Clin. Immunol. Allergy, Feb., Vol. 2, No. 1, 1982.
59. Vane, J. R. Inhibition of prostaglandin synthesis as a mechanism of action for aspirin-like drugs. *Nature New Biol., 231*:232-235, 1971.

8
Arthritis and Food Allergy

RICHARD S. PANUSH
College of Medicine, University of Florida, and Veterans Administration Medical Center, Gainesville, Florida

LAWRENCE P. ENDO and ELLA M. WEBSTER
College of Medicine, University of Florida, Gainesville, Florida

For many years physicians and patients alike have been intrigued with the possibility that certain foods or food-related products might cause rheumatic diseases and others might ameliorate arthritis. If this were so, then arthritis might be responsive to appropriate nutritional modulation. Diet therapy for rheumatic disease has generally been considered as a form of "quackery." The notion that nutritional manipulations might have a relationship to symptoms of rheumatic disease has never achieved credibility among the mainstream of contemporary rheumatologists and clinical immunologists. However, these conclusions have been based on inadequate data. A number of recent observations are of interest; the hypothesis that rheumatic diseases or their symptoms may relate to food or food-related products in some patients is plausible. We shall review certain historical observations, broadly consider nutrition and rheumatic disease, and finally comment on recent evidence that food allergy may be expressed as rheumatic disease.

HISTORICAL PERSPECTIVE

Earlier in this century, a considerable amount of literature accumulated on diet, nutrition, and rheumatic diseases. Most students of the problem were unimpressed that any dietary approaches had consistent effects on outcome of rheumatic diseases.

For example, Weatherbee carried out a clinical analysis of 350 cases of arthritis. He concluded, "Dietary treatments of all types had been tried in many cases . . . little definite improvement from dietary management alone was reported" [1]. Minot stated, "There exist many peculiar facts concerning diets for arthritis and these patients will often have fanciful ideas regarding what they can and cannot eat . . . there is, of course, no standard diet for arthritis" [2]. Bauer wrote, "there exists no unanimity of opinion concerning the correct diet for an arthritic patient," although he believed that allergy to certain foods may provoke arthritis in certain patients [3]. However, an authoritative and comprehensive review of the English language rheumatology literature in its time concluded, "The incidence of food allergy among rheumatic patients is not significant" [4]. This same group had previously written, "We cannot approve the emphasis laid on the factor of food allergy in cases of atrophic arthritis; it is neither common nor do we consider it important. Variations in articular systems are so common from day to day that it is easy to blame erroneously some food for the day's ill-feeling. Cases of atrophic arthritis with undoubted and repeatable articular exacerbations from foods are few and far between" [5]. Indeed, based on this literature, one of the last textbooks of rheumatology to extensively consider the relationship between diet and arthritis stated, "It is almost universally acknowledged that rheumatoid arthritis cannot be overcome by any dietary manipulations which have thus far been proposed" [6]. The Arthritis Foundation, in its informational pamphlets for patients, The Truth About Diet and Arthritis, summarized, "The possible relationship between diet and arthritis has been thoroughly and scientifically studied. The simple proven fact is: no food has anything to do with causing arthritis and no food is effective in treating or 'curing' it" [7].

Yet, there were provocative observations supporting the notion that specific dietary manipulation ameliorated arthritis, based on the hypothesis that foods or food-related products are noxious and cause and/or perpetuate arthritis. Much of the older data may be inadequate, in that controlled, prospective, blinded experimental studies were not carefully conducted in the past as would be expected today. Also, different types of arthritis were lumped together, making conclusions about any specific disease difficult to interpret. Although considered uncommon, Hench and Rosenberg acknowledged that food allergy was related to occasional cases of "atrophic arthritis" (rheumatoid arthritis) [5]. Moreover, in describing palindromic rheumatism [8], they suggested that allergy may be an etiological factor in certain of the cases.

Several allergists considered the issue of allergy and "rheumatism" at length. Zeller presented four case reports to illustrate his thesis that ingested foods may exacerbate rheumatoid arthritis and dietary exclusions may improve its course [9]. Some of his patients failed to improve on exclusion diets. Zussman also presented a number of patients whose histories suggested an exacerbation of their musculoskeletal problems with certain food ingestions [10]. Of 1000 consecutive adults with allergic complaints (e.g., asthma, hay fever, and urticaria), 20% had rheumatic complaints. Most of these had allergic symptoms attributable to food, although only 27 (of the original 1000) had rheumatic symptoms exacerbated by ingestion of specific foods. In a review of literature from 1917 through 1972, Rowe concluded, "Food allergy as a cause of arthritis pain or arthralgia and swelling occurs not infrequently." He included substantiating literature and personal cases [11].

FOOD AND RHEUMATIC DISEASE

If there is indeed a relationship between nutrition and rheumatic diseases, this could occur through two possible mechanisms that are not mutually exclusive. First, nutritional modification might alter immune responsiveness and thereby affect manifestations of rheumatic diseases. Second, rheumatic disease may be a manifestation of food allergy or hypersensitivity. In this view, articular or rheumatic symptoms might reflect allergic hypersensitivity, in the same manner as we recognize more traditional forms of food allergies (eczema, urticaria, asthma, or gastrointestinal problems).

NUTRITION AND MODIFICATION OF THE IMMUNE RESPONSE

Considerable experimental evidence has accumulated indicating that nutritional status exerts a profound effect on immune responsiveness. Protein-calorie malnutrition and caloric restriction affect immunologic responsiveness. Fats and lipids have important roles in prostaglandin and leukotriene pathways, as well as less defined roles. Abnormal zinc and copper metabolism may relate to abnormal immune responses.

Protein (or protein-calorie) malnutrition has been associated with impaired antibody production, decreased development of antibody-forming cells, increased allograft rejection, heightened delayed hypersensitivity, augmented in vitro cellular responsiveness, and elevated lymphokine production in both experimental animals and humans [12-16]. Fasting also has been associated with notable changes in immune responsiveness in both experimental animals and humans — increased immunoglobulin levels, increased neutrophil bacteriocidal activity, depressed lymphocyte blastogenesis, heightened monocyte killing and bacteriocidal function, and augmented natural killer cell activity [17-19].

Zinc deficiency in certain animals or disease states was associated with impaired T-cell-mediated immune responses and immunodeficiency syndromes; in some instances immune responsiveness could be restored with zinc [20, 21]. Copper and ceruloplasmin levels are elevated in rheumatoid arthritis and correlate with serum antioxidant activity. It has been suggested that this may have a protective effect in the presence of tissue damage [22, 23].

Several interesting studies have examined the effect of modifying dietary lipids on experimental systemic lupus erythematosus in NZB/NZW F_1 hybrid mice [24-29]. Hurd et al. noted that animals fed coconut oil (an essential fatty acid deficient diet) or given prostaglandin E_1 (PGE_1) survived longer than control animals or those fed a safflower oil-rich diet (rich in essential fatty acids) [24]. Prickett et al. observed that lupus mice fed a Menhaden oil diet (rich in eicosapentaenoic acid, a naturally occurring 20-carbon polyunsaturated fatty acid, precursor to various leukotrienes) experienced prolonged survival and that benefit could be achieved if dietary manipulation was instituted after onset of clinical lupus [27]. These experiments suggested that dietary factors that could modify the generation of arachidonic acid-derived prostaglandins and/or leukotrienes might affect inflammatory and immunologic responses and ultimately clinical manifestations of rheumatic disease. Certainly this form of nutritional therapy — if clinically feasible, acceptable, and effective — would provide a novel, nontoxic, and potentially exciting therapeutic alternative to our current approaches for certain systemic rheumatic diseases in humans.

FOOD ALLERGY AND RHEUMATIC DISEASE

If arthritis is the result of hypersensitivity to foods, then food antigens must cross the gastrointestinal barrier and circulate in antigenic form until they are recognized by effector or intermediary cells in the immune system. There are experimental data for considering that food antigens may cross the gastrointestinal barrier and circulate both as food antigen and as immune complexes [30-33].

In immunologically abnormal persons, the intrinsic abnormalities of the gastrointestinal mucosa may permit the transport of larger quantities of different sorts of antigenic material. Selective IgA deficiency is associated with both gastrointestinal disorders and immunologic diseases. Cunningham-Rundles and colleagues showed that antibodies to cow's milk in IgA-deficient subjects correlated with the presence of circulating immune complexes [34]. They also found a correlation with serologically defined autoimmune disease [30]. Those patients with hypogammaglobulinemia had both increased absorption of bovine milk antigens and prolonged persistence of these antigens in the circulation [35].

Some studies have suggested that patients with rheumatic disease may have abnormal digestive and absorptive function. Abnormal fecal fat excretion and vitamin A and D xylose absorption have been demonstrated [36, 37]. Further, some have considered that the gastrointestinal tract in patients with rheumatoid arthritis (RA) may be more penetrable to food antigens than normal individuals, although this has not been confirmed [38, 39]. In fact, it has been suggested that the abnormal intestinal permeability may be due to effects of nonsteroidal antiinflammatory drugs [40]. Antigens of the intraluminal contents, other than food antigens, also have been demonstrated to stimulate lymphocyte transformation and production of leukocyte inhibiting factor in patients with spondyloarthropathies [41]. Patients with jejunoileal bypass for obesity may develop an arthritis indistinguishable from rheumatoid arthritis. They also may evince immunologic abnormalities, including immune complexes of which the antigen is intraluminal.

In addition to experimental and laboratory data, there are a number of clinical observations suggesting relationships between food intake and rheumatic diseases [4, 5, 8-11, 42-49]. Recent reports include a case report wherein a dermatologist documented his own palindromic rheumatism to be due to sodium nitrate hypersensitivity [50]. Black walnut ingestion was linked to clinical exacerbations of Behcet's syndrome and abnormal cellular hypersensitivity responses [51].

Alfalfa seed and sprout ingestion has been associated with systemic lupus erythematosus in both humans and monkeys [52, 53]. The disease induced in the primate model was characterized by an autoimmune hemolytic anemia with low complement levels, positive ANA, anti-DNAs, positive lupus erythematosus (LE) preparations, and the deposition of immunoglobulin and complement in the skin. Induction of the disease was attributed to a nonprotein amino acid component of alfalfa, L-canavanine. Antibody to the alfalfa seed cross-reacted with DNA and may have activated B lymphocytes [54].

Fasting seems to ameliorate disease in a portion of patients with rheumatic disease. Of 15 patients with classic rheumatoid arthritis who fasted 7-10 days, 5 benefited, whereas only one of ten controls improved. Fasting patients showed lessened pain, stiffness, medication requirements, Ritchie index, and finger size. Continuation of a lactovegetarian diet was without consistent benefit [55]. The improvement demonstrated may be because gastrointestinal permeability is reduced during fasting [39] or may be related to decreased neutrophil function, depressed lymphocyte response to mitogen, or increased cortisol concentration during fasting [19, 56].

A well-described challenge study in a single patient with rheumatoid arthritis was reported by Parke and Hughes in 1981 [57]. Challenge with dairy products produced marked exacerbation of her arthritis as measured by increased pain, increased Ritchie index, morning stiffness, decreased grip strength, and swelling as measured by ring size. Stroud and coworkers, in another uncontrolled study, confirmed the antirheumatic effect of fasting and also found that chemical or food challenges, particularly wheat, corn, and beef, caused deterioration of grip strength and dolorimeter and arthrocircameter scores [58].

Preliminary report of a prospective study of patients with definite or classic rheumatoid arthritis indicated that withdrawal of allergenic substance identified by an elimination diet resulted in a rather varied response, from "complete success with total abolishing of all rheumatic symptoms to deterioration" [59]. A double-blind provocation test study, also reported in preliminary fashion, found that challenges "with food extracts and other incitants including alternaria, house dust, tobacco smoke and petrochemicals" induced " 'rheumatic' joint and muscle reactions, indistinguishable from presenting complaints . . . in . . . (87.5% of 40) . . . subjects" [60].

We carried out a prospective, controlled, randomized study of a particular prescription diet (eliminating red meat, fruit, dairy products, herbs and spices, preservatives and additives, and alcohol) for rheumatoid arthritis [61]. This diet, followed for 10 weeks by a group of outpatients with long-standing, progressive, active rheumatoid arthritis, was of no demonstrable benefit compared with placebo diet.

However, 2 of our 11 patients on the experimental diet improved on the experimental diet, elected to continue this diet, and experienced recurrence of symptoms when deviating from it. We have confirmed in recent controlled, double-blind encapsulated challenges carried out under clinical research center protocol that food and chemicals can indeed exacerbate symptoms of inflammatory arthritis [62].

CONCLUSIONS

The observations reviewed support the hypothesis that individualized dietary manipulations may be beneficial for certain, selected patients with rheumatic disease. Further controlled, careful studies are needed to resolve this issue and are underway. Until such data are available, nutritional therapy for rheumatic disease must be considered experimental.

ACKNOWLEDGMENTS

Supported by the Florida Chapter, Arthritis Foundation, Veterans Administration, National Institutes of Health Clinical Research Grant RR82, Society for Clinical Ecology, and International Foundation for the Promotion of Nutrition Research and Education. The authors appreciate the assistance of Barbara Gibbs in typing this manuscript. Portions of this material appear in similar forms in Panush, R. S., and Webster, E. M., Nutrition and arthritis. In *Rehabilitation Management of Rheumatic Conditions,* editor G. E. Ehrlich, (Williams and Wilkins, 1985, pp. 290-303) and Panush, R. S., Controversial arthritis remedies, *Bull. Rheumatic Dis.* (*34*:1-10, 1985).

REFERENCES

1. Weatherbee, M. Chronic arthritis. The clinical analysis of three hundred and fifty cases. *AMA Arch. Intern. Med. 50*:926–944, 1932.
2. Minot, G. R. General aspects of the treatment of chronic arthritis. *N. Engl. J. Med. 208*:1285–1290, 1933.
3. Bauer, W. What should a patient with arthritis eat? *JAMA 104*:1-6, 1935.

4. Hench, B. S., Bauer, W., Boland, E., Dawson, M. H., Freyberg, R., Holbrook, W. P., Key, J. A., Locke, L. N., and McEwen, C. Rheumatism and arthritis. Review of the American and English literature, for 1940 (8th Rheumatism Review). *Ann. Intern. Med.* *15*:1002–1108, 1941 (p. 1039).

5. Hench, B. S., Bauer, W., Dawson, M. H., Hall, F., Holbrook, W. P., Key, J. A., and McEwen, C. The problem of rheumatism and arthritis. Review of American and English literature, 1938 (6th Rheumatism Review). *Ann. Intern. Med.* *13*:1838–1990, 1940 (p. 1859).

6. Rosenberg, E. F. Diet and vitamins in rheumatoid arthritis. In Comroe's *Arthritis and Allied Conditions.* Fifth edition. Edition by J. L. Hollander. Lea and Febiger, Philadelphia, 1954, pp. 542–546.

7. Arthritis Foundation, *Arthritis: The Basic Facts,* Atlanta, Georgia, 1976.

8. Hench, P. S., and Rosenberg, E. F. Palindromic rheumatism. *Proc. Staff Meetings Mayo Clinic.* *16*:808–815, 1941.

9. Zeller, M. Rheumatoid arthritis – food allergy as a factor. *Ann. Allergy 7*: 200–239, 1949.

10. Zussman, B. M. Food hypersensitivity simulating rheumatoid arthritis. *South. Med. J.* *59*:935–939, 1966.

11. Rowe, A. H. Food allergy and the arthropathies. In *Food Allergy: Its Manifestation and Control.* Charles C. Thomas, Springfield, Illinois, 1972, pp. 435–443.

12. Good, R. A. Nutrition and immunity. *J. Clin. Immunol.* *1*:3–11, 1981.

13. Good, R. A., West, A., and Fernandes, G. Nutritional modulation of immune response. *Fed. Proc.* *39*:3048–3104, 1980.

14. Hansen, M. A., Fernandes, G., and Good, R. A. Nutrition and immunity: The influence of diet on autoimmunity and the role of zinc in the immune response. *Annu. Rev. Nutr.* *2*:151–177, 1982.

15. Weindruch, R., Gottesman, S. R. S., and Walford, R. L. Modification of age-related immune decline in mice dietarily restricted from or after mid-adulthood. *Proc. Natl. Acad. Sci. USA 79*:898–902, 1982.

16. Weindruch, R., and Walford, R. L. Dietary restriction in mice beginning at 1 year of age: Effect on life-span and spontaneous cancer incidence. *Science 215*:1415–1418, 1982.

17. Wing, E. J., Barczynski, L. K., and Boehmer, S. M. Effect of acute nutritional deterioration on immune function in mice. I. Macrophages. *Immunology 48*:543–550, 1983.

18. Wing, E. J., Stanko, R. T., Winkelstein, A., and Adibi, S. A. Fasting-enhanced immune effector mechanisms in obese subjects. *Am. J. Med. 75*:91–96, 1983.

19. Uden, A. M., Trang, L., Venizelos, N., and Palmbad, J. Neutrophil functions and clinical performance after total fasting in patients with rheumatoid arthritis. *Ann. Rheum. Dis. 42*:45–51, 1983.

20. Fernandez, G., Nair, M., Onoe, K., Tunake, T., Floyd, R., and Good, R. A. Impairment of cell-mediated immunity in dietary zinc deficiency in mice. *Proc. Natl. Acad. Sci. USA 76*:457–461, 1979.

21. Duchateau, J., Delepesse, G., Vrijens, R., and Collet, H. Beneficial effects of oral zinc supplementation on the immune response of old people. *Am. J. Med. 70*:1001–1004, 1981.
22. Scudder, P. R., Al-Timini, D., McMurray, W., White, A. G., Zoob, B. C., and Dormandy, T. L. Serum copper and related variables in rheumatoid arthritis. *Ann. Rheum. Dis. 37*:67–70, 1978.
23. Scudder, P. R., McMurray, W., White, A. G., and Dormandy, T. L. Synovial fluid copper and related variables in rheumatoid and degenerative arthritis. *Ann. Rheum. Dis. 37*:71–72, 1978.
24. Hurd, E. R., Johnston, J. M., Okita, J. R., MacDonald, P. C., Ziff, M., and Gilliam, J. N. Prevention of glomerulitis and prolonged survival in New Zealand Black/New Zealand White F_1 hybrid mice fed an essential fatty acid-deficient diet. *J. Clin. Invest. 67*:476–485, 1981.
25. Zurier, R. B., Sayadoff, D. M., Torrey, S. B., and Rothfield, N. F. Prostaglandin E_1 treatment of NZB/NZW mice. I. Prolonged survival of female mice. *Arthritis Rheum. 20*:723–728, 1977.
26. Kelley, V. E. Fish oil diet decreases prostaglandin (PGE) production in auto-immune lupus in MRL-lpr mice, (abstract). *Fed. Proc. 42*:1211, 1983.
27. Prickett, J. D., Robinson, D. R., and Steinberg, A. D. Effects of dietary enrichment with eicosapentaenoic acid upon autoimmune nephritis in female NZB X NZW/F_1 mice. *Arthritis Rheum. 26*:133–139, 1983.
28. Ziff, M. Diet in the treatment of rheumatoid arthritis. *Arthritis Rheum. 26*: 457–461, 1983.
29. Levy, J. A., Ibrahim, A. B., Shirai, T., Ohta, K., Nagasawa, R., Yoshida, H., Estes, J., and Gardner, M. Dietary fat affects immune response, production of antiviral factors, and immune complex disease in NZB/NZW mice. *Proc. Natl. Acad. Sci. USA 79*:1974–1978, 1982.
30. Walker, W. A., and Isselbacher, K. J. Uptake and transport of macromolecules by the intestine. Possible role in clinical disorders. *Gastroenterology 67*:531–550, 1974.
31. Paganelli, R., Levinsky, R. J., Brostoff, J., and Wraith, D. G. Immune complexes containing food proteins in normal and atopic subjects after oral challenges and effect of sodium cromoglycate on antigen absorption. *Lancet 1*:1270–1272, 1979.
32. Cunningham-Rundles, C., Brandeis, W. E., Pudifin, D. J., Day, N. K., and Good, R. A. Autoimmunity in selective IgA deficiency: Relationship to anti-bovine protein antibodies, circulating immune complexes and clinical disease. *Clin. Exp. Immunol. 45*:299–304, 1981.
33. Paganelli, R., Levinsky, R. J., and Atherton, D. J. Detection of specific antigen within circulating immune complexes: Validation of the assay and its application to food antigen-antibody complexes formed in healthy and food-allergic subjects. *Clin. Exp. Immunol. 46*:44–53, 1981.
34. Cunninghan-Rundles, C., Brandeis, W. E., Good, R. E., and Day, N. K. Bovine antigens and the formation of circulating immune complexes in selective immunoglobulin A deficiency. *J. Clin. Invest. 64*:272–279, 1979.

35. Cunningham-Rundles, C., Carr, R., and Good, R. A. Dietary protein antigenemia in humoral immunodeficiency: Correlation with splenomegaly. *Am. J. Med.* 76:181-185, 1984.

36. Siurala, M., Julkuven, H., Torvoneu, S., Selkoveu, R., Saxen, F., and Pithaven, F. Digestive tract in collagen disease. *Acta Med. Scand.* 178:13, 1965.

37. Peterson, T., Wegelius, U., and Skrifrans, B. Gastrointestinal disturbances in patients with severe rheumatoid arthritis. *Acta Med. Scand.* 188:139, 1970.

38. Rooney, P. J., Jenkins, R. T., Goodacre, R. L., and Sivakumaran, T. Gut permeability of small molecules in rheumatoid disease (abstract). *Clin. Res.* 31:160A, 1983.

39. Sundqvist, T., Lindstrom, F., Magnusson, K. E., Skoldstom, L., Stjernstom, I., and Tagesson, C. Influence of fasting on intestinal permeability and disease activity in patients with rheumatoid arthritis. *Scand. J. Rheum.* 11: 33-38, 1982.

40. Bjarnason, I., So, A., Levi, A. J., Peters, T., Williams, P., Zanelli, G., Gumpel, J., and Ausell, B. Intestinal permeability and inflammation in rheumatoid arthritis. Effects of non-steroidal antiinflammatory drugs. *Lancet* 2:1171, 1984.

41. Gross, W. L., Ludemann, G., Ullman, U., and Schmidt, K. L. *Klebsiella* induced LIF response in *Klebsiella* infection and ankylosing spondylitis. *Br. J. Rheum.* 22 (Suppl. 2):50-52, 1983.

42. Turnbull, J. A. Changes in sensitivity to allergenic foods in arthritis. *Am. J. Dig. Dis.* 15:182-190, 1944.

43. Pottenger, R. T. Constitutional factors in arthritis with special reference to incidence and role of allergic disease. *Ann. Intern. Med.* 12:323-333, 1928.

44. Kaufman, W. Food induced allergic musculoskeletal syndromes. *Ann. Allergy* 11:179-184, 1953.

45. Millman, M. An allergic concept of the etiology of rheumatoid arthritis. *Ann. Allergy* 30:135-141, 1972.

46. Lewin, P., and Taub, S. J. Allergic synovitis due to ingestion of English walnuts. *JAMA* 106:2144, 1936.

47. Berger, H. Intermittent hydroarthrosis with an allergic basis. *JAMA* 112: 2402-2405, 1939.

48. Vaughn, W. T. Palindromic rheumatism among allergic persons. *J. Allergy* 14:256-263, 1943.

49. Randolph, T. G. Ecologically oriented rheumatoid arthritis. In *Clinical Ecology*, edited by L. D. Dickey. Charles C. Thomas, Springfield, Illinois, 1976, pp. 201-212.

50. Epstein, S. Hypersensitivity to sodium nitrate: A major causative factor in cases of palindromic rheumatism. *Ann. Allergy* 27:343-349, 1969.

51. Marquardt, J. L., Snyderman, R., and Oppenheim, J. J. Depression of lymphocyte transformation and exacerbation of Behcet's syndrome by ingestion of English walnuts. *Cell. Immunol.* 9:263-272, 1973.

52. Malinow, M. R., Bardana, E. J., Pirofsky, B., Craig, S., and McLoughlin, P. Systemic lupus erythematosus-like syndrome in monkeys fed alfalfa sprouts: Role of a nonprotein amino acid. *Science* 216:415-417, 1982.

53. Roberts, J. L., and Hayashi, J. A. Exacerbation of SLE associated with alfalfa ingestion (letter). *N. Engl. J. Med. 308*:1361, 1983.
54. Bardana, E. J., Malinow, M. K., Craig, S., and McLoughlin, P. Cross-reaching antibody to alfalfa seed and deoxyribonucleic acid in systemic lupus erythematosus (abstract). *J. Allergy Clin. Immunol. 71*:102, 1983.
55. Skoldstam, L., Larsson, L., and Lindstrom, F. D. Effects of fasting and lactovegetarian diet on rheumatoid arthritis. *Scand. J. Rheum. 8*:249–255, 1979.
56. Palmbad, J., Cantell, K., Holm, G., Norberg, R., Strander, H., and Sundblad, L. Acute energy deprivation in man: Effect on serum immunoglobulins, antibody response, complement factors 3 and 4, acute phase reactants and interferon capacity of lymphocytes. *Clin. Exp. Immunol. 30*:50–55, 1977.
57. Parke, A. L., and Hughes, G. R. V. Rheumatoid arthritis and food: A case study. *Br. Med. J. 282*:2027–2029, 1981.
58. Stroud, R. M. The effect of fasting followed by specific food challenge on rheumatoid arthritis. In *Current Topics in Rheumatology*, edited by B. H. Hahn, F. C. Arnett, T. M. Zizic, and M. C. Hochberg, Upjohn, 1983, pp. 145–157.
59. Darlington, L. E., and Mansfield, J. R. Food allergy and rheumatoid disease (abstract). *Ann. Rheum. Dis. 42*:219, 1983.
60. Mandell, M., and Conte, A. The role of allergy in arthritis, rheumatism, and associated polysymptomatic cerebro-viscero-somatic disorders: A double-blind provocation test study. *Ann. Allergy 44*:51, 1980.
61. Panush, R. S., Carter, R. L., Katz, P., Kowsari, B., Longley, S., and Finnie, S. Diet therapy for rheumatoid arthritis. *Arthritis Rheum. 26*:462–471, 1983.
62. Panush, R. S., Stroud, R. M., and Webster, E. M. Food-induced (allergic) arthritis. I. Inflammatory arthritis exacerbated by milk. *Arthritis Rheum.* (in press).

9

Non-IgE-Mediated and Delayed Adverse Reactions to Food or Additives

WILLIAM T. KNIKER and L. MARIA RODRIGUEZ
University of Texas Health Science Center, San Antonio, Texas

One of the most controversial areas in medicine is the subject of adverse reactions to foods. There is disagreement on incidence and prevalence, possible clinical manifestations, and diagnostic criteria, as well as considerable ignorance of likely pathogenic mechanisms. Expanded research by critical clinical and laboratory investigators is necessary to shed further light on the darkness surrounding the subject.

In considering disorders that follow the ingestion of foods, it is helpful to understand the steps that lead to any acquired disease (Fig. 1). A pathogenic reaction always involves the activation of host mediators or biologic amplification systems; it is the actions of these activated cells and/or noncellular factors that lead to deranged function or inflammation. The process begins when a particular triggering agent activates one or more mediators by one of several pathways. If the trigger, such as food, serves as an antigen and specifically interacts with antibodies or lymphocytes, the triggering mechanism is "immune." On the other hand, the triggering food may activate mediators directly ("nonimmunologically"), via a chemical or idiosyncratic reaction. Other possible triggering pathways, such as physical or neurogenic, are not as likely to be as relevant in food-associated disorders.

To diagnose adverse reactions to foodstuffs, the clinician chiefly needs to be satisfied that ingestion of a food predictably and repeatedly causes disease. It is not necessary to know the precise triggering mechanism or which mediators of inflammation are activated. Such information is difficult to obtain, often requiring considerable laboratory investigation beyond the scope of clinical practice.

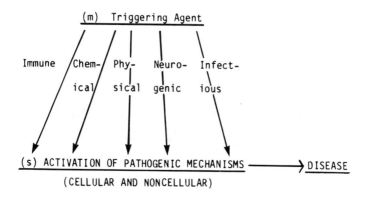

Figure 1   General equation for acquired disease. (m) = Modifying influences, such as climatological change, total "load" of triggering agents, or effect of medications. (s) = Susceptibility factors, such as genetic predisposition, psychologic/metabolic state, antecedent infection.

It is useful to remember that there are two levels at which adverse reactions to foods may occur [1-4]. The first is the gastrointestinal tract itself; in some instances, the entire reaction is limited to that organ system. The second level, probably accounting for the bulk of clinically relevant reactions, is extragastrointestinal. Intact food, digested food, or chemical additives are absorbed, circulate in the blood, and gain access to virtually any part of the body where the opportunity for sensitization and triggering of adverse reactions exists.

CLASSIFICATION OF ADVERSE REACTIONS TO FOODS OR ADDITIVES

In many papers and reviews, various pathogenic and clinical classifications have been proposed [1-9]. Generally consistent with these authors, we will use the following terminology. "Adverse reaction" is the preferred term for any pathologic reaction following exposure to the food. (Although skin or mucous membrane contact with food or inhalation of food molecules can cause disease, the discussion will be limited to those reactions following ingestion of foodstuffs.)

Adverse reactions conveniently can be divided into two groups based on triggering mechanisms (Fig. 2). The first is the true food "allergy" group, in which immunologic triggering is assumed (but rarely proved); a further subdivision into IgE-mediated (reaginic) or non-IgE-mediated (other hypersensitivity mechanisms) can be made. The second major category is the food "nonallergic" group, in which no relevant immune sensitization exists. The reactions are variously described as toxic, pharmacological, idiosyncratic, or intolerant; unfortunately these terms sometimes are used interchangeably.

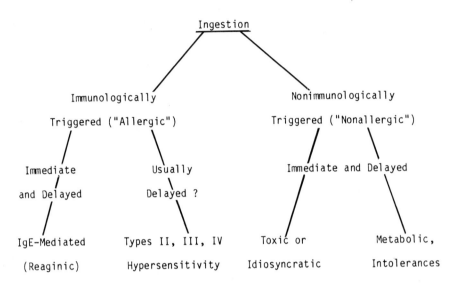

Figure 2 Possible mechanisms for adverse reactions to ingested foods and additives.

A most useful clinical differentiation between patients having adverse reactions is based on the time elapsed since ingestion of the offending food [3, 8, 10-12] (see Table 1).

Immediate Reactions

Symptoms occur up to 2 hr following ingestion of a food or chemical. The patient usually recognizes the food-symptom relationship and prevents further reactions by avoiding the offending foodstuff. The reactions are generally classically allergic and include

Anaphylaxis
Abdominal pain, cramping
Vomiting, diarrhea
Urticaria, angioedema
Atopic eczema
Rhinitis, asthma

Most of these individuals are atopic, and the presumed triggering mechanism is IgE mediated, involving activation of mast cells or basophils. For diagnosis, the history alone is often sufficient; immediate skin tests or radioallergosorbent tests (RAST) are usually positive for the provoking food.

Table 1 Temporal Comparison of Adverse Reactions to Foods

	Immediate (<2 hr)[a]	Delayed (>2 hr)
Triggering mechanisms	IgE in atopic individuals	Types I (IgE), II, III, and IV hypersensitivity; nonimmune
Pathogenic mechanisms	Mast cell/basophil release of mediators	Variable; any mediator of inflammation; metabolic aberration
Clinical manifestations	Classical allergic disorders	Classic allergic disorders; variable presentations involving single or multiple organ systems
Diagnostic approaches	History usually identi identifies agent; specific IgE (skin tests, RAST) tests usually positive	History is of limited help; in vitro tests and skin tests generally of little help
	Elimination and challenge positive, often to relatively small dose of food	Elimination and challenge is the definitive test; relatively large doses often required

[a]This classification excludes idiosyncratic reactions that provoke reactions by nonimmune mechanisms; their prevalence is unknown.

Various foodstuffs and additives may cause immediate or delayed reactions by nonimmune mechanisms that are poorly understood (Fig. 2 and Table 2). Some of these are covered elsewhere in this book; others will be discussed more fully in this chapter.

Delayed Reactions

(See Table 1 and Fig. 2).

Clinical Reactions

Symptoms occur at least 2 hr after ingestion of the offending agent, even up to several days afterward. Because there is such a delay between eating and subsequent disease, the patient usually is unaware of the etiological relationship, and the medical history for dietary causation is unclear. The prevalence of such reactions generally is unknown; diagnosis depends upon a high level of suspicion followed by elimination and challenge studies. It is likely that delayed reactions to food outweigh immediate reactions in terms of overall prevalence and importance; many epidemiological studies are required to settle the issue.

Table 2 Some Foodstuffs and Additives Reported to Trigger Nonallergic (Nonimmune) Adverse Reactions

	Agent	Reaction	Comment
Toxic or idiosyncratic	Monosodium glutamate	Chinese restaurant syndrome	Mechanism unknown
	Bisulfites	Asthma, urticaria	Converts to SO_2
	Dyes, preservatives, and salicylates	Asthma, urticaria, hyperactivity	Variable mechanisms
	Nutmeg	Hallucinations	LSD-like psychotrope
	Histamine	Flushing, urticaria, "allergic reactions"	Dose related
	Sucrose	Hypertension	Mechanism unknown
	Yeast products, sugar, alcohol, etc.	Variable	Unknown
Metabolic, intolerance	Sugars (mono- or disaccharidase)	Gastrointestinal and variable	Deficiency of digest, enzyme
	Glutens, gliadins	Celiac disease	Mechanism unclear
	Tyramine, tryptophan	Migraine headache, hypertension	Lowered MAO levels

Delayed adverse reactions to foods are exceedingly varied and may involve virtually any organ system [1, 3, 8, 9, 10-15]. Some reactions are classically allergic (the same list described for immediate reactions alone) and at times may reflect delayed IgE-mediated mechanisms. Others involve a single organ system (e.g., the gastrointestinal tract) or multiple organ systems (e.g., the central nervous system, respiratory system, skin, musculoskeletal apparatus, gastrointestinal system, or cardiovascular system) with puzzling combinations of symptoms.

Types of Triggers

Foodstuffs. Foodstuffs themselves clearly are important triggers of delayed reactions, in the native form, cooked or processed form, or a partially digested state [6, 15-17]. In some individuals, food appears only to cause disease when acting in concert with another trigger factor, as when there is exposure seasonally to large amounts of inhalant antigens or when vigorous exercise takes place within 2 hr of eating [18]. Besides nutrients of fairly large molecular size, smaller molecular weight carbohydrates, amino acids, minerals, vitamins, and purines may induce disease [17, 19, 20].

Additives. Hundreds, perhaps thousands of chemicals are added to foods and drugs; some of these have been implicated in causing untoward effects (Table 2). These include dyes, preservatives, flavoring, salicylates, and stiffeners [21-24]. Some, like tartrazine and sodium benzoate, physiologically cross-react with aspirin and cause similar reactions, such as asthma or urticaria [21, 22, 25-30]. Bisulfites, used to freshen foods and preserve their color, also have been shown to cause the same sort of pseudoallergic reactions, even anaphylaxis [31-34]. Even such simple chemicals as ethanol and acetic acid have been implicated in some patients [35, 36].

Pathogenic Mechanisms

For most adverse reactions to foods, the nature of the triggering mechanism and kinds of mediators of inflammation that are activated are not well understood. Although antibody or lymphocyte sensitization to specific food antigens may be demonstrated, it is difficult to *prove* that the interaction of immune reactant with antigen in vivo actually initiates disease. Inability to demonstrate immunologic sensitization to a food antigen may mean that (1) the test is falsely negative (e.g., insensitive); (2) the test is inappropriate and immune sensitization can be shown by a different assay; or (3) no immune sensitization exists, and any adverse reaction is triggered by nonimmune means.

Immunologic Activation or Triggering of Mediators of Inflammation by Food Antigens. (See Fig. 2.) A variety of reports suggest that many reactions to foods are immunologically triggered; every known hypersensitivity mechanism has been implicated [5, 37]. Delayed type I IgE-mediated reactions have been suggested in asthma, eczema, and migraine, for instance [1-9, 37]. Type II cytotoxic reactions involving food antibodies of various classes can be represented by milk-induced thrombocytopenia [5, 38] or villous epithelial cell damage seen in intestinal biopsies from cases of food-allergic disease [39, 40].

In type III hypersensitivity, food antigen-antibody complexes localize in tissues by one of two possible mechanisms [41]. The first is the Arthus phenomenon, whereby relatively high levels of food antigen combine with relatively large numbers of antibody molecules in the walls of small vessels to form precipitates de novo. The gastrointestinal tract is a likely site for such reactions, associated subsequently with gastritis, enteritis or colitis; malabsorption; bleeding; ulceration; and other disorders [4, 40, 42-44].

The second type III mechanism is the deposition of circulating food antigen-antibody complexes from the blood into vascular structures of target tissue. Antigenic food molecules are regularly absorbed after meals; abnormally increased amounts are absorbed from the immature gut or the inflamed gut or when there is a state of immune dysfunction or deficiency [42, 45-47]. Antibody sensi-

Table 3   Mediator Systems Implicated in Adverse Reactions to Foods

Cellular	Noncellular
Mast cells	Complement
Basophils	Classic
Eosinophils	Alternative
Polymorphonuclear neutrophils	Hageman factor cascade
	Coagulation (fibrin)
Platelets	Fibrinolysis (plasmin)
Lymphocytes	Kinins
	Complement
	Arachidonic acid metabolites
	Prostaglandins
	Leukotrienes
	Other

tization to food antigens is normal and common; many healthy people have food antigen-antibody complexes (e.g., IgG) circulating for hours or days after a meal. In some instances the presence of IgE food antibodies or rheumatoid factors or anti-idiotypic antibodies to IgE are associated with type III hypersensitivity reactions, such as arthritis, eczema, and perhaps migraine [48–53].

Type IV mechanisms would depend upon sensitization of T lymphocytes by food antigens and subsequent release of lymphokines, development of delayed hypersensitivity responses, and emergence of cytotoxic cells after exposure to the specific food. T-cell sensitization to allergenic foods is common, and the likelihood for participation in subacute or chronic pathologic responses in the gut, lung, skin, and other organs is high [47, 54–61].

Activation of Mediators of Inflammation (Biologic Amplification). Because all four hypersensitivity mechanisms have been implicated in the triggering of adverse reactions to food, it is likely that most if not all biologic amplication systems can participate. Indeed, each of the mediator systems listed in Table 3 has been reported to be activated in one or more types of adverse reaction to food.

Mast cells or basophils can be triggered by IgE-antigen interactions on their membranes, by unattached antigen-antibody complexes, by inflammatory mediators (e.g., complement C3a and C5a) and by various chemicals or drugs [41, 62]. Patients with food allergy exhibit heightened spontaneous histamine release in vitro [63–65] and release of histamine into plasma after food challenge [6, 66–68]. Other cellular events include the activation of phagocytic cells (neutrophils and macrophages) [69, 70], eosinophilia and tissue accumulation of eosinophils [71–73], platelet aggregation with potential release of thrombokines [38, 74], and lymphocyte activation as previously described. During adverse reactions and after food challenge, numbers of circulating neutrophils, lymphocytes, eosinophils, or platelets may drop or their function become altered [6, 75–79].

Noncellular mediator systems also are involved in adverse reactions to foods or additives. These include both the classic and alternative pathways of complement activation [79–84], the Hageman (factor XII) factor cascade, which includes coagulation, plasmin activation, kinin generation, and complement activation [84, 85], and the arachidonic acid pathways in cell membranes with production of such metabolites as prostaglandins and leukotrienes [6, 25, 68, 86–89].

Toxic or Idiosyncratic Reactions (Table 2). When foodstuffs or chemical additives produce disease, immune triggering usually cannot be demonstrated. In some instances the substance acts as a "first signal" on the cell membrane, as does histamine. In others, the agent has been shown to influence one or more mediators, such as aspirin's effect on mast cells, complement, and prostaglandin synthesis. Most of the time the pathogenic mechanism is unknown. In Table 2 a variety of disorders are listed in which some foodstuff or additive leads to a reaction in one or more organ systems in susceptible individuals.

Metabolic Derangements Leading to Food-Induced Disease (Table 2). A common example is the gastrointestinal disorder (bloating, malabsorption, diar‑ rhea, and so on) associated with intolerance to lactose in milk, secondary to lactase deficiency [90, 91]. Intolerance to other carbohydrates is far less common. Celiac disease is due to intolerance of glutens and gliadins found in wheat that leads to the classic gastrointestinal and systemic manifestations [40, 58, 92]. In migrainous individuals there is a statistically significant lowered level of mono-amine oxidase (MAO); ingestion of foods high in tyramine or tryptophan may thereupon trigger migraine attacks [93, 94].

VARIOUS CLINICAL DISORDERS

General Manifestations of Adverse Reactions to Foods

Subjective responses associated with food reactions are listed in Table 4. These are symptoms recognized only by the patient that have no measurable functional or inflammatory parameters. Clearly, they might be on a neurotic or psychoso-matic basis and are easily discounted unless accompanied by historical, physical, or laboratory findings that support food-related disease.

Functional changes in tissues or organs are stronger evidence of food-related disease, particularly when they follow provocative food challenge (see Table 5). Examples of smooth muscle dysfunction include the bladder detrusor muscle (enuresis), bronchioles (asthma), and the small intestine (hyperperistalsis) [5, 25, 95–97]. Increased vascular permeability is observed locally (e.g., perioral angioedema), in increased glomerular permeability seen in milk-induced nephrotic

Table 4 Adverse Reactions to Foods and Chemicals: Some Subjective Responses

Head	Headache, giddiness, sensitivity to odors
Abdominal	Bloating, pain, colic, cramping
Musculoskeletal	Myalgia, arthralgia, weakness
Mental	Anxiety, tension
General	Fatigue, fever

Table 5 Adverse Reactions to Foods and Chemicals: Some Examples of Tissue and Organ Dysfunction

Smooth muscle spasm	Bladder, bronchioles, gut
Increased vascular permeability	Edema, proteinuria, shock
Gastrointestinal	Hyperperistalsis, malabsorption
Cardiovascular	Tachycardia, arrhythmia, hypertension
Exocrine activity	Sweat, mucus
Immunologic	Lymphocytes, phagocytic leukocytes, mediators of inflammation
Central nervous system	Hyperactivity, depression, seizures, behavioral changes, psychotic manifestations

syndrome [98], and in systemic anaphylactic reactions. In the cardiovascular system, adverse reactions to food have been said to cause tachycardia, arrhythmia, and even hypertension [79]. In patients suffering from multiple food and chemical sensitivities, reversible immunologic aberrations, such as leukopenia, lymphopenia, decreased chemotaxis, increased complement utilization, and decreased lymphocyte blastogenesis, have been described [48, 55, 75, 77, 78, 99, 100]. There are many reports of central nervous system (CNS) dysfunction, ranging from irritability, sleep disturbances, and behavioral changes to hyperactivity, seizures, lethargy, depression, and psychotic manifestations [8, 82, 101-104]. Certainly many instances of dysfunctions associated with food ingestion are "anecdotal" and not convincingly demonstrated in the literature; the most compelling proofs occur when a quantifiable abnormality in function (e.g., reduced spirometric measurements) follows a double-blind food challenge.

Morphological and inflammatory changes in tissues, as observed in biopsies, that are present during food challenge and that disappear during clinical remission

Table 6   Adverse Reactions to Foods and Chemicals: Some Examples of
Morphological and Inflammatory Changes

Respiratory	Rhinitis, asthma, Heiner's syndrome
Cardiovascular	Arteritis, thrombophlebitis, vasculitis
Gastrointestinal	Gasteroenteritis, ulceration, celiac syndrome, chronic granulomatous reactions
Dermatological	Urticaria, eczema, dermatitis herpetiformis
Musculoskeletal	Arthritis, myositis
Hematological	Dyscrasias involving lymphocytes, phagocytes, platelets, erythrocytes

on elimination of an offending food can be strong evidences of food-induced
disease (see Table 6). There are many well-documented examples involving
different organ systems. In Heiner's syndrome, immune complexes containing
specific IgG antibody and cow's milk antigens become localized in pulmonary
vascular structures leading to pneumonitis, hemorrhage, and hemosiderosis [105,
106]. Arteritis, thrombophlebitis, and vasculitis involving small vessels at times
are food related [77, 79, 107]. Some instances of thrombocytopenia, with or
without the absent radius syndrome, appear to be manifestations of food allergy
[5, 38, 74]. Other blood dyscrasias, sometimes with lupuslike syndromes, have
uncommonly been seen in conjunction with food allergy [5, 78]. Gastrointestinal,
dermatological, and musculoskeletal examples of food-associated pathologic
changes are discussed in detail later.

Selected Disorders Related to Age

Infants

Probably 1-3% of infants suffer from food allergy, cow's milk being the leading
offender, far and away [5, 96]. Gerrard has emphasized that there are two
reaction patterns: one in which the baby is exquisitely sensitive, developing
immediate classic allergic (IgE-mediated) reactions after ingesting small amounts
of milk, and another in which delayed reactions of a wider spectrum are seen
after ingestion of relatively large amount of antigens [10, 108]. In the first 6
months of life, a number of factors predispose the infant to sensitization and
disease; these include a relatively indiscriminate absorption of macromolecules
(including antigenic food molecules) from the gut, an immature surface immunity
with lessened IgA "gatekeeper" function, and low levels of digestive enzymes,
which are in the process of maturation [5, 109-111].

Symptoms of food allergy most commonly appear in the first 2 months of life and are frequently overlooked [96, 112-114]. The gastrointestinal system is most commonly involved, with colic, vomiting, distention, diarrhea (frequently chronic, sometimes bloody), malabsorption, and failure to thrive. Next, in order of frequency, is the respiratory system, upper manifestations including rhinitis ("frequent colds," chronic obstruction), sinusitis and otitis media, and lower manifestations, including bronchitic reactions (congestion, coughing), bona fide asthma, and pneumonitis, exemplified by the Heiner syndrome [105, 106, 115].

The latter occurs in atopic infants who chronically ingest large quantities of cow's milk and develop extremely high levels of IgE and precipitating antibodies (e.g., IgG) to multiple milk antigens. The babies are chronically ill, fail to thrive, and have repeated bouts of gastrointestinal distress and migratory pneumonitis, with fever and dyspnea. Milk antigen-antibody complexes localize in the lungs (and presumably the gut), leading to acute and chronic inflammation. Anemia is often severe, due to both gastrointestinal blood loss and iron malabsorption and bleeding in lung sites (pulmonary hemosiderosis). Affected babies in remission can develop systemic symptoms, fresh radiological evidence of pneumonitis, and a sudden drop in blood hemoglobulin within several hours of a single cow's milk challenge.

In babies with food allergy, the skin is next most often involved, usually with atopic eczema and sometimes with urticaria or angioedema. Central nervous system symptoms follow in frequency, with a spectrum including irritability, behavioral changes, hyperactivity, and sleep disturbances (e.g., insomnia). Systemic anaphylaxis is relatively uncommon.

Toddlers and Preschool Children

Food allergy continues from infancy into the toddler ages, apparently falling off in the frequency of "typical" manifestations thereafter.

A varied spectrum of manifestations has been reported from around the world [114, 116, 117], typified by the findings in a study by Hill and others in Australia [117]. When over 100 infants and toddlers with cow's milk allergy were followed, three broad groupings appeared (Table 7). Group I, with almost half the subjects, had immediate (1-hr) reactions after milk challenge, mainly involving the skin (not eczema) and usually involving IgE mediation. In group II, slightly over a thrid of the children reacted later in the first 24 hr, mainly with gastrointestinal symptoms, especially chronic diarrhea and failure to thrive. Half had serological evidence of rotavirus infection and reduced levels of serum IgA; less than a third showed IgE-specific sensitization to milk antigen. Group III contained 17% of the cases; they tended to be older than the others and developed symptoms as late as a day or longer after relatively large challenge doses of milk. Gastrointestinal symptoms and respiratory symptoms (rhinitis, asthma) were most prominent. IgE sensitization to milk was present in only a fourth; elevated IgM and IgE were seen in a fourth, the latter usually in conjunction with eczema.

Table 7 Varying Manifestations of Cow's Milk Allergy in 118 Infants and Toddlers

	Type I (N = 54)	Type II (N = 44)	Type III (N = 20)
Time of onset	<1 hr	1–24 hr	>24 hr
Milk dose required	Smallest	Intermediate	Largest
Manifestations			
Skin	Angioedema, urticaria +++	Pallor; eczema ±	Eczema +
Respiratory	Wheeze +	–	Rhinitis, asthma ++
Gastrointestinal	Vomiting; diarrhea ±	Vomiting; diarrhea, failure to thrive ++	Diarrhea, failure to thrive +++
Central nervous system	Irritable, etc. +	Irritable, etc. +	Irritable, etc. +
Immunologic phenomena	Immediate skin tests or RAST to milk positive 90% of time, serum IgE ↑ in a third	Immediate skin tests or RASTs to milk positive 30% of time, serum IgA ↓ in a half	Immediate skin tests or RASTs to milk positive 25% of time (always with eczema), serum IgM ↑ in a fourth; if serum IgE ↑, eczema usually present

Source: Adapted from Hill, et al., Australia.

Chronic rhinitis and persistent otitis media with effusion (OME) is one of the most common causes of morbidity in pediatrics. Although anatomic factors, dysfunction of the eustachian tube spiral muscle, viral and bacterial infection, and allergy have been recognized as contributory to rhinitis and OME, the relative role role of food allergy has been controversial [117-122]. Many children with OME have systemic symptoms that go far beyond the eustachian tube and contiguous middle ear; they have a recurring cyclic pattern of disease beginning with upper respiratory "cold" symptoms, pallor, irritability, and loss of appetite, progressing to ear symptoms, often with fever, and sometimes with lower respiratory and gastrointestinal symptoms. With or without antibiotics, each bout lasts several days to a week or so, only to recur within days or weeks. In our clinic we have found that some of these affected children are sensitive to common food allergens, such as milk, often without evidence of atopy or IgE sensitization, and that elimination of these foods from the diet leads to remission. At present we are carrying out a study at the University of Texas Health Science Center at San Antonio to determine the incidence of food allergy in OME and to learn more about the pathogenic mechanism and range of clinical features.

Atopic eczema is most common in the first few years of life, with the prevalence and severity falling off markedly in the young adult years. It is a complex, multifactorial disorder chiefly characterized by itchy dry skin that shows abnormal whealing and flare reactions to a variety of physiologic and pharmacological stimuli [123]. Most cases are atopic, with IgE sensitization present to many or most environmental and dietary antigens; many have evidence of cell-mediated (T-cell) immune dysfunction and abnormalities in phagocyte movement or phagocytosis [51, 100, 123, 124]. Although most dermatologists have denied a pathogenic role for food allergy, allergists have long supported the notion based on the following reasons: (1) IgE sensitization to foods is commonly demonstrated, (2) after challenge with a presumed "unsafe" food, immediate flaring [120] or delayed flaring [117, 123-128] of eczema has been observed, (3) amelioration of chronic eczema may follow elimination diets [123, 126, 127], (4) incidence of eczema is reduced by prophylactic dietary regimens in atopic infants, and (5) oral cromolyn prevents appearance of food antigen-antibody complexes and flaring of eczema after challenge with proven offending food.

In San Antonio, we have recently completed an epidemiological study of 30 unselected cases of chronic moderate to severe eczema [129]. Of these, 60% achieved significant remission of eczema after 3-12 days on an elemental diet (Vivonex) and maintained some or all of the improvement when later placed on a rotary elimination diet, avoiding the multiple foods to which they were found allergic. (This was true for 75% of the 16 children and 43% of the 14 adults studied.) The 13 worst food offenders are listed in Table 8; it should be noted that soy, peanut, and corn are not prominent on European lists; fish, which are common in continental diets, do not appear on the Texas list. Of the food-

Table 8 Worst Food Offenders Causing
Symptoms on Repeated Open Challenge
During Rotary Elimination Diet in 13
Vivonex Responders

Food	% Reacting
Egg	77
Soy	69
Peanut	61
Chocolate	61
Milk	54
Wheat	54
Potato	54
Corn	46
Oat	46
Chicken	31
Beef	31
Orange	23
Pork	23

allergic subjects, 12 were challenged double blind; none reacted to a "placebo" safe food, but all reacted to one or more known unsafe foods, usually with flaring of eczema, and uncommonly with gastrointestinal or respiratory symptoms. Half of the reactions were immediate, and the other half were delayed, occurring 2 hr or more after challenge. Studies from England [126–128], Italy [123, 130], and Australia [117, 124, 131] have noted that eczema responses after unsafe food challenge are delayed much or most of the time, rather than immediate. One recent U.S. study unequivocally demonstrated food allergy in the causation of atopic eczema in the majority of studied children but found that all positive reactions after double-blind challenge were immediate [120]. One possible explanation is that the study population was highly selected and extremely atopic, with an average serum total IgE of 8463 IU/ml.

The so-called tension-fatigue syndrome represents a constellation of food-allergic symptoms, often with non-IgE-mediated mechanisms and with delayed onset [14, 56, 102, 103]. It has been described in preschool children and those in the early school years. CNS symptoms are prominent, alternating between "tension" (hyperkinesis, irritability, and so on) and "fatigue" (lethargy, achiness, depression and so on) in association with a wide variety of non-CNS allergic symptoms in other organ systems. There is controversy about the prevalance or validity of the diagnosis [104], and many clinicians decline the use of the term, preferring to diagnose adverse reactions to foodstuffs in relation to the major organ systems involved.

Older Children and Adults

Although some of the disorders listed below have been described mostly in young children, they may occur at all ages or can be anticipated to do so.

Many observers have noted that some individuals develop altered CNS activity in relation to foodstuffs, a phenomenon that gained national prominence with the advancement of the Feingold hypothesis and diet in the 1970s. It seems clear that learning disabilities, hyperkinesis, and torpor (features of the tension fatigue syndrome) are at times unquestionably caused by adverse reactions to foods or additives, generally by non-IgE mechanisms. The main question concerns incidence or prevalence. Some have claimed a rate approaching 25% or more [103, 132, 133], but some investigators and a recent NIH consensus panel conclude that childhood hyperactivity can be related to foodstuffs in a relatively small percentage of cases [101, 104, 134, 135]. Clearly, more carefully designed controlled studies are needed.

Many of the previously cited review articles mention muscle aches, "growing pains," and myofascitis syndromes as manifestations of food allergy. Recurrent or chronic arthralgia, usually without serological evidence of rheumatoid arthritis or permanent joint changes, seems to be a frequent manifestation of delayed food reactions, often in association with bowel disease, headaches, and other "allergic" symptoms [51, 136-139]. Some of these patients have circulating immune complexes containing food, specific IgE antibody, and rheumatoid factor (IgG anti-IgE); both the appearance of complexes and joint symptoms can be prevented by pretreatment with oral cromolyn before unsafe food challenge [51]. Some workers have demonstrated that classic adult or juvenile rheumatoid arthritis may be associated with food allergy, but the incidence so far appears to be quite low [136, 138, 140].

Chronic urticaria has been causally associated with many foods, additives, and chemicals and is often associated with many other "allergic" manifestations in various tissues, usually on a non-IgE-mediated basis [27, 31, 32, 128, 141]. The commonest offenders appear to be dyes, flavorings, salicylates, and preservatives, which can cause, upon challenge, similar pathologic reactions in spite of their lack of chemical structural similarity. The majority of studies suggest that a third to a half of patients with chronic urticaria have demonstrable sensitivity to foodstuffs or additives and that stringent diets eliminating the offending substances may be ameliorative [57, 142-145].

It has been reported that some individuals with small-vessel vasculitis (edema, petechiae, bruising, and peripheral cyanosis) and idiopathic thrombophlebitis clear their vascular disease upon a stringent dietary elimination program and comprehensive environmental control [107, 146, 147]. The disease recurred upon challenge with a variety of foods and chemicals. The same group reported similar finding for cardiac disease (abnormal pulse rate, arryhthmias, and chest pain) [79]. Tobacco and possibly cross-reacting foodstuffs in the Solanacaeae family (e.g., potato, tomato, and eggplant) may be immunologically implicated in a variety of cardiovascular diseases [148]. Internists recognize an ill-defined syndrome including vasculitis, urticaria, arthralgias, myositis, and hypocomplementemia that may constitute a distinct category of collagen-vascular disease [149, 150]; an etiological role for foodstuff deserves exploration.

Chronic and recurrent headaches of the cluster, migraine, or other types have long been associated with adverse reactions to foodstuffs. Although trigger factors are multiple (exhaustion, tension, and so on) headaches following ingestion of trigger substances account for many attacks, perhaps the majority in sufferers [93, 151-155]. Immunologic mechanisms, both IgE and otherwise (e.g., immune complex associated, preventable by oral cromolyn pretreatment before unsafe food challenge), have clearly been demonstrated in some patients [51, 152, 155]. In other cases, foodstuffs trigger headaches by nonimmune mechanisms, such as chocolate, cheese, and beer, in susceptible subjects with low serum MAO levels [94, 93, 154]. Elimination diets can successfully reduce the number and intensity of headaches and even reduce the occurrence of other associated phenomena, such as convulsions or hypertension [93, 151-153, 155].

Because the gastrointestinal tract is the first site where ingestants interact with body constituents, it is no surprise that vomiting, diarrhea, distention, and hyperistalsis are common manifestations of foodstuff sensitivity at all ages. It could also be predicted that adverse reactions involving different levels of the gastrointestinal tract would occur, and that is the case. Moving downward from the mouth, there are reports of aphthous ulcers, eosinophilic gastroenteritis, peptic ulcer, colic, celiac disease, Crohn's disease, enterocolitis, irritable bowel syndrome, and ulcerative colitis [4, 8, 13, 42, 58, 92, 40, 43, 95, 156-166]. Intestinal biopsies in appropriate patients make it clear that inflammatory changes, alterations in T cells and B cells, and activation of mediators are common events, even in those food-allergic patients who do not have clinically evident gastrointestinal disease [39, 72, 92, 167-171]. Increased intestinal permeability and malabsorption are common, and the acquisition of carbohydrate intolerance secondary to gut allergic inflammation is well documented [13, 46, 114, 156, 157, 166, 170, 172-175].

The occurrence of bronchial asthma following ingestion of foods is well documented in all ages [36, 69, 120, 121, 128, 176, 177]. It is particularly common in infancy and tends to wane as inhalant sensitization increases [116, 121]. It should be emphasized that many asthmatic reactions are delayed, either due to IgE-mediated mechanisms or others that are not [128, 171, 178]. Foodstuffs suspended in dust, such as wheat or soybean flour, also may induce immediate or late-onset asthma [179, 180]. As previously mentioned, asthma also is caused by a variety of food additives, including salicylates, sulfites, dyes, and preservatives; even alcohol has been implicated [25, 28, 31, 32, 34].

In 1977, Sandberg et al reported six older children with nephrotic syndrome and cow's milk allergy [98]. Elimination of milk from the diet was associated with remission and reintroduction with exacerbation. Enuresis on the basis of food allergy is mentioned in this chapter's introductory review [1-9]; we have seen it disappear when children with OME were placed on a diet eliminating common food offenders. An association between Henoch-Schonlein purpura and food allergy has been reported [181].

Many patients are appearing who manifest a host of intolerances to endogenous (self), dietary, and environmental factors that largely incapacitate them [77, 99, 182-185]. Most are adults, and females are predominant. In many, some stressful event (e.g., surgery, injury, infection, chemical exposure, or psychological trauma) is followed by a progressive deterioration of their health and increasing intolerance of foods, medications, and inhaled substances. Laboratory derangements of some immune parameters, increased levels of autoantibodies, and and endocrinopathies are sometimes seen. Recurrent symptoms in many unrelated organ systems occur, and profound changes in CNS function (behavior, alertness, mood, and so on) are frequent, raising the question: whether this whole "disease" is essentially a massive psychoneurotic reaction or the CNS dysfunction is part of a systemic pathologic process [182, 186-189].

Because these patients manifest a picture that has not been widely appreciated or defined, it is a dilemma for physicians and patients alike. Patients make the rounds of various specialists, usually including a psychiatrist or two, and are likely to try a variety of "controversial" and "unproven" therapies [190-192]. It is possible that this group of unfortunate people reflects a breakdown in self-non-self-recognition and homeostatic control, involving the highly integrated CNS, immune, and endocrine systems [193]. Careful study of patients with this complex syndrome is required to better define and recognize the disorder and to understand how such profound dysregulation of bodily functions can come about.

DIAGNOSTIC APPROACHES TO DELAYED FOOD REACTIONS

Many aspects of diagnosis of adverse reactions to foods are covered elsewhere in this book, so only those points relevant to non-IgE and delayed reactions will be emphasized here. Strategies for diagnosis and the advantages or disadvantages of various tests are discussed in several reviews [2, 12, 194, 195]; points about individual approaches will be covered in additional references.

In Vitro Tests or Techniques

Immunologic, Specific for Food

Some individuals with delayed adverse reactions to food will have elevated levels of specific IgE, IgG_4 (type I hypersensitivity mechanisms?) [12, 128, 154, 196–205]. Sometimes this evidence of specific antibody sensitization correlate with delayed positive food challenges, but there is an unacceptably high rate of false-positive and false-negative results, making the tests largely unreliable for diagnosis. Circulating immune complexes are commonly found in allergic diseases, and their presence per se means little. There is some suggestion that the presence of food antigen and specific IgE and the presence of rheumatoid factor to IgE in complexes tends to have diagnostic and pathogenic importance [48, 49, 52, 206]. Extremely high levels of precipitating antibodies to milk antigens strongly support the diagnosis of Heiner's syndrome [105, 106, 115]. Specific lymphocyte sensitization to foodstuffs and chemical additives is readily demonstrated in patients with clinical hypersensitivity to the products, but once again false-positive and false-negative tests are common. Measurement of the lymphokine (LIF) released upon incubation with the offending food extract may offer more promise [54–57, 60, 75, 207].

Specific Tests Without Demonstrable Immune Mechanisms

Elevated plasma or urinary histamine is found spontaneously in individuals with food allergy or after oral challenge with a known offending food [63, 64, 66, 205]. The test does not necessarily indicate IgE mediation but rather mast cell or basophil activation, by whatever means. The so-called cytotoxic assay involves incubation of living buffy coat leukocytes with food extract dried on microscopic slides [80, 208–210]. A positive test seems to reflect activation of phagocytes (e.g., PMN) by food in the presence of cations and complement. It has little utility in diagnosis because of poor clinical correlations and problems with reproducibility [118, 209].

In Vivo Tests or Techniques

Skin Tests

Immediate IgE-mediated reactions to foods (but not chemical additives) are often associated with diagnostically reliable immediate skin test responses to the same foods; the rate of false-positive reaction tends to be a problem [7, 120, 200, 211, 212]. Clinically delayed reactions to foods or chemicals simply do not correlate well with immediate, late (6–8 hr) or delayed (24–48 hr) skin test responses to the same substances [200, 205, 213]. Patch tests, using food extracts with or without DMSO carrier, have shown some promise for diagnostic utility when read at 24–72 hr [214–216].

Dietary Techniques and Provocative Challenge

Because all the tests so far mentioned are by and large unsuitable or unreliable, there is general agreement that definitive diagnosis rests upon a positive provocative challenge, the reproduction of typical symptoms upon challenge with a possible offending food [205, 217–220]. Performing the oral challenge is prolonged and cumbersome. The following steps should prove helpful [221].

Preparatory Phase. As stated before, the clinical history (as usually obtained) may provide little suggestion that foods or chemicals play a causative role in producing a patient's symptoms. A detailed and lengthy further history often is quite productive, when carried out by a physician or nutritionist who has the training and who takes the time. A "food frequency" questionnaire can be helpful; foods most suspect are those that are eaten every day, those that are most craved, and those that are least liked. It is helpful for the patient to keep a diet diary at home for a few weeks, recording all foods, snacks, medications, and clinical events; a careful scrutiny of foodstuffs in the 12 hr or so preceding bouts of illness may uncover some possible offenders.

Elimination Phase. Before attempting a food challenge it is necessary to eliminate all or enough offending foods from the diet that the patient becomes partially or completely asymptomatic. This is easy if only one or two allergenic foods are strongly suggested by history or diary, and clinical remission occurs within a week or two of their elimination. Usually one is forced to select a so-called oligoantigenic diet in which multiple commonly allergic foodstuffs are eliminated for 1–3 weeks (see Table 9). We have evolved such a list of omitted foodstuffs (Table 10); during the period the patient's nutritional needs are adequately supplied by generally nonallergenic foods, which are rotated so that none are taken more often than every 4 days.

Some individuals appear to be sensitive to so many foods that it may be more efficient to remove all or virtually all of them during the elimination phase (Table 9). Fasting for such a long period (water is permitted) is extremely difficult to carry out, and resultant metabolic derangements confuse the picture. In infants it is relatively simple to interdict all solid foods and cow's milk formulas, permitting only breast milk or a non-allergenic cow's milk substitute, such as a casein hydrolysate or meat-based formula. Beyond infancy, an elemental diet, such as Vivonex, is preferred to fasting since it provides adequate nutrition [222a, 222b, 223]. Because Vivonex is so unpalatable, compliance will be poor unless patient motivation is high and a nutritionist spends considerable time in explanations and frequent follow-up calls or visits.

Challenge Phase. Remission of symptoms during food elimination only is suggestive that the patient had been sensitive to foodstuffs; proof that foods or chemicals cause adverse reactions is dependent upon a symptomatic response to oral challenge (Table 11). When multiple foods have been eliminated, they are

Table 9 Comparison of Diagnostic Approaches that Eliminate Food from the Diet

	Advantages	Disadvantages
Fasting	No potential allergens, inexpensive, convenient	Requires strict supervision or self-discipline, metabolic derangements
Elemental diet (e.g., Vivonex)	Provides adequate nutrition, hypoallergenic	Poor compliance due to unpalatibility, expensive
Elimination diet excluding multiple foods	Best compliance, provides adequate nutrition	Offending foods may not be excluded, difficulty in finding and preparing "pure" foods

Table 10 Foods Omitted from Basic Rotary Elimination Diet (University of Texas Health Sciences Center, San Antonio)

Milk, cheese, dairy products	
Egg	
Wheat, corn	
Legumes	Peas, beans (including soy), peanut
Citrus fruits	Lemon, lime, orange, grapefruit, tangerine
Lily family	Garlic, onion, chives, leeks, asparagus
Cane/beet sugar	
Stercula family	Chocolate, cocoa, colas
Coffee/tea	
Yeast-containing products	Vitamins, breads, beer, wines

reintroduced separately (one each day or two), beginning with the least allergenic and ending with the most allergenic. Because adverse reactions may be intensified after an elimination period, a tiny amount of diluted food is first offered and the dose rapidly incrementally increased so that meal-size portions are offered within several hours. At any sign of a reaction, the challenge is halted. Because subjective responses are so hard to quantify and are prone to conditioning or bias, it is always preferable to employ objective measures of altered function (e.g., pulmonary function tests) following oral challenge.

The simplest procedure for challenge is "open," in which the patient knows what is being offered and can readily consume meal-sized portions. It works well

Table 11 Oral Provocative Challenge Testing with Food

Logistics	Patient must be symptom-free; a prepratory elimination period generally is necessary
	Challenge begins with tiny dose followed by incremental amounts to reduce likelihood of severe reactions
	Because of varying levels of reactivity, large portions given daily may be required
	Open challenge	Double-blind challenge
Advantages	Relatively easy and convenient, meal-sized portions readily reached	Unbiased, no conditioning effect, scientifically acceptable
Disadvantages	Very subjective, conditioning phenomenon, scientifically unacceptable	Difficult to do, inconvenient, dose effect, capsules versus bolus amounts

in clinical practice, the patient obtaining and preparing the food and carrying out all challenges at home (Table 11). There are many disadvantages, though, including the opportunity for mistakes, dependence on the patient's acuity, and a conditioning phenomenon leading to an unduly high number of positive responses. Although the double-blind challenge procedure is more difficult and inconvenient, it is the more accurate. For relatively small challenge doses, "hiding" the food in opaque capsules or in a carrier food or Vivonex is useful. For many non-IgE-mediated delayed reactions, relatively large meal-sized portions are required to obtain a positive challenge. In that case, it may be more efficient to make a slurry of challenge food with water or Vivonex to be sipped while blindfolded and with the nose clamped (to prevent tasting of food). After a water chaser, the blind fold and clamp are removed.

MANAGEMENT OF DELAYED ADVERSE REACTIONS TO FOODSTUFFS

Prophylaxis of Allergic Disease in Infants

It is possible to forestall allergic disease in infants, at least for a few years, by instituting a prophylactic regimen in the newborn [224-227]. In the first year of life, cow's milk, soy formula, and common allergic foods are interdicted. The major source of nutrition is breast milk or hypoallergic formula, such as casein hydrolysate. "Safe" foods are added after 6 months. Reduction in inhalant sensitization is accomplished by dust and mold control and absence of pets in the home.

Table 12 Problems That May Arise During Dietary Management of Foods and Chemical Intolerance

"Hidden" foods/chemicals in processed products

Poor compliance with dietary restrictions

Suboptimal nutrition, dependent on degree of restrictions

Apparent "sensitization" to many or most common foods, precluding a satisfactory elimination or rotary diet

Treatment of Diagnosed Food or Additive Adverse Reactions

Dietary Manipulation

Prevention is clearly the best medicine, logically accomplished by eliminating offending foods from the diet. There is relatively little displacement of life-style when one or two foods are eliminated. If many foods are eliminated, severe stresses are placed on the patient and family. A nutritionist needs to provide guidance about food families, sources of foods, shopping practices, recipes, and diet plans. We prefer a rotary elimination diet (no particular food is ingested more often than every 4 days), which maximizes exposure to safe food groups (better compliance), optimizes nutrition, and may reduce the likelihood for sensitization to new foods.

There are still potential problems (Table 12) that compromise the success of any long-term dietary program. "Hidden" unsafe foods or chemicals in processed food products or in restaurant servings will sporadically trigger disease. The dietary restrictions at times lead to rebellion and poor compliance. If many foods are eliminated it becomes almost impossible to maintain optimal nutrition; supplements with hypoallergic foodstuffs, such as Vivonex, may become necessary.

Pharmacological Agents

Pharmaceutical agents should not be the mainstay in treatment of food allergy but may be considered as an adjunct to the dietary elimination regimen. Medications can be considered, for instance, when an unacceptable level of disease persists while on the diet or when the dietary exclusions are so profound that compliance or adequate nutrition is difficult to achieve. Powdered cromolyn can be dissolved in warm water and given orally before each meal or snack. Taken prior to oral challenge with unsafe food, it reduces absorption from the gut, prevents appearance of circulating immune complexes, and abolishes the expected positive response (e.g., migraine, arthritis, and eczema) [50, 52, 228]. Oral cromolyn with elimination diet has been found to be efficacious in the chronic management of these diseases; not only is disease ameliorated but patients are able to increasingly tolerate foods previously found to be unsafe [50, 51, 53,

123, 130, 152, 229, 230]. Unfortunately, oral cromolyn is not commercially available in the United States; newer related compounds and ketotifen [231, 232], which also stabilizes mast cell membranes, deserve consideration.

Various clinicians anecdotally have found that oral administration of enteric-coated slow-release pancreatic enzymes may increase toleration of foods and further reduce symptomatology, perhaps by further digesting allergenic foodstuffs before absorption from the gut. Nonsteroidal antiinflammatory agents (e.g., aspirin and indomethacin) have been observed to benefit some food-allergic subjects by altering mediator metabolism and preventing the expected adverse reaction to food challenge [86, 88, 89, 232]. Controlled studies are necessary to determine if such drugs (which can cause adverse reactions themselves) have a role in the long-term management of some patients. Administration of small amount of food extracts or chemicals by sublingual or injected (subcutaneous or intradermal) routes that "neutralize" the pathogenic effects of the same foodstuffs in the diet is practiced by some clinicians [191, 209, 233–236]. This approach is considered controversial, and further studies are needs to determine its efficacy, if any.

CONCLUDING COMMENTS

In the last few years, adverse reactions to foods and chemicals increasingly have been taken seriously by the medical community. Immediate reactions to foodstuffs often are IgE mediated, and are relatively easy to diagnose, study, and document. On the other hand, delayed reactions, by their very nature, are more difficult to suspect, recognize, and prove. Pathogenic mechanisms may be immunologic or nonimmunologic, and possible clinical manifestations run the gamut of much of the known disease spectrum. A great stumbling block to the acceptance of delayed reactions to foodstuffs is the lack of epidemiological data establishing the incidence (and thereby importance) of adverse reactions to foodstuffs in such disorders as asthma, arthritis, inflammatory bowel diseases, and chronic urticaria. When such data accumulate, it is likely that adverse reactions to ingestants will rival or surpass the importance of adverse reactions to inhalants (e.g., seasonal and perennial allergens) in clinical immunology and allergy.

REFERENCES

1. Denman, A. M. Nature and diagnosis of food allergy. *Proc. Nutr. Soc. 38*: 391–403, 1979.
2. Bock, S. A. Food sensitivity: A critical review and practical approach. *Am. J. Dis. Child. 134*:973–982, 1980.
3. Bierman, C. W., and Furukawa, C. T. Food allergy. *Pediatr. Rev. 3*(7):213–220, Jan. 1982.

4. Aiuti, F., and Paganelli, R. Food allergy and gastrointestinal diseases. *Ann. Allergy 51*:275–280, Aug. 1983.
5. Bahna, S. L., and Gandhi, M. D. Milk hypersensitivity. I. Pathogenics and symptomatology. *Ann. Allergy 50*(4):218–223, Apr. 1983.
6. Buckley, R. H., and Metcalfe, D. Food allergy. *JAMA 248*(20):2627–2631, Nov. 26, 1982.
7. Golbert, T. M. Food allergy. *J. Med. Soc. N. J. 77*(13):895–899, Dec. 1980.
8. McCarty, E. P., and Frick, O. L. Food sensitivity: Keys to diagnosis. *J. Pediatr. 102*(5):645–652, May 1983.
9. AAAI and NIAID, *Adverse Reactions to Foods*, U.S. Dept. of Health and Human Services, Public Health Services NIH, July 1984.
10. Gerrard, J. W. The diagnosis of the food allergic patient. In *The Mast Cell: Its Role in Health and Disease*, edited by J. Pepys and A. M. Edwards, Pitman, London, 1979.
11. Deamer, W. C. Unrecognized allergy: Milk and other food allergies. *Consultant*, pp. 55–64, June 1980.
12. Galant, S. P., Bullock, J., and Frick, O. L. In immunological approach to the diagnosis of food sensitivity. *Clin. Allergy 3*:363–373, 1973.
13. May, C. D., and Bock, S. A. Adverse reactions to food due to hypersensitivity. In *Principals and Practice*, edited by Eliott Middleton, Charles E. Reed, and Elliot F. Ellis, Vol. 62, pp. 1159–1171, 1978.
14. Crook, W. C. Food allergy – the great masquerader. *Pediatr. Clin. North Am. 22*(1):227–238, Feb. 1975.
15. Speer, F. Multiple food allergy. *Ann. Allergy 34*(12):71–76, Feb. 1975.
16. Schwartz, H. B., Lata, S., Nerurkai, S., et al. Milk hypersensitivity: Rast studies using new antigens generaled by pepsin hydrolysis of beta-lactoglobulin. *Ann. Allergy 45*:242–245, Oct. 1980.
17. Herman, R. H., and Hagler, L. Food intolerance in humans. *Western J. Med. 130*(2):95–116, Feb. 1979.
18. Maulitz, R. M., Pratt, D. S., and Schocket, A. L. Exercise-induced anaphpylactic reaction to shellfish. *J. Allergy Clin. Immunol. 63*(6):433–434, June 1979.
19. NIH, *Adverse Reactions to Foods*, Chap. II, Chemistry of selected food antigens. U.S. Dept. of Health and Human Services, Public Health Service, July, 1984, pp. 7–16.
20. Atkins, F. M., and Metcalfe, D. D. Diagnostic approaches to food allergy. *Immunol. Allergy Pract. 5*(3):37–43, March 1983.
21. Lockey, Sr., S. D. Reactions to hidden agents in foods and drugs can be serious. *Ann. Allergy 35*:239–243, Oct. 1975.
22. Juhlin, L. Incidence of intolerance to food additives. *Int. Soc. Dermatol. 19*(10):548–551.
23. MacCara, M. E. Tartrazine: A potentially hazardous dye in Canadian drugs. *Can. Med. Assoc. J. 126*:910–914, April 1982.
24. NIH, *Adverse Reactions to Foods*, Chap. V, Adverse food reactions that do not involve immunologic reactions. U.S. Dept. of Health and Human

Services, Public Health Service, July 1984, pp. 103–121.
25. Settipane, G. A. Adverse reactions to aspirin and related drugs. *Arch. Intern. Med. 141*:328–332, Feb. 23, 1981.
26. Speer, F., Denison, T. R., and Baptist, J. E. Aspirin allergy. *Ann. Allergy 46*:123–126, March 1981.
27. Settipane, R. A., Constantine, H. P., and Settipane, G. A. Aspirin intolerance and recurrent urticaria in normal adults and children. *Allergy 35*:149–154, 1980.
28. Tarlo, S. M., and Broder, I. Tartrazine and benzoate challenge and dietary avoidance in chronic asthma. *Clin. Allergy 12*:303–312, 1982.
29. Schlumberger, H. D. Pseudo-allergic reactions to drugs and chemicals. *Ann. Allergy 51*:317–324, Aug. 1983.
30. Ortolani, C., Pastorello, E., Luraghi, M. T., Gattei, G., and Zanussi, C. Acetylsalicylic acid and food additive intolerance. *Adv. Pediatr. Allergy,* Int. Allergy Workshop, editor Luisa Businco. Rome, Oct. 23, 1982, pp. 251–262.
31. Habenicht, H. A., Preuss, L., and Lovell, R. G. Sensitivity to ingested metabisulfites: Cause of bronchospasm and urticaria. *Immunol. Allergy Pract. 5*(8):25–27, Aug. 1983.
32. Schwartz, H. J. Sensitivity to ingested metabisulfite variations in clinical presentation. *J. Allergy Clin. Immunol. 71*(5):487–489, May 1983.
33. Baker, G. J., Collett, P., and Allern, D. H. Bronchospasm induced by metabisulphite-containing foods and drugs. *Med. J. Aust. 2*:614–616, Nov. 28, 1981.
34. Stevenson, D. D., and Simon, R. A. Sensitivity to ingested metabisulfites in asthmatic subjects. *J. Allergy Clin. Immunol. 68*(1):26–32, July 1981.
35. Przybilla, B., and Ring, J. Anaphylaxis to ethanol and sensitisation to acetic acid. *Lancet* 483, Feb. 26, 1983.
36. Gong, Jr., H., Tashkin, D. P., and Calvarese, B. M. Alcohol-induced bronchospasm in an asthmatic patient. *Chest 80*(2):167–173, Aug. 1981.
37. Haddad, Z. H. Clinical and immunological aspects of food hypersensitivity. *Ann. Allergy 49*:29–39, July 1982.
38. Whitfield, M. F., and Barr, D. G. D. Cow's milk allergy in the syndrome of thrombocytopenia with absent radius. *Arch. Dis. Child. 51*:337–343, Aug. 1975.
39. Fontaine, J. L., and Navarro, J. Small intestinal biopsy in cow's milk protein allergy in infancy. *Arch. Dis. Child. 50*:357–362, 1975.
40. Scott, H., Brandtzaeg, P., Thorsby, E., Baklien, K., Fausa, O., and Ek, J. Mucosal and systemic immune response patterns in celiac disease. *Ann. Allergy 51*:233–239, Aug. 1983.
41. Kniker, W. T. Diseases of the immune response, Chap. 36. In *Principles of Pediatrics: Health Care of the Young,* edited by R. A. Hoekelman, S. Blatman, P. S. Brunnel, S. B. Friedman, and H. M. Seidel, McGraw-Hill, New York, 1978, pp. 1053–1096.
42. Aiuti, F., and Paganelli, R. Food allergy and gastrointestinal diseases. *Ann. Allergy 51*:275–280, Aug. 1983.

43. Siegel, J. Immunologic approach to the treatment and prevention of gastro-intestinal ulcers. *Ann. Allergy 38*(1):27–41, Jan. 1977.
44. Andre, C., Moulinier, B., Andre, F., and Daniere, S. Evidence for anaphylactic reactions in peptic ulcer and varioliform gastritis. *Ann. Allergy 51*: 325–328, Aug. 1983.
45. Walker, W. A., and Bloch, K. J. Gastrointestinal transport of macromolecules in the pathogenesis of food allergy. *Ann. Allergy 51*:325–328, Aug. 1983.
46. Reinhardt, M. C., Paganelli, R., and Levinsky, R. J. Intestinal antigen handling at mucosal surfaces in health and disease: Human and experimental studies. *Ann. Allergy 51*(2):311–314, Aug. 1983.
47. Saavedra–Delgado, A. M., and Metcalfe, D. D. Gastrointestinal defense mechanisms: Their role in the pathogenesis of food allergy. *Immunol. Allergy Pract. 5*(4):52–57, April 1983.
48. Paganelli, R., Atherton, D. J., and Levinsky, R. J. Differences between normal and milk allergic subjects in their immune responses after milk ingestion. *Arch. Dis. Child. 58*:201–206, 1983.
49. Delire, M. Detection of circulating immune-complexes in infants fed on cow's milk. 375–379.
50. Brostoff, J., Cairni, C., Wraith, D. G., Paganelli, R., and Levinsky, R. J. Immune-complexes in atopy. In *The Mast Cell,* edited by J. Pepys and A. M. Edwards, Pitman, London, 1979, pp. 380–393.
51. Brostoff, J., Carini, C., and Wraith, D. G. The presence of immune complexes containing IgE following food challenge and the effect of sodium cromoglycate. *Proceedings of The Second Fisons Food Allergy Workshop,* Fisons Corp., Jan. 1983, pp. 30–34.
52. Carini, C., and Brostoff, J. An antiglobulin: IgG anti-IgE occurrence and specificity. *Ann. Allergy 51*:251–254, Aug. 1983.
53. Brostoff, J., Carini, C., Wraith, D. G., and Johns, P. Production of IgE complexes by allergen challenge in atopic patients and the effect of sodium cromoglycate. *Lancet* 1268–1269, June 1979.
54. Ashkenazi, A., Levin, S., Idar, D., Or, A., Rosenberg, I., and Handzel, Z. T. In vitro cell-mediated immunologic assay for cow's milk allergy. *Pediatrics 66*(3):399–402, Sept. 1980.
55. Minor, J. D., Tolber, S. G., and Frick, O. L. Leukocyte inhibition factor in delayed-onset food allergy. *J. Allergy Clin. Immunol. 66*(4):314–321, Oct. 1980.
56. Valverde, E., Vich, J. M., Garcia-Calderon, J. V., and Garcia-Calderon, G. In vitro response of lymphocytes in patients with allergic tension-fatigue syndrome. *Ann. Allergy 45*:1885–188, Sept. 1980.
57. Valverde, E., Vich, J. M., Garcia-Calderon, J. V., and Garcia-Calderon, P. A. In vitro stimulation of lymphocytes in patients with chronic urticaria induced by additives and food. *Clin. Allergy 10*:691–698, 1980.
58. Auricchio, S., Buffolano, W., Ciccimarra, E., et al. In vitro proliferation of lymphocytes from celiac children and their first-degree relatives in response to wheat gliadin-derived peptides. *J. Pediatr. Gastroenterol. Nutr. 1*(4): 515–524, 1984.

59. Clinical nutrition: Lymphocyte hypersensitivity in cow's milk protein intolderance. *Nutr. Rev. 35*(2):39–41, Feb. 1977.
60. Stafford, H. A., Polmar, S. H., and Boar, T. F. Immunologic studies in cow's milk-induced pulmonary hemosiderosis. *Pediatr. Res. 11*:898–903, 1977.
61. Ferguson, A., McImowat, A., Strobel, S., and Barnetson, R. S. T-cell mediated immunity in food allergy. *Ann. Allergy 51*:246-248, Aug. 1983.
62. Saavedra-Delgado, A. M., and Metcalf, D. D. The gastrointestinal mast cell in food allergy. *Ann. Allergy 51*:185–189, Aug. 1983.
63. May, C. D. High spontaneous release of histamine in vitro from leukocytes of persons hypersensitive to food. *J. Allergy Clin. Immunol. 58*(3): 432–437, Sept. 1976.
64. May, C. D., and Remigio, L. Observations on high spontaneous release of histamine from leucocytes in vitro. *Clin. Allergy 12*:229–241, 1982.
65. Reiman, H. J., Ring, J., Ultsch, B., Wendt, P., et al. Release of gastric histamine in patients with urticaria and food allergy. *Agents Actions 12*(13): 111–113, 1982.
66. Bellanti, J. A., Nerurkar, L. S., and Willoughby, J. W. Measurement of p plasma histamine in patients with suspected food hypersensitivity. *Ann. Allergy 47*:260–263, Oct. 1981.
67. Sampson, H. A., and Jolie, P. L. Increased plasma histamine concentrations after food challenges in children with atopic dermatitis. *N. Engl. J. Med. 311*:372–376, Aug. 9, 1984.
68. Bellanti, J. A., Tate, S. M., Liu, W. J., Guillen, M., et al. The role of histamine and prostaglandins in food allergy. In *Advances Pediatric Allergy,* editor Luisa Businco, Rome, Oct. 23, 1982, pp. 242–248.
69. Papageorgiou, N., Lee, T. H., Nagakura, T., Cromwell, O., et al. Neutrophil chemotactic activity in milk-induced asthma. *J. Allergy Clin. Immunol. 72*(1):75–82, July 1983.
70. Butler, H. L. Cow's milk intolerance. *Pediatr. Rev. 77*(8):329–333, Jan. 1981.
71. Winqvist, I., Olsson, I., Werner, S., and Stanstam, M. Variations of cationic proteins from eosinophil leukocytes in food intolerance and allergic rhinitis. *Allergy 36*:419–423, 1981.
72. Perkkio, M. Immunohistochemical study of intestinal biopsies from children with atopic eczema due to food allergy. *Allergy 35*:573–580, 1980.
73. Church, J. A., Wang, D. W., Swanson, V., Thomas, D., and Sinatra, F. Cow's milk allergy in a premature infant with hypereosinophilia and hyperimmunoglobulinemia E. *Ann. Allergy 41*:307–310, Nov. 1978.
74. Caffrey, E. A., Sladen, G. E., Isaaca, P. E. T., and Clark, K. G. A. Thrombocytopena caused by cow's milk. *Lancet,* 316, Aug. 8, 1981.
75. Kuperman, S. W. O., Ilfeld, D., Fienlt, M., and Freier, S. Specific suppressor cell activity and lymphocyte response to B-lactoglobulin in cow's milk protein hypersensitivity. *J. Pediatr. Gastroenterol. Nutr. 1*(3):389–393, 1982.

76. Sandilands, G. P., Reid, F. M., Galbraith, I., Peel, M. G., and Lewis, C. J. In vivo modulation of human lymphocyte Fcγ-receptior in response to oral antigen (cow's milk) challenge. *Int. Arch. Allergy Appl. Immunol.* 67:344–350, 1982.

77. Rea, W. J. Diagnosing food and chemical susceptibility. *Cont. Ed. 57:* 47–59, Sept. 1979.

78. Anderson, J. A., Weiss, L., Rebuck, J. W., Cabal, L. A., and Sweet, L. C. Hyperactivity to cow's milk in an infant with LE and tart cell phenomenon. *J. Pediatr. 84*(1):59–67, Jan. 1974.

79. Rea, W. J. Environmentally triggered cardiac disease. *Ann. Allergy 40:* 243–251, April 1978.

80. Trevino, R. J. Immunologic mechanisms in the production of food sensitivities. *Laryngoscope 91:*1913–1936, Nov. 1981.

81. Berrens, L., Van Dijk, A. G., and Weemaes, C. M. R. Complement consumption in eggwhite and fish sensitivity. *Clin. Allergy 11:*101–109, 1981.

82. Strunk, R. C., Pinnas, J. L., John, T. J., Hansen, R. C., and Blazovich, J. L. Rich hypersensitivity associated with serum complement depression. *Clin. Allergy 8:*51–58, 1978.

83. Olenchock, S. A., Mull, J. C., and Major, P. C. Complement activation by commercial allergen extracts of cereal grains. *Clin. Allergy 10:*395–404, 1980.

84. Neuman, I., Elian, R., Nahum, H., Shaked, P., and Creter, D. The danger of "yellow dyes" (tartrazine) allergic subjects. *Clin. Allergy 8:*65–68, 1978.

85. Theorell, H., Blomback, M., and Kockum, C. Demonstration of reactivity of airborne and food allergens in cutaneous vasculitis by variations in fibrofibrinopeptide A and other blood coagulation, fibrinolysis and complement parameters. *Thrombos. Haemostas. (Stuttg.) 36:*593–604, 1976.

86. Buisseret, P. D., Heinzelmann, D. I., Youlten, L. J. F., and Lessof, M. H. Prostaglandin-synthesis inhibitors in prophylaxis of food intolerance. *Lancet* 906–908, April 19, 1978.

87. Asad, S. I., Youlten, L. J. F., and Lessof, M. H. Specific desensitization in "aspirin sensitive" urticaria; plasma prostaglandin levels and clinical manifestations. *Clin. Allergy 13:*459–466, 1983.

88. Lessof, M. H., Anderson, J. A., and Youlten, L. J. F. Prostaglandins in the pathogenesis of food intolerance. *Ann. Allergy 51:*249–250, Aug. 1983.

89. Buissert, P. D., Youlten, L. J., Heinzelman, D., and Lessof, M. H. Prostaglandin synthetase inhibitors and food intolerance. *Monogr. Allergy 14:* 197–202, 1979.

90. Mitchell, K. J., Boyless, T. M., Paige, D. M., Goodgame, R. W., and Huang, S. S. Intolerance of eight ounces of milk in healthy lactose-intolerant teenagers. *Pediatrics 56*(5):718–721, Nov. 1975.

91. Kwon, Jr., P. H., Rorick, M. H., and Scrimshaw, N. S. Comparative tolerance of adolescents of differing ethnic backgrounds to lactose-containing and lactose-free dairy drinks. II. Improvement of a double-blind test. *Am. J. Clin. Nutr. 33:*22–26, Jan. 1980.

92. Scott, H., Brandtzaeg, P., Thorsby, E., Baklien, K., et al. Mucosal and

systemic immune response patterns in celiac disease. *Ann. Allergy 51*: 233–239, Aug. 1983.

93. Hanington, E. Diet and migraine. *J. Hum. Nutr. 34*:175–180, 1980.
94. Glover, V., Sandler, M., Grant, E., Rose, F. C., et al. Transitory decrease in platelet monoamine-oxidase activity during migraine attacks. *Lancet* 391–393, Feb. 1977.
95. Bahna, S. L., and Heiner, D. C. Cow's milk allergy: Pathogenesis, manifestations, diagnosis and management. *Adv. Pediatr. 25*:1–37, 1978.
96. Heiner, D. C. Intolerance to milk. *Immunol. Allergy Pract. 5*(7):17–22, July 1983.
97. Eastham, E. J., and Walker, W. A. Effect of cow's milk on the gastrointestinal tract: A persistent dilemma for the pediatrician. *Pediatrics 60*(4): 477–481, 1977.
98. Sandberg, D. H., Bernstein, C. W., McIntosh, R. M., Carr, R., and Strauss, J. Severe steroid-responsive nephrosis associated with hypersensitivity. *Lancet* 388–391, Feb. 19, 1977.
99. McGovern, Jr., J. J., Lazaroni, J. A., Hicks, M. F., Adler, J. C., and Cleary, F. Food and chemical sensitivity: Clinical and immunologic correlates. *Arch. Otolaryngol. 109*:292–297, May 1983.
100. Furukawa, C. T. Recent immunologic findings relating food allergy to atopic dermatitis. *Ann. Allergy 42*:207–210, April 1979.
101. Weiss, B. Food additives and environmental chemicals as sources of childhood behavior disorders. *J. Am. Acad. Child Psychiatr. 21*(2):144–152, 1982.
102. Hall, K. Allergy of the nervous system: A review. *Ann. Allergy 36*:49–64, Jan. 1976.
103. Crook, W. G. Can what a child eats make him dull, stupid or hyperactive? *J. Learning Disabilities 13*(5):53–58, May 1980.
104. Johnson, J. T. Eat, drink, and be merry – or argue about food "allergy." *JAMA 250*(6):701–711, Aug. 12, 1983.
105. Heiner, D. C., Sears, J. W., and Kniker, W. T. Multiple precipitins to cow's milk in chronic respiratory disease. *Am. J. Dis. Child. 103*:40–60, May 1962.
106. Lee, S. K., Kniker, W. T., Cook, C. D., and Heiner, D. C. Cow's milk-induced pulmonary disease in children. *Adv. Pediatr. 25*:39–57, 1978.
107. Rea, W. J., Peters, D. W., Smiley, R. E., Edgar, R., et al. Recurrent environmentally triggered thrombophlebitis: A five-year follow-up. *Ann. Allergy 47*:338–344, Nov. 1981.
108. Gerrard, J. W., and Shenassa, M. Food allergy: Two common types as seen in breast and formula fed babies. *Ann. Allergy 50*:375–379, June 1983.
109. Kleinman, R. E. Relationship of uptake and transport of protein by the immature intestine to antigenicity of infant formulas. In *The Mast Cell: Its Role in Health and Disease*, edited by J. Pepys and A. M. Edwards, Pitman, London, 1979, pp. 371–374.
110. Eastman, F. J., Lichauco, T., Grade, M. I., and Walker, W. A. Antigenicity of infant formulas: Role of immature intestine on protein permeability. *J. Pediatr. 93*(4):561–564, Oct. 1978.

111. Businco, L., and Cantani, A. Prevention of atopy – current concepts and personal experience. *Clin. Rev. Allergy* 2:107–123, 1984.

112. Goldman, A. S., Anderson, Jr., D. W., Sellers, W. A., Saperstein, S., et al. Milk allergy. I. Oral challenge with milk and isolated milk proteins in allergic children. *Pediatrics* 32(3):425–443, Sept. 1963.

113. Kibort, P. M., and Ament, M. E. Cow's milk and soy protein intolerance in childhood. *Pediatr. Ann.* 11(1):71–75, 1975.

114. Holael, A. Cow's milk allergy – some clinical and immunological aspects. *Postgrad. Med. J.* 51(3):71–75, 1975.

115. Boat, T. F., Polmar, S. H., Whitman, V., Kleinerman, J. I., et al. Hyperreactivity to cow milk in young children with pulmonary hemosiderosis and cor pulmonale secondary to nasopharyngeal obstruction. *J. Pediatr.* 87(1):23–29, July 1975.

116. Minford, A. M. B., MacConald, A., and Littlewood, J. M. Food intolerance and food allergy in children: A review of 68 cases. *Arch. Dis. Child.* 57: 742–747, 1982.

117. Hill, D. J., Ford, P. K., Shelton, M. J., and Hosking, C. S. A study of 100 infants and young children with cow's milk allergy. *Clin. Rev. Allergy 2*: 125–142, 1984.

118. Ruokonen, J., Paganus, A., and Lehti, H. Elimination diets in the treatment of secretory otitis media. *Int. J. Pediatr. Otorhinolaryngol.* 4:39–46, 1982.

119. Viscomi, G. J. Allergic secretory otitis media: An approach to management. *Laryngoscope* 751–758, Dec. 27, 1973.

120. Sampson, H. A. Role of immediate food hypersensitivity in the pathogenesis of atopic dermatitis. *J. Allergy Clin. Immunol.* 71(5):473–480, May 1983.

121. Ogle, K. A., and Bullock, J. D. Children with allergic rhinitis and/or bronchial asthma treated with elimination diet: A five-year follow-up. *Ann. Allergy 44*:273–278, May 1980.

122. Saarinen, U. M., Savilahi, E., and Arjomaa, P. Increased IgM-type beta-lactoglobulin antibodies in children with recurrent otitis media. *Allergy 38*:571–576, 1983.

123. Businco, L., Benicori, N., and Cantani, A. Clinical and immunological aspects of atopic dermatitis: A review and update. *Adv. Pediatr. Allergy*, editor Luisa Businco, Rome, Oct. 23, 1982, pp. 195–236.

124. Van Asperen, P. P., Lewis, M., Rogers, M., and Kemp, A. S. Experience with an elimination diet in children with atopic dermatitis. *Clin. Allergy 13*:479–485, 1983.

126. Atherton, D. J. Allergy and atopic eczema. II. *Clin. Exp. Dermatol. 6*: 317–325, 1981.

127. Atherton, D. J. The role of foods in atopic eczema. *Clin. Exp. Dermatol. 8*:227–232, 1983.

128. Wraith, D. G., Merrett, J., Roth, A., Yman, L., and Merrett, T. G. Recognition of food-allergic patients and their allergens by the RAST technique and clinical investigation. *Clin. Allergy 9*:25–36, 1979.

129. Ratner, P. H., Davis, S. H., Rodriguez, L. M., DeVillez, R. L., and Kniker, W. T. The efficacy of rotary elimination diet and of oral cromolyn in the management and prevention of atopic eczema. *Abstract presented at the International Symposium of Prevention of Allergic Diseases, Florence, Italy,* June 1984.

130. Businco, L., Benincori, N., Businco, E., Infussi, R., and DeAngelis, M. Double-blind crossover study with an oral solution of sodium cromoglycate in children with atopic dermatitis due to food allergy. *The Second Fisons Food Allergy Workshop,* Jan. 1983, pp. 116–119.

131. Hill, D. J., and Lynch, B. C. Elemental diet in the management of severe eczema in childhood. *Clin. Allergy 12*:313–315, 1982.

132. Williams, J. L., and Cram, D. G. Diet in the management of hyperkinesis. *Can. Psychiatr. Assoc. J. 23*:241–248, 1978.

133. Hughes E. C., Weinstein, R. C., Gott, P. S., Binggeli, R., and Whitaker, K. L. Food sensitivity in attention deficit disorder with hyperactivity (Add/Ha): A procedure for differential diagnosis. *Ann. Allergy 49*(5):276–280, Nov. 1982.

134. Ribon, A., and Joshi, S. Is there any relationship between food additives and hyperkinesis? *Ann. Allergy 48*:275–278, May,1982.

135. NIH Consensus Development Conference, Defined diets in childhood hyperactivity. *Clin. Pediatr. 21*(10):627–630, Oct. 1982.

136. Denman, A. M., Mitchell, B., and Ansell, B. M. Joint complaints and food allergic disorders. *Ann. Allergy 51*:260–263, Aug. 1983.

137. Editorial, Aging, arthritis and food allergies: A research opportunity revisited. *Growth 44*:155–159, 1980.

138. Zeller, M. Rheumatoid arthritis – food allergy as a factor. *Ann. Allergy* 200–205, Mar.–Apr. 1949.

139. Stroud, R. M., Kroker, G., Marshall, R., Carroll, M., Bullock, T., et al. Comprehensive environmental control and its effect on rheumatoid arthritis. I. Food and chemical challenges. (Abstracts) Presented at American College of Allergists Third International Food Allergy Symposium, Boston, Massachusetts, October 1980.

140. Parke, A. L., and Hughes, G. R. V. Rheumatoid arthritis and food: A case study. *Br. Med. J. 282*:2027–2029, June 20, 1981.

141. Fisherman, E. W., and Cohen, G. N. Chronic and recurrent urticaria: New concepts of drug-group sensitivity. *Ann. Allergy 39*(6):404–414, Dec. 1977.

142. Rudzki, E., Czubalski, K., and Grzywa, Z. Detection of urticaria with food additives intolerance by means of diet. *Dermatologica 161*:57–62, 1980.

143. Gibson, A., and Clancy, R. Management of chronic idiopathic urticaria by the identification and exclusion of dietary factors. *Clin. Allergy 10*:699–704, 1980.

144. Chronic urticaria. *Br. Med. J. 283*(6295):805–806, Sept. 1981.

145. Michaelsson, G., and Juhlin, L. Urticaria induced by preservatives and dye additives in food and drugs. *Br. J. Dermatol. 88*:525–532, Mar. 1973.

146. Rea, W. J. Environmentally triggered small vessel vasculitis. *Ann. Allergy* *38*(4):245–251, Apr. 1977.
147. Rea, W. J. Environmentally triggered thrombophlebitis. *Ann. Allergy 37*(2): 101–109, Aug. 1976.
148. Becker, C. G., and Dubin, T. Tobacco allergy and cardiovascular disease. *Cardiovasc. Med.* 851–854, Aug. 1978.
149. Marder, R. J., Rent, R., Choi, E. Y. C., and Gewurz, H. Clq deficiency associated with urticarial-like lesions and cutaneous vasculitis. *Am. J. Med. 61*:560–565, Oct. 1976.
150. Feig, P. U., Soter, N. A., Yager, H. M., Caplan, L., and Rosen. W. Vasculitis with urticaria, hypocomplementemia and multiple system involvement. *JAMA 236*(18):2065–2068, Nov. 1976.
151. Egger, J., Wilson, J., Carter, C. M., Turner, M. W., and Soothill, J. F. Is migraine food allergy? *Lancet* 865–868, Oct. 1983.
152. Monro, J., Carini, C., Brostoff, J., and Zilkha, K. Food allergy in migraine. *Lancet* 1–4, July 1980.
153. Monro, J. A. Food allergy in migraine. *Proc. Nutr. Soc. 42*:241–246, 1983.
154. Merrett, J., Peatfield, R. C., Rose, F. C., and Merrett, T. G. Food related antibodies in headache patients. *J. Neurol. Neurosurg. Psychiatry 46*:738–742, 1983.
155. Grant, E. C. G. Food allergies and migraine. *Lancet* 966–968, May 5, 1979.
156. Powell, G. K. Milk- and soy-induced enterocolitis of infancy. *J. Pediatr. 93*(4):553–560, Oct. 1978.
157. Butler, H. L. Cow's milk intolerance. *Pediatr. Rev. 77*(8):329–333, Jan. 1981.
158. Wilson, C. W. M. Food sensitivities, taste changes, aphthous ulcers and atopic symptoms in allergic disease. *Ann. Allergy 44*:302–307, May 1980.
159. Bentley, S. J., Pearson, D. J., and Rix, K. J. B. Food hypersensitivity in irritable bowel syndrome. *Lancet* 295–296, Aug. 6, 1983.
160. Bahna, S. L., Tateno, K., and Heiner, D. C. Elevated IgD antibodies to wheat in celiac disease. *Ann. Allergy 44*:146–151, Mar. 1980.
161. Haeney, M. R., Goodwin, B. J. F., Barratt, M. E. J., Mike, N., and Asquith, P. Soya protein antibodies in man: Their occurrence and possible relevance in coeliac disease. *J. Clin. Pathol. 35*:319–322, 1982.
162. Liebman, W. M. Infantile colic: Association with lactose and milk intolerance. *JAMA 245*(7):732–733, Feb. 20, 1981.
163. Lothe, L., Lindberg, T., and Jakobsson, I. Cow's milk formula as a cause of infantile colic: A double-blind study. *Pediatrics 70*(1):7–10, July 1982.
164. Caldwell, J. H., Tennenbaum, J. L., and Bronstein, H. A. Serum IgE in eosinophilc gastroenteritis. *N. Engl. J. Med. 292*(26):1388–1390, June 26, 1975.
165. Hunter, J. O., Jones, V. A., Freeman, A. H., Shorthouse, M., Workman, E., and McLaughan, P. Food intolerance in gastrointestinal disorders. *The Second Fisons Food Allergy Workshop,* Jan. 1983, pp. 69–72.

166. Aivti, F., and Paganeli, R. Food allergy and gastrointestinal disease. In *Advances in Pediatric Allergy*, editor Luisa Businco, Rome, Oct. 23, 1982, pp. 34–50.

167. Perkkio, M., Savilahti, E., and Kuitunen, P. Morphometric and immuno-histochemical study of jejunal biopsies from children with intestinal soy allergy. *Eur. J. Pediatr. 137*:63–69, 1981.

168. Halpin, T. C., Byrne, W. J., and Ament, M. E. Colitis, persistent diarrhea, and soy protein intolerance. *J. Pediatr. 91*(3):404–407, Sept. 1977.

169. Shiner, M., Ballard, J., Brook, C. G. D., and Herman, S. Intestinal biopsy *Br. Med. J.* Feb 19, 1977, pp. 510–511.
     Lancet 1060–1063, Nov. 29, 1975.

170. Kuitunen, P., Visakorpi, J. K., Savilanti, E., and Pelkonen, P. Malabsorption syndrome with cow's milk intolerance: Clinical findings and course in 54 cases. *Arch. Dis. Child. 50*:351–356, 1975.

171. Lessof, M. H. An overview of diagnostic techniques. *The Second Fisons Food Allergy Workshop,* Jan. 1983, pp. 56–58.

172. Jackson, P. G., Baker, R. W. R., Lessof, M. H., and Ferrett, J. Intestinal permeability in patients with eczema and food allergy. *Lancet* 1285–1286, June 13, 1981.

173. Goel, K., Lifshitz, F., Kahn, E., and Teichberg, S. Monosaccharide intolerance and soy-protein hypersensitivity in an infant with diarrhea. *J. Pediatr. 93*(4):617–619, Oct. 1978.

174. Iyngkaran, N., Abdin, Z., Davis, K., Boey, C. G., et al. Acquired carbohydrate intolerance and cow milk protein-sensitive enteropathy in young infants. *J. Pediatr. 95*(3):373–378, Sept. 1979.

175. Manuel, P. D., Soeparto, P., and Walker-Smith, J. A. Cow's-milk allergy in chronic diarrhoeas and malnutrition in Indonesian infants. *The Second Fisons Food Allergy Workshop,* Jan. 1983, pp. 66–68.

176. Podell, R. N. Food allergy and asthma. *Postgrad. Med. 73*(5):287–289, May 1983.

177. Burr, M. L., Merrett, T. G., Fehily, A. M., and Stott, N. C. H. Epidemiological studies. *The Second Fisons Food Allergy Workshop,* Jan. 1983, pp. 61–65.

178. Arroyave, C. M., Stevenson, D. D., Vaughan, J. H., and Tan, E. M. Plasma complement changes during bronchospasm provoked in asthmatic patients. *Clin. Allergy 7*:173–182, 1977.

179. Bush, K., and Cohen, M. Immediate and late onset asthma from occupational exposure to soybean dust. *Clin. Allergy 7*:369–373, 1977.

180. Sutton, R., Hill, D. J., Baldo, B. A., and Wrigley, C. W. Immunoglobulin E antibodies to ingested cereal flour components: Studies with sera from subjects with asthma and eczema. *Clin. Allergy 12*:63–74, 1982.

181. Robinson, B. W. S. Henoch–Schonlein purpura due to food sensitivity. *Br. Med. J.* Feb. 19, 1977.

182. Mike, N., and Asquith, P. Total allergy syndrome: What evidence can be established? *The Second Fisons Food Allergy Workshop,* Jan. 1983, pp. 79–83.

183. Lessof, M. Food and environmental factors in human disease. *Lancet* 1308, June 9, 1984.

184. Randolph, T. G. The scope of food and chemical allergy/addiction. *Cont. Educ.* 63–76, Sept. 1979.

185. Randolph, T. G. Specific adaptation. *Ann. Allergy 40*:333–345, May 1978.

186. May, C. D. Food allergy: Lessons from the past. *J. Allergy Clin. Immunol. 69*(3):255–259, March 1982.

187. May, C. D. Immunologic versus toxic adverse reactions to foodstuffs. *Ann. Allergy 51*:267–268, Aug. 1983.

188. Pearson, D. J., Rix, K. J. B., and Bentley, S. J. Food allergy: How much in the mind? A clinical and psychiatric study of suspected food hypersensitivity. *Lancet* 1259–1261, June 4, 1983.

189. Finn, R., and Cohen, H. N. "Food allergy": Fact or fiction? *Lancet* 426–428, Feb. 25, 1978.

190. Truss, C. O. The role of *Candida albicans* in human illness. *J. Orthomol. Psy. 10*(4):1–11, 1981.

191. Miller, J. B. A double-blind study of food extract injection therapy: A preliminary report. *Ann. Allergy 38*:185–191, March 1977.

192. Crook, W. G. *The Yeast Connection.* Second Edition. Professional Books, Jackson, Tennessee, 1983, 1984.

193. Talal, N., Dauphinee, M., and Christadoss, P. Immune and endocrine factors in autoimmune disease. In *Stress, Immunity, and Aging,* (Edwin K. Cooper, ed.). Marcel Dekker, New York, 1984, Chapt. 12, pp. 187–193.

194. Bahna, S. L., and Gandhi, M. D. Milk hypersensitivity. II. Practical aspects of diagnosis, treatment and prevention. *Ann. Allergy 50*:295–301, May 1983.

195. NIH, Methods for diagnosis of adverse reactions to foods, Chapt. VI. In *Adverse Reactions to Foods.* U.S. Department of Health and Human Services, Public Health Service, July 1984, pp. 123–160.

196. Galant, S., Nussbaum, E., Wittner, R., DeWeck, A. L., and Heiner, D. C. Increased IgD milk antibody responses in a patient with Down's syndrome, pulmonary hemosiderosis and corpulmonale. *Ann. Allergy 51*:446–449, Oct. 1983.

197. Bjorksten, B., Ahlstedt, S., Bjorksten, F., Carlsson, B., et al. Immunoglobulin E and immunoglobulin G_4 antibodies to cow's milk in children with cow's milk allergy. *Allergy 38*:119–124, 1983.

198. Dannaeus, A., Johansson, S. G. O., Foucard, T., and Ohman, S. Clinical and immunological aspects of food allergy in childhood. *Acta. Paediatr. Scand. 66*:31–77, 1977.

199. Aas, K. The diagnosis of hypersensitivity to ingested foods. *Clin. Allergy 8*:39–50, 1978.

200. Lessof, M., Wraith, D. G., Merrett, T. G., Barrett, J. M., and Buisseret, P. D. Food allergy and intolerance in 100 patients – local and systemic effects. *Q. J. Med. (New Series XLIX) 195*:259–271, 1980.

201. May, C. D., Remigio, I., and Bock, S. A. Usefullness of measurement of

antibodies in serum in diagnosis of sensitivity to cow milk and soy proteins in early childhood. *Allergy 35*:301–310, 1980.

202. Gavani, U. D., Hyde, J. S., and Moore, B. S. Hypersensitivity to milk and egg with skin tests, RAST results and clinic intolerance. *Ann. Allergy 40*: 314–318, May 1978.

203. Ford, R. P. K., and Fergusson, D. M. Egg and cows' milk allergy in children. *Arch. Dis. Child. 55*:608–610, 1980.

204. Kemeny, D. M., Parkes, P., and Lessof, M. H. Setting up RAST to measure IgE antibodies to foods. *The Second Fisons Food Allergy Workshop*, Jan. 1983, pp. 45–47.

205. Bernstein, M., Day, J. H., and Welse, A. Double-blind food challenge in the diagnosis of food sensitivity in the adult. *J. Allergy Clin. Immunol. 70*(3): 205–210, Sept. 1982.

206. Paganelli, R., Levinsky, R. J., and Atherton, D. J. Detection of specific antigen within circulating immune complexes: Validation of the assay and its application to food antigen-antibody complexes formed in healthy and food-allergic subjects. *Clin. Exp. Immunol. 46*:44–53, 1981.

207. Ashkenazi, A., Idar, D., Barzilai, N., Levin, S., Or, A., and Handzel, Z. T. Effect of gluten-free diet on an immunological assay for coeliac disease. *Lancet* 914–916, April 25, 1981.

208. Ulett, G. A., and Perry, S. G. Cytotoxic testing and leucocyte increase as an index to food sensitivity. II. Coffee and tobacco. *Ann. Allergy 34*: 150–160, March 1975.

209. Lehman, C. W. The leukocytic food allergy test: A study of its reliability and reproducibility. Effect of diet and sublingual food drops on this test. *Ann. Allergy 45*:150–158, Sept. 1980.

210. Holopainen, E., Palva, T., Stenberg, P., Backman, A., et al. Cytotoxic leukocyte reaction. *Acta Otolaryngol.* (*Stockh.*) *89*:222–226, 1980.

211. Bock, S. A., Lee, W. Y., Remigio, L., Holst, A., and May, C. D. Appraisal of skin tests with food extracts for diagnosis of food hypersensitivity. *Clin. Allergy 8*:559–564, 1978.

212. Lessof, M., Buisseret, P. D., Merrett, J., Merret, T. G., and Wraith, D. Assessing the value of skin prick tests. *Clin. Allergy 10*:115–120, 1980.

213. Kniker, W. T. Relationship of immunologic sensitization and pathogenic mechanisms in food intolerance. 13. *Presented at The American College of Allergists International Food Allergy Symposium IV, Vancouver, British Columbia*, Canada, July 1982.

214. Walsh, W. E. Food allergy in atopic dermatitis: Diagnosis of food sensitivity using patch tests. *Minn. Med.* 310–312, Apr. 1975.

215. Breneman, J. Patch test for diagnosis of food allergy. *Presented at The American College of Allergists International Food Allergy Symposium IV, Vancouver, British Columbia*, Canada, July 1982.

216. Boonk, W. J., and van Ketel, W. G. Skin testing in chronic urticaria. *Dermatologica 163*:151–159, 1981.

217. NIH, Treatment of food allergy, Chap. VII. In *Adverse Reactions to Foods*, U.S. Department of Health and Human Services, Public Health Service, July 1984, pp. 161–174.

218. Rowe, A. H. The elimination diets, Chapt. V. In *Elimination Diets and Patients Allergies,* Lea and Febiger, Philadelphia, 1941, pp. 141–155.
219. Ford, R. P. K., and Fergusson, D. M. Egg and cows' milk allergy in children. *Arch. Dis. Child.* 55:608–610, 1980.
220. Atherton, D. J., Soothill, J. F., Sewell, M., and Wells, R. S. A double-blind controlled crossover trial of an antigen-avoidance diet in atopic eczema. *Lancet* 401–403, Feb. 25, 1978.
221. Kniker, W. T., Rodriguez, L. M., and Olejer, V. L. The utility of food elimination and provocation challenge in diagnosis of adverse reactions to foods. Presented at the 5th International Food Allergy Symposium, American College of Allergists, Atlanta, Gerogia, Oct. 1984.
222a. Hughes, E. C. Use of a chemically defined diet in the diagnosis of food sensitivities and the determination of offending foods. *Ann. Allergy 40*(6): 393–398, June 1978.
222b. Dockhorn, R. J., and Smith, T. C. Use of a chemically defined hypoallergenic diet (Vivonex). *Ann. Allergy 47*(4):264–266, Oct. 1981.
223. Galant, S. P., Franz, J. L., Walker, P., Wells, I. D., and Lundak, R. L. A potential diagnostic method for food allergy: Clinical application and immunogenicity evaluation of an elemental diet. *Am. J. Clin. Nutr. 30*: 512–516, Apr. 1977.
224. Gruskay, F. L. Comparison of breast, cow and soy feedings in the prevention of onset of allergic disease. *Clin. Pediatr.* 486–491, Aug. 1982.
225. NIH, Avoidance of specific foods, prior to known sensitization, in potentially susceptible infants, Chap. VIII. In *Adverse Reactions to Foods,* U.S. Department of Health and Human Services, Public Health Service, July 1984, pp. 175–190.
226. Saarinen, U. M. Prophylaxis for atopic disease: Role of infant feeding. *Clin. Rev. Allergy 2*:151–167, 1984.
227. Hamburger, R. N., Heller, S., Mellow, M. H., O'Connor, R. D., and Zeiger, R. S. Current status of the clinical and immunological consequences of a prototype allergic disease prevention program. *Ann. Allergy 51*:281–290, Aug. 1983.
228. Dahl, R. Oral and inhaled sodium cromoglycate in challenge test with food allergens or acetylsalicylic acid. *Allergy 36*:161–165, 1981.
229. Moneret-Vautrin, D. A., and Claudot, N. Allergie alimentaire de type I et pseudo-allergies alimentaires chez l'adulte. *Lancet* 1065–1068, May 20, 1978.
230. Kocoshis, A., and Gryboski, J. D. Use of cromolyn in combined gastrointestinal allergy. *JAMA 242*(11):1169–1173, Sept. 14, 1979.
231. Ellul-Micallef, R. Effect of oral sodium cromoglycate and ketotifen in fish-induced bronchial asthma. *Thorax 38*:527–530, 1983.
232. Zanussi, C., Ortolani, C., and Pastorello, E. Dietary and pharmacologic management of food intolerance in adults. *Ann. Allergy 51*:307–310, Aug. 1983.
233. A.A.A. position statements, Provocative and neutralization testing (subcutaneous). *J. Allergy Clin. Immunol.* 336–337, May 1981.

234. Todd, S., and Mackarness, R. Allergy to food and chemicals. 2. Investigation and treatment. *Nursing Times* 506–510, Mar. 23, 1978.
235. Green, M. Sublingual provocative testing for foods and FD&C dyes. *Ann. Allergy 33*:274–281, Nov. 1974.
236. Lehman, C. W. A double-blind study of sublingual provocative food testing: A study of its efficacy. *Ann. Allergy 45*:144–149, Sept. 1980.

10
Laboratory Tests for Food Hypersensitivity

ROBERT J. DOCKHORN
University of Missouri School of Medicine, Kansas City, Missouri

Before one can determine a specific laboratory test for the diagnosis of food allergy or food hypersensitivity, one must define the common term "food allergy." It seems to mean different things to different people. One of the reasons for the confusion lies in the definition of the broad term "allergy."

Early this century, Coca and Cooke [1] stated that to make the diagnosis of an allergic state, common criteria must be determined. They suggested three criteria: (1) the identification of the antigen, (2) the establishment of a causal relationship between exposure to the antigen and occurrence of the lesion, and (3) the identification of the immunologic mechanism involved in the reaction causing a specific illness. More recently, Spector and Farr [2] defined "allergy" as an untoward physiologic event mediated by a variety of different immunologic reactions.

"Antibodies" and "antigens" are frequently used immunologic terms, but what about "reagins" and "allergens"? It was not until 1966, when Ishizakas et al. [3] and Johanssen discovered IgE antibodies, that the mysterious terms reagin and reaginic antibody could be discraded in favor of IgE antibody or atopic antibody. Allergens are those antigens that react with IgE antibody. Today the definition of atopy has been described as reaction associated with but not necessarily caused by IgE antibodies. In order to bring order to this confusion, Coombs and Gell developed a classification of allergic or hypersensitivity reactions [4].

Tissue alterations caused by various allergic reactions may be inflammatory in nature. Since more than one organ system may be involved in the same allergic process and since the alterations in different organ systems caused by the same process have pathologic similarities, the lesions produced by allergic reactions are best classified according to the particular type of allergic mechanism involved. Four types of allergic reactions have been described by Coombs and Gell [4].

Type I allergic reactions, dependent upon IgE antibodies, are anaphylactic in nature. The reaction, which is initiated by an allergen reacting with tissue cells, passively sensitized by the antibody produced elsewhere, results from the release of pharmacologically active substances, such as vasoactive amines.

Type II reactions are known as cytotoxic reactions. They are initiated by an antibody reacting with either an antigenic component on a cell or tissue element or an antigen or hapten that has become immediately associated with these tissues. Complement is usually but not always necessary to effect the cellular damage.

Type III reactions, known as immune complex reactions, are initiated when an antigen reacts in the tissue spaces with potentially precipitating antibody, forming microprecipitates in and around the small vessels, causing damage to the tissues. Another mechanism in connection with type III reactions is excess antigen reacting in the bloodstream with potentially precipitating antibody forming soluble circulating complexes, which are deposited in the blood vessel walls or in the basement membrane, causing local inflammation.

Type IV reactions, also known as delayed or cell-mediated reactions, essentially are initiated by the reaction of specifically modified lymphocytes containing substances capable of responding specifically to allergens deposited at a local site.

There may even be a type V reaction, known as a systemic mediator reaction. Certain studies have shown that not all food allergy reactions are necessarily produced by the allergen contacting antibody at the shock organ. It is now apparent that the immune creations in the wall of the gut may also be produced in situ, with only the mediators traveling to the shock organ [5].

TYPE I REACTIONS

The presence of specific factors responsible for immediate hypersensitivity reactions were first demonstrated by Prausnitz and Kustner [6] in the early 1920s. It was almost 50 years before the chemical identity of these factors, called reaginic antibodies, was established. In 1967, two independent research teams purified immunoglobulin E (IgE) in the laboratory. Ishizakas et al. [7] and their collaborators in the United States isolated IgE from the serum of allergic patients and demonstrated that it was the carrier of reaginic activity. Johansson and associates [8] recognized a patient with an IgE myeloma and isolated IgE (originally called IgND) from this patient's sera.

IgE exists in monomeric form and is produced primarily by plasma cells in the mucous membranes and regional lymphy nodes of the respiratory and gastrointestinal tracts [9]. It is found free in the serum and in secretions and bound to tissue mast cells and blood basophils. The higher the serum IgE level, the more IgE is bound to mast cells.

When polyvalent allergens interact with cell-bound IgE antibodies, bridging occurs between adjacent IgE molecules. This can result in basophil and mast cell degranulation and liberation of histamine, slow-reacting substance of anaphylaxis (SRS-A), now called leukotrienes, and the eosinophilic chemotactic factor of anaphylaxis (ECF-A). These chemical mediators cause increased vascular permeability, contraction of bronchiolar smooth muscle, and influx of eosinophils, giving rise to the characteristic clinical manifestations of immediate hypersensitivity reactions [10].

There is evidence to show that the basophilic leukocyte and the mast cell are not, as was formerly thought, lysed in reactions of tissue, fixed IgE, and specific antigen. It has also been demonstrated that agents capable of increasing the intracellular level of cyclic 3, 5-adenosine monophosphates (cAMP) will inhibit the release of mediators from mast cells sensitized with human IgE [11]. Catecholamines, such as epinephrine, activate a membrane-bound enzyme adenylcyclase, which in turn mediates the reaction of adenosine triphosphate to cAMP with concomitant inhibition of mediator release. Certain drugs, such as methylxanthines, block the action of the enzyme phosphodiesterase, which breaks down cAMP to 5-AMP. These agents have been shown to work synergistically to inhibit the IgE-specific release of mediators.

Studies of the immunoglobulin IgE have shown that serum IgE levels are elevated with extrinsic asthma and other atopic diseases, suggesting that quantitation of serum IgE might be significant in the diagnosis of allergic disorders, such as food allergies [12]. IgE is present in nanograms quantities in serum. Even in the sera of patients with marked IgE elevations, the concentration is only 1/1000 that of IgG. Serum IgE levels in unselected populations of adult humans vary from less than 1 unit per milliliter to more than 10,000 units per milliliter. Conventional test procedures, such as the single radiodiffusion method, were neither specific nor sensitive enough to use in clinical diagnosis of atopic disease. Isolation of IgE in the preparation of anti-IgE opened the way for development of a suitable test based on a radioimmunoassay.

Radioimmunosorbent Tests

Two radioimmunoassays for IgE currently in use are the radioimmunosorbent test (RIST) and the double-antibody radioimmunoassay. Both procedures depend on the inhibition of binding of radioiodinated purified IgE myeloma protein to specific IgE antibody.

A commercially available kit utilizing the RIST principle, the Phadebas IgE test, is available from Pharmacia Laboratories, Piscataway, NJ. This test uses specific anti-IgE antibodies covalently linked to Sephadex particles as a solid phase. Standards of known IgE concentration and the unknown serum are incubated with Sephadex-anti-IgE and purified $[^{125}I]$ IgE for anti-IgE binding sites. Reaction mixtures are then washed by centrifugation and the insoluble Sephadex-anti-IgE-^{125}I complexes are counted in a γ spectrometer. The higher the concentration of unlabeled IgE in the standard or unknown, the lower is the radioactivity of the Sephadex complexes. The limit of sensitivity of this assay is approximately 2–5 ng/ml [13].

Double-Antibody Radioimmunoassay

The double antibody radioimmunoassay for total IgE, known commercially as the Phadebas IgE PRIST (paper radioimmunosorbent test), is a "sandwich-type" modification of the solid-phase radioimmunoassay. This test is a direct radioimmunoassay using paper disks as a solid phase. Anti-IgE covalently coupled in the paper disk reacts during the first incubation with the IgE in the serum sample. After washing, radioactively labeled immunosorbent-purified antibodies against IgE are added, forming a complex. The radioactivity of this complex is measured in a γ counter. The more bound radioactivity found, the more IgE is present in the serum sample [14].

The correlation between serum IgE levels and atopic disease in older children and adults has been confirmed in a large number of studies. However, in infants and children under 1 year of age, measurements of total serum IgE levels have not contributed significantly to the diagnosis, predictive value, or treatment of atopic disorders. Only about 60% of patients with allergic rhinitis and 75% of patients with allergic asthma have elevated total serum IgE levels. Radioimmunoassays for total IgE lack the necessary specificity. They may be valuable, however, in screening for other diseases associated with abnormal IgE levels.

Serum IgE levels are elevated in a number of parasitic infections, including paragonimiasis, visceral larva migrans, capillariasis, ascariasis, fascioliasis, and bronchopulmonary aspergillosis. Elevated serum IgE levels also have been reported in some dermatological conditions, including chronic acral dermatitis, bullous pemphigoid, and the dermatitis associated with the Wiskott-Aldrich syndrome. Low levels of IgE have been reported in conjunction with variable or combined immunodeficiency states, hypogammaglobulinemias, macroglobulinemia and multiple myeloma, isolated IgA deficiency, and ataxia telangiectasia. It has also been shown that some healthy individuals may have an isolated serum IgE deficiency [15].

Radioallergosorbent Test

A large quantity of the IgE of atopic individuals is specifically reactive with identifiable environmental allergens. Measurement of these antigen-specific IgE antibodies is essential for the diagnosis of atopic disorders, but a suitable test must be able to handle the minute quantities involved as well as wide ranges in quantities.

The radioallergosorbent test (RAST) fulfills these requirements and was described first in 1967 [16]. The suspected allergen is coupled to solid-phase particles, such as Sephadex or cellulose, or to filter paper disks by cyanogen-bromide linkage. Reaginic or antigen-specific IgE antibodies, as well as other antibodies, react with the allergen and are bound to the allergen-polymer complex. When excess serum protein is washed away, the presence of bound IgE-antibody is determined by addition of ^{125}I-labeled anti-IgE. The radioactive anti-IgE bound to the antigen-polymer complex is measured in a γ scintillation counter after excess labeled antiserum has been removed by washing.

The concentration of IgE-antibody in the serum sample is proportional to the radioactivity of the processed complex. The γ-count rate is expressed as a percentage of a reaginic reference serum, a numerical score related to the IgE allergen-polymer complex.

The introduction of antigen-coupled filter-paper disks by Pharmacia Laboratories is a practical implementation. One disk is incubated with 50 μl of serum at room temperature for at least 3 hr. No rotation or shaking is necessary; the tube rack is simply placed on the laboratory bench with a cover. The three required washings involve only addition of saline and use of a water suction device; no centrifugation is necessary. The ^{125}I-labeled anti-IgE is added — 50μl represents approximately 80,000 cpm (counts per minute) — for a second incubation overnight. This anti-globulin reaction is relatively slow; 80% saturation is not reached for at least 6 hr. Following the incubation period, the disks are washed again and the radioactivity is counted in a γ counter.

The critical reagents in the RAST are the anti-IgE and the allergen. Two non-cross-reacting antigenic determinants have been identified on the ϵ chain of IgE. The D_1 antigen is located in the hinge region of the IgE immunoglobulin and is heat stable. The D_2 antigen, located on the F_c fragment, is heat labile. Heating serum to 56°C for 30 min destroys approximately 85% of D_2 antigenic activity. An antiserum of D_2 seems to give the best technical results for the RAST, probably because the D_2 antigen is easily accessible when an IgE molecule is involved in an allergen-reagin complex. Because of the ability of the D_2 antigen, however, it is recommended that the antiserum used in the RAST contain activity against both D_1 and D_2 specificities. The animal origin of the antiserum is also important. Rabbit anti-IgE is preferable because anti-sera raised in sheep or goats tend to give false-positive results in a RAST with animal dander allergen-polymer complexes. These false positives occur because almost 70% of the population have antibodies to bovine gammaglobulin.

The RAST is used in conjunction with histories and challenge tests to diagnose a variety of allergies. Specifically, the RAST has been adapted to measure measure serum IgE antibodies to pollens, animal danders, housedust and housedust mites, foods, stinging insects, molds, and, recently, penicillin.

RAST results have been correlated with findings from challenge tests for a variety of allergens. Agreement between these procedures has ranged from 59% for allergies to housedust to 93% for fish allergies. Using a highly purified allergen from cod, Aas and Lundkvist found in 100% correlation between results of RAST and challenge tests in 112 allergic children [17].

High correlations also have been obtained between the RAST and measures of leukocyte sensitivity, such as the leukocyte histamine-release test, and between the RAST and symptom indices of patients who are highly sensitive to foods [18].

A negative RAST does not definitely exclude a low-grade allergy, defined as a positive intradermal skin test combined with a positive challenge test obtained with the strongest available allergen.

RAST Scoring System

One of the difficulties with RAST has been the confusing scoring systems for determining the results of the RAST test. The Phadebas RAST scoring system utilizes four reaginic reference standards: standard A, which is pooled serum from patients highly sensitive to birch pollen allergens; standard B, which is a fivefold dilution of standard A; standard C, which is a fivefold dilution of standard B; and standard D, which is a twofold dilution of standard C. Each of these reference standards has been assigned an arbitrary number of Phadebas RAST units, known as PRU. The Phadebas RAST units are based on the observation that the Phadebas reference B had binding ability similar to 10 units of IgE in the PRIST system and, therefore, was assigned 10 Phadebas RAST units. The PRU is only a relative term and does not quantitate specific IgE.

In the Phadebas RAST scoring system, sera with bound radioactivity less than that obtained with standard D when tested against its homologous birch disk are considered to have a nondetectable level of allergen-specific IgE. Therefore, by dividing the counts for each unknown serum sample by the mean count for reference serum D, one can determine multiples of reference serum D. Values of 0.5 and above represent progressive increased binding of allergen-specific IgE antibodies. Multiples of reference D values below 0.5 are not differentiable from nonspecific background binding values and thereby represent absent or undetectable levels of allergen-specific IgE antibody. To determine Phadebas RAST units or PRU per milliliter, one must assign reference A, B, C, and D the PRU per milliliter values of 17.5, 3.5, 0.7, and 0.35. Following this assignment, the counts are plotted for each reference serum on a logarithmic diagram. The PRU per milliliter values are then read for each unknown sample from the reference curve. PRU per milliliter values of 0.1 and above represent progressive increased relative concentration of allergen-specific IgE antibodies, and therefore, PRU per milliliter values of less than 0.1 represent absent or undetectable values of allergen-specific antibodies.

Another difficulty in RAST scoring seems to be arriving at a cutoff level. At the present time, the cutoff point for the Phadebas RAST is 0.35 PRU. The separation of positive from negative results in most laboratory tests is an arbitrary and difficult matter. Because of concerns over cutoff points in scoring systems, a modified RAST scoring system has been suggested by Fadal and Nalebuff. Changes in test procedures were necessary. First it required an initial incubation period of 18 hr rather than the 3 hr utilized in the original RAST. Second, it increased the test serum volume from 50 to 100 μl, and third, disks are removed from the original tubes and placed in fresh tubes before counting. Then to develop the modified scoring system, the fivefold changes in serum concentration were maintained; however, in order to keep counts constant from day to day despite variations in temperature and isotope decay, a time control was incorporated using 25 units of IgE reacted with the RAST isotope and determining the time required to reach 25,000 counts. In this type of scoring system, the lower limit of detectable levels of allergen-specific IgE (or the cutoff level) is 1.5 times the binding of negative control. Therefore, the cutoff point is 750 counts. Consequently, sera with counts between 250 and 750 are recorded as negative, indicating allergen-specific IgE antibody below detectable levels. This system would then have the cutoff point at levels as low as 0.02 or 0.04 PRU. From this information, one can see the physician's dilemma in determining the significance of the laboratory test in relationship to the clinical condition of the patient. These RAST classes, cutoff points, PRU, and arbitrary scores tend more to confuse the physician while they try to show that one particular procedure is superior to another. It is only important to remember that each of these tests is a radioimmunoassay for detection of allergen-specific IgE antibody. It is also quite clear that the most important aspect of scoring is that the greater of number the counts, the more allergen-specific IgE antibody is present in the patient's sera. It is the physician who must finally determine the severity of the patient's problems by a carefull history and physical examination and by having the radioactive counts for a specific allergen — regardless of the scoring system. If the physician is furnished with a positive and negative control from that run and if the test is based on a specific amount of IgE, then the physician should be able to determine the significance of the laboratory test without reference to company names or physician names.

Enzyme-Linked Immunosorbent Assay

The enzyme-linked immunosorbent assay (ELISA) described by Engvall and Perlmann, is an in vitro test in which the allergens are adsorbed onto the inside surface of a plastic tube. Antibodies in the patient's serum will bind to the allergen on the tube wall, and reagins are then detected by adding enzyme-labeled anti-IgE. In a preliminary study in selected material, Ahlstedt and collaborators found rather good agreement between results obtained with ELISA and clinical allergy, but the clinical value of ELISA has not been completely evaluated in representative patient samples [20].

Diazo Allergen Specific Assay (DASA)

The diazo allergen specific assay (DASA) utilizes a solid-phase carrier of aminophenylthioether-APT-activated paper, which then is subjected to diazotization. This new material, then, is an activated diazotized paper that can then be cut into disks. The attachment of proteins to the activated diazotized paper disks provides an especially strong protein attachment that is not a harsh chemical reaction attachment, such as that found with the use of cyanogen-bromide.

This strong attachment does not damage the antigenic material, and once the attachment process with the diazotized APT paper disk has occurred, further binding by nonspecific proteins does not readily occur.

The diazo allergen specific assay is basically an improved radioimmunoassay to determine the presence of allergen-specific IgE anti-bodies. The technique for performing the DASA in evaluation in vitro consists of utilizing the specially prepared solid-phase carrier with allergens attached through the chemical coupling of the APT disk with diazotization. The diazo allergen disks are incubated with human serum containing IgE antibodies specific for the allergens. After careful washing of the solid-phase carrier, anti-IgE antibodies labeled with a radioisotope are added. These are capable of binding to the antibodies of IgE attached to the diazo allergen disk. The radioactivity of the complex is determined. The patient's IgE antibodies specific for the allergens being tested are directly proportional to the level of radioactivity.

Positive and negative controls are necessary to determine the accuracy of each test run. The negative controls should have very low counts, measured in the range of 150 to 250 counts per minute (cpm). This low background count demonstrates the very minimal nonspecific binding of this type of solid-phase carrier [21].

The ultimate place of the various new diagnostic tests in clinical allergy is still being established. Such factors as cost, convenience, safety, and diagnostic precision must be taken into consideration when choosing among the methods of diagnosis.

Clinical Application in Food Allergy

The use of antigen-specific radioimmunoassays should be an adjunct to conventional procedures in the diagnosis of food allergies when clinical signs suggest an IgE-mediated response. IgE-mediated food hypersensitivity is characterized by a variety of symptoms, including anaphylaxis, angioedema, urticaria, asthma, atopic eczema, allergic rhinitis, gastrointestinal upset, diarrhea, headache, and tension-fatigue syndrome. This diversity of symptoms, combined with the complex mechanisms involved in food allergy, makes definitive diagnosis a laborious task.

The first step in diagnosis of food allergy is a careful history. This record is much more subjective than a corresponding history for pollen or animal dander allergies, however. Elimination diets and provocative rechallenge diets for a large number of foods are complicated, time consuming, and often cumbersome for the patient. Conventional diagnostic skin tests with food allergens are known to be unreliable. High frequencies of false-negative as well as false-positive wheal-and-flare skin test reactions have been reported [22]. Also, intracutaneous tests can cause severe systemic reactions in some patients with food allergies. Use of the radioimmunoassay for diagnosis of food allergies has been most successful in patients with the classic symptoms of immediate hypersensitivity. For patients who are allergic to frequently ingested foods, such as cow's milk, cereals, and eggs, radioimmunoassay results may augment a case history that has been difficult to establish. Allergic reactions to grains may require special documentation, however, because of the known cross-reactivity between different cereals and grasses. A positive radio-immunoassay for potent allergens, like nuts, peas, peanuts, shellfish, and fish, is highly significant and confirms the diagnosis, especially in cases in whom a provocative challenge test could result in a severe systemic reaction.

Basic understanding of the mechanisms of food allergy is still limited. IgE-binding capacity may differ from allergen to allergen. IgE antibodies may be present only in the skin and shock tissues and not in the circulation. Circulating IgE antibodies may remain undetected despite a convincing clinical history of food allergy because the antibodies may be directed against allergens that are modified during industrial processing, cooking, or digestion. Some atopic children produce IgE antibodies to cereal grains, eggs, or milk but do not exhibit any overt symptoms associated with ingestion of these foods. Finally, many food allergies are not IgE mediated. Results from the radioimmunoassay must be evaluated in perspective; they should never be used as the single diagnostic criterion in food allergy.

TYPE II CYTOTOXIC OR CYTOLYTIC REACTION

Type II food hypersensitivity reactions involve tissue-fixed antigens, in which the tissue is really an innocent bystander that becomes involved in an immune reaction when complement is activated on the tissue cell surface. Cytotoxic antibodies with pathogenic potential bind to the surface of cells by means of antigen-specific configurations on the Fab portion of the immunoglobulin molecules rather than by the F_c-related binding postulated for IgE antibodies, which is antigen independent and not immunologically specific. Cytolytic antibodies generally belong to the IgG class. The antigen may be an intrinsic component of the cell, or it may be an antigen or hapten that has become intimately associated with the cell.

The coating of circulating blood cells by cytolytic antibodies renders them more susceptible to intra- and extravascular destruction. Destruction may result directly from complement activation on the cell surface or indirectly as a consequence of phagocytosis of such cells by the mononuclear-phagocyte (reticulo-endothelial) system. This depends on the presence of specific receptors for IgG and the third component of complement (C3) on the phagocytes [23]. Certain drugs and one particular food, the Mexican fava bean, seems to have predilection for this type of reaction with red blood cells deficient in glucose-6-phosphate dehydrogenase (G-6-PD). The red cell involved is lysed. For type II reactions, a radioimmunoassay, such as the RAST for human IgG food-specific antibodies, is unsatisfactory because of interference from the large amounts of IgG antibody present in human sera. Therefore, we have developed a double-antibody assay that utilized a solid-phase carrier (an APT-activated disk) with various food antigens attached. It had several advantages. (1) The APT or diazo-allergen-specific disk provides a strong bond between the solid-phase carrier and the food antigen. (2) It was not a harsh chemical bond that alters the food antigen, and (3) because of the diazotization reaction, there is very little nonspecific binding, leading to a very low background count.

The procedure is as follows. Human sera from the allergic individual is applied to this disk containing the food allergens. Both IgG and IgE food-specific antibodies will attach to the disk. The disk is then washed free of excess sera, and a goat anti-human IgG antibody will attach to the IgG that is attached to the APT food allergen disk. This complex is then washed three times, and to this disk is applied rabbit anti-goat IgG radioactively tagged with ^{125}I. The rabbit anti-goat IgG will then attach to the goat antigen portion of the goat anti-human IgG. This complex is then washed and counted in a γ counter. The purpose for using the double-antibody assay is to avoid interference from human IgG that would be present if one used a radioactively tagged anti-human IgG antibody.

By using this technique, we have been able to demonstrate circulating IgG antibodies to food allergens in a number of patients suffering from a variety of complaints.

TYPE III IMMUNE COMPLEX DISEASE

Type III food hypersensitivity reactions involve circulating food antigens and circulating IgG antibodies. For the most part, these IgG antibodies are precipitating antibodies that can form toxic immune complexes. Toxic complexes are formed by antigen and precipitating antibodies in the zone of moderate antigen excess. Immune complexes formed in tissue spaces precipitate around small blood vessels, fixing complement and producing a local inflammatory response.

The model of a local type III reaction was described by Arthus in 1903 and bears his name. He injected rabbits with several doses of a foreign protein over a period of 1-2 weeks. The initial doses were innocuous, but later injections produced a severe local inflammatory reaction that eventually led to necrosis. The antigen introduced by the challenging injections diffused toward the antibody generated by the earlier sensitizing doses. At the point where antigen and antibodies meet in the zone of moderate antibody excess, an inflammatory reaction occurs. Serum sickness, a type III reaction, is produced by circulating immune complexes. However, it must be remembered that in the actual clinical state usually more than one type of allergic response is operative. Toxic complexes formed in the circulation localize in the vessels themselves.

The mechanisms of tissue injury once the complexes have been formed, irrespective of their location, are similar. The complement system is activated, and the cascade progresses through C3, C5, C6, and C7, with a production of several fractions. This enhances the inflammatory response by increasing vascular permeability, producing leukocyte and platelet thrombi, and attracting polymorphonuclear leukocytes into the area. Tissue injury is produced largely by the action of the polymorphonuclear leukocyte [24].

Coombs and Gell consider that the primary point in differentiating type III reactions from type I and type II reactions is that the initiating antigen-antibody reaction proceeds independently of cells or tissue. They are only secondarily involved, either by the irritant action of the complexes or by the inflammatory response initiated by complement activation.

A typical food type III reaction can be demonstrated in patients with Heiner's syndrome who develop precipitating antibodies to milk protein. Testing for this type of precipitating antibody is conveniently carried out by double diffusion in agar. The antigen (skim milk or purified milk protein fractions) is usually placed in the central well, and the patient's sera to be tested for antibody is placed in the peripheral wells. As antigen and antibody diffuse through the agar and react with one another, complexes form that appear as precipitate lines, one for each antigen and its corresponding precipitating antibody. These lines can be analyzed visually.

Though the technique is relatively simple and inexpensive, it requires considerable experience for proper interpretation. All conditions, such as the percentage and amount of agar used, distance between the reservoirs, time of incubation, and the use of positive and negative controls and other variables, must be carefully standardized if comparable results are to be expected. Antibodies of the IgG or IgA class can be detected when present in concentrations of approximately 50 μg/ml or more and of IgM antibodies in concentrations of about 200 μg/ml.

In Heiner's study of children with milk-induced gastrointestinal bleeding, anti-milk precipitants were detected in 62% of patients, compared with 1 or 2% in an unselected population. High precipitin titers or multiple precipitin bands are rare in normal persons and are infrequent in adults with milk allergy. One shortcoming of this test is that it only detects the presence of circulating antibodies before they have formed immune complexes [25].

To overcome this, a new assay was developed to measure antigen-specific immune complexes in food-allergic patients. This new test is an allergen- and isotype-specific assay to quantify the presence of complexes in the serum. The assay is based on a two-site recognition system so that only molecular complexes containing both antigen and antibody are counted. In the original development of the test, affinity-purified antibodies to egg and milk whey were used in conjunction with a soluble. labeled anti-immunoglobulin of the IgG-, IgE-, or IgA-specific class.

To evaluate the assay, immune complexes were prepared in vitro by mixing antigen at different concentrations from serum from a patient with high levels of antibody. Complexes were detected over a 5-log range of antigen concentration. The lower limit of sensitivity of the assay is about 4.8 ng of complexed IgG per milliliter of patient's serum. Sera from patients with positive RAST scores to egg white or milk were selected as the preliminary study. Only three of the nine egg white-positive sera and two of the nine milk-positive sera were found to contain significant levels of IgE-immune complexes [26]. In the second study, 45 patients were selected for study on the basis of history and physical examination that indicated a possible food sensitivity. Only 10 of these 45 patients had a positive RAST for milk. However, IgG-milk immune complexes were found in 25 of these patients. Of these 45 patients, 15 had symptoms that included hives and/or eczema, and all of these (15 of 15) had circulating IgG-milk complexes. The incidence of IgG complexes was much lower in patients with other symptoms and absent in normal controls. Only 2 patients had milk IgE-immune complexes. The majority of these patients with skin disease did not have milk-specific IgE, suggesting that a type III hypersensitivity reaction might be important in patients with hives and/or eczema [27].

TYPE IV CELL-MEDIATED IMMUNE REACTION

Type IV food hypersensitivity reactions involve food antigens and sensitized circulating lymphocytes. The food antigen causes the sensitized lymphocyte to release lymphokines. These lymphokine substances have recently been shown to possess a variety of biologic activities that are thought to be the in vitro correlates of cell-mediated immunity.

Following the in vitro interaction of the sensitized lymphocyte with its specific antigen, a substance is released that has the capacity to transfer delayed hypersensitivity to another nonreactive individual. This substance is referred to as transfer factor and has been described in humans and primates.

Migration inhibitory factor (MIF) inhibits the migration of normal macrophages in vitro. When cells from a peritoneal exudate of animals are put into a capillary tube, the macrophage migrates peripherally from the end of the tube. If one adds to the medium small quantities of antigen to which the animal exhibits cell-mediated immunity, the macrophage fails to migrate from the tube. "Lymphotoxin" is the term for a series of molecules liberated from specifically sensitized lymphocytes or nonspecific stimulants, such as phytohemagglutinin. Lymphotoxin seems to be associated with target cell injury and inhibits the capacity of cells to divide. Skin-reactive factor is a material produced by the interaction of specifically sensitized lymphocytes with antigens and mitogens. When introduced into the skin of normal guinea pigs, skin-reactive factor or factors produced an indurated and erythematous lesion within 3 hr. Several chemotactic factors have been described that are released from the reaction of specific antigen and sensitized lymphocytes and can also be generated by nonspecific mitogens. Another substance that may be released is mitogenic factor or blastogenic factor, which has the capacity to cause blast cell transformation and increased tritiated thymidine uptake.

In general, cell-mediated immunity includes those manifestations of the specific immune response expressed by a variety of cells and cell products. The hallmarks of these reactions, which differentiate them from humeral antigen-antibody reactions, are their delayed onset, the requirement of living lymphocytes or their products to elicit their response, and the recently discovered effector molecules with relatively low molecular weights, which appear to be the in vitro correlate of the in vivo response. This type of immunologic mechanism appears to be particularly well suited to antigens that are cell bound or in other ways inaccessible to the antibody mechanism [28].

Laboratory tests for evaluation of delayed hypersensitivity reaction to foods foods have been difficult and limited. The in vitro antigen-induced lymphocyte stimulation procedure has been used in recent years to study patients with milk allergy. Cultures of patient peripheral blood lymphocytes are prepared. In predetermined amounts, skim milk or isolated milk protein is added. Control cultures must be tested, including unstimulated lymphocytes, lymphocytes stimulated by mitogens, and antigen stimulation of lymphocytes of healthy subjects. Tritiated thymidine is added on day 5, and a day later the lymphocytes are harvested. The counts of incorporated radioactivity indicating the amount of DNA that is synthesized is a measure of lymphocyte proliferation. The degree of antigen-induced proliferation is indicated by the ratio of the count of the antigen-stimulated culture to the mean count of unstimulated cultures. The incorporated count of mitogen-stimulated cultures indicates maximal degree of incorporation; it also demonstrates the viability of the cells.

A few observers utilizing this test have reported high reliability. However, some other observers have shown the converse. Lymphocytes of allergic patients may show an increased proliferation in vitro without the addition of the specific antigen. Another limitation of the test is that β-lactoglobulin preparations may have a significant nonspecific mitogenic activity even on lymphocytes of normal subjects [29].

It is known that contact dermatitis is a type of cell-mediated immunity or delayed hypersensitivity and that this type of sensitivity can be diagnosed by patch testing. It has been postulated that patch testing with foods might serve as a reliable source for evaluating several types of food hypersensitivity reactions, including type IV cell-mediated immunity. Breneman has developed a patch test for food allergy diagnosis. His study consisted of using food patch tests applied to patients with known ingestant intolerance that had been previously determined by elimination diet and challenge techniques. The patch test materials were pure, sterile, freeze-dried foodstuffs suspended in DMSO (dimethylsulfoxide). His initial studies were done in a blinded technique in which the technicians applying the patches were unaware of the patient's particular intolerance. The patient was unaware of the results of the patch test results (read both 20 min and 3 days later). Besides elimination diet, RAST was also used as a basis for comparison of both sensitivity and reliability of the patch test. A total of 75 unselected cases were used for the statistics. Sensitivity of RAST for correlation of the elimination diet and challenge intolerance was 5.38%; using the same standards, sensitivity of the patch test was 74.41%. Reliability for RAST was 23.08%; however, the reliability for the patch test was 34.08%.

Biopsies of positive patch tests showed T-lymphocyte invasion perivascularly in proportion to the positivity of the patch test. Light-chain invasion also paralleled the positiveness of the patch response. Complement invasion followed the same pattern; prostaglandins (PGE_2, PGF_2, and prostacyclin) were decreased, a phenomenon reported to be due to DMSO.

Preliminary data suggest that food allergy involving all four Coombs and Gell types of hypersensitivity is being measured by these patch tests. A high degree of clinical correlation is achieved, suggesting that these inexpensive, safe, and simple methods might be helpful in the diagnosis of food allergy [30].

CONCLUSION

It is quite evident with the recent development of new laboratory tests that the diagnosis of food allergy by specific laboratory procedures is becoming closer to a reality. For type I hypersensitivity, food allergy of the anaphylactic or IgE-mediated reaction, the RAST test is quite reliable. However, the implementation of new techniques, such as the use of the APT or diazo-allergen-specific disk, as well as the removal of IgG-interfering substances with staphylococcal protein A, makes the test much more useful [31]. Type II food hypersensitivity reactions, which involved tissue-fixed antigens and circulating IgG antibodies, can now be evaluated using the double-antibody radioimmunoassay for antigen-specific IgG. Type III food hypersensitivity reactions, involving circulating food antigens and circulating IgG antibodies, can now be diagnosed by the use of the allergin-isotype-specific assay to quantify for the presence of complexes in the serum of food allergy pateints. And finally, with the Dimsoft or the DMSO food antigen patch test, the evaluation of all four types of Coombs and Gell hypersensitivity reactions to foods may be measured. However, the food patch test may be most useful in the diagnosis of type IV or cell-mediated immunity.

The use of laboratory tests in confirmation of the diagnosis of food allergy is still in its infancy. A number of other procedures are being developed at present that will continue to enhance the ability of the laboratory to be helpful in determining specific food sensitivities in allergic patients.

REFERENCES

1. Coca, A. F., and Cooke, R. A. The classification of the phenomena of hypersensitiveness. *J. Allergy 8*:163, 1927.
2. Spector, S. L., and Farr, R. S. Aspirin idiosyncrasy: Asthma and urticaria. In *Allergy Principles and Practice*, ed. 2, E. Middleton, Jr., C. E. Reed, and E. F. Ellis (eds.), C. V. Mosby, Co., St. Louis, 1983, p. 1249.
3. Ishizaka, K., Ishizaka, T., and Hornbrook, M. H. Correlation of reaginic activity with E. globulin antibody. *J. Immunol. 97*:840, 1960.
4. Coombs, R. R. A., and Gell, P. G. H. Classification of allergic reactions responsible for clinical hypersensitivity and disease. In *Clinical Aspects of Immunology*, ed. 2, R. R. A. Coombs and P. G. H. Gell (eds.), F. A. Davis, Philadelphia, 1968, p. 575.
5. Breneman, J. C. *Basics of Food Allergy*, Charles C Thomas, Springfield, Illinois, 1978, p. 163.
6. Prausnitz, C., and Kustner, H. Studien uber Uberempfindlichkeit. *Zentralbl. Bakteriol. 1 86*:160, 1921.
7. Ishizaka, K., Ishizaka, T., and Hornbrook, M. M. Physio-chemical properties of human reaginic antibody. IV. Presence of a unique immunoglobulin as a carrier of reaginic activity. *J. Immunol. 97*:75, 1966.
8. Johansson, S. G. O., Bennich, H., and Wide, L. A new class of immuno-globulin in human serum. *Immunology 14*:265, 1968.
9. Bennich, H., and Johansson, S. G. O. Structure and function of human immunoglobulin E. *Adv. Immunol. 13*:1, 1971.
10. Orange, R. P., and Austen, K. F. *Progress in Immunology*, B. Amos (ed.), Academic Press, New York, 1971, p. 173.

11. Orange, R. P., and Austen, K. F. Chemical mediators of immediate hypersensitivity. In *Immunobiology,* R. A. Good and D. W. Fisher (eds.), Sinauer, Stamford, 1971, p. 115.

12. Bazaral, M., Orgal, H. A., and Hamburger, R. N. IgE levels in normal infants and mothers and an inheritance hypothesis. *J. Immunol. 107:*794, 1971.

13. Wide, L., and Porath, J. Radioimmunoassay of proteins with the use of Sephadex-coupled antibodies. *Biochem. Biophys. Acta 130:*257, 1966.

14. Ceska, M., and Lundkvist, U. A new and simple radioimmunoassay method for the determination of IgE. *Immunochemistry 9:*1021, 1972.

15. Yunginger, J. W., and Gleich, G. J. The impact of the discovery of IgE on the practice of allergy. *Pediatr. Clin. North Am. 22:*3, 1975.

16. Wide, L., Bennich, H., and Johnasson, S. G. O. Diagnosis of allergy by an in vitro test for allergen antibodies. *Lancet 2:*1105, 1967.

17. Aas, K., and Lundkvist, U. The radioallergosorbent test with a purified allergen from codfish. *Clin. Allergy 3:*255, 1973.

18. Johansson, S. G. O. Comparison of in vivo and in vitro tests for diagnosis of immediate hypersensitivity. In *Laboratory Diagnosis of Immunologic Disorders,* G. N. Vyas, D. O. Stites, and G. Brecher (eds.), Grune and Stratton, New York, 1975, p. 231.

19. Dockhorn, R. J. Using the RAST and PRIST with an overview of clinical significance. *Ann. Allergy 49:*4, 1982.

20. Engvall, E. and Perlmann, P. Enzyme-linked immunosorbent assay, ELISA. III. Quantitation of specific antibodies by enzyme-labeled anti-immunoglobulin in antigen-coated tubes. *J. Immunol. 109:*129–135, 1972.

21. Dockhorn, R. J. Using the RAST and PRIST with an overview of clinical significance. *Ann. Allergy 49:*6, 1982.

22. Tapay, N. J. Diagnostic tests for allergy. In *Allergy and Immunology in Children,* F. Speer and R. J. Dockhorn (eds.), Charles C Thomas, Springfield, Illinois, 1973, p. 363.

23. Knogshavn, P. A. L., Hawkins, D., and Shuster, J. The biology of the immune response. In *Clinical Immunology,* S. O. Freedman and P. Gold (eds.), 2 ed., Harper and Row, New York, 1976, p. 48.

24. Biondi, R. M. Damage by toxic complexes. In *Allergy and Immunology in Children,* F. Speer and R. J. Dockhorn, (eds.), Charles C Thomas, Springfield, Illinois, 1973.

25. Bahna, S. C., and Heiner, D. C. Diagnosis of milk allergy by the precipitation test. In *Allergies to Milk,* Grune and Stratton, New York, 1980, p. 96.

26. Leary, Jr., H. L., Dockhorn, R. J., and Halsey, J. F. An assay to measure antigen-specific immune complexes in food allergic patients. Abstract Am. Assoc. Clin. Immunol. and Allergy, Orlando, Florida, 1983.

27. Necessary, P. C., Leary, H. L., Dockhorn, R. J., and Halsey, J. F. Allerginspecific immune complexes in food sensitive patients. Abstract Am. Coll. Allergists, San Francisco, 1984.

28. Bellanti, J. A., and Rocklin, R. E. Cell-mediated reaction. In *Immunology II,* J. A. Bellanti (ed.), W. B. Saunders, Philadelphia, 1978, p. 233.

29. Bahna, S. L., and Heiner, D. C. Diagnosis of milk allergy by the lymphoblast transformation test. In *Allergies to Milk,* Grune and Stratton, New York, 1980, p. 100.

30. Breneman, J. C. Preliminary report on patch test for food (Abstract). Allergy Diagn., Southwest Allergy Forum, 1983.

31. Oggel, J. D., and Dockhorn, R. J. Staphylococcal protein A and enhancement of disc RAST sensitivity. *Ann. Allergy 50*:178, 1983.

11
Today's Approved Diagnostic and Treatment Methods

CECIL COLLINS–WILLIAMS
University of Toronto, Toronto, Ontario, Canada

LAURENT V. CONSTANTIN*
The Hospital for Sick Children, Toronto, Ontario, Canada

HISTORY

One of the best methods for diagnosing a food allergy is a detailed history. This shows whether the signs and symptoms the patient reports could reasonably have been caused by a food allergy and is useful in ruling out other conditions (for example, lactose intolerance in a patient with suspected milk allergy) as the source of the problem.

The dietary history must go back to infancy, looking for signs and symptoms that might have been caused by food allergy in early life. It should include an exact description of the reactions, the time of onset after food ingestion, and an estimate of the amount of the food required to cause a reaction. Since many foods (with the notable exception of fish and nuts) are less allergenic when cooked, it is also important to find out whether the foods appearing to cause problems were heated before they were eaten [1].

History taking is very straightforward when signs and symptoms appear immediately after a food is eaten. For example, generalized urticaria and angioedema a few seconds after ingestion of peanut clearly classify the peanut as an important allergen. Often, however, the symptoms are neither so immediate nor is the cause so obvious. The physician must then ask the right questions to obtain enough detailed information to make a correct diagnosis.

*Present affiliation: A. H. Robins Canada

To take a good history, the physician must have extensive knowledge of biologic food families since patients often have symptoms from two or more foods in the same family. In addition, the physician must know the constituents of various foods and have access to detailed information about where minute amounts of foods, such as milk or egg, may occur in a hidden form in other foods. Familiarity with food additives and access to information about what foods contain them are also necessary.

When taking the history, it is important to find out whether the reaction claimed is based on an observation by another physician or a family friend or on the results of previous skin tests. Frequently, one is given a list of foods that allegedly cause allergic symptoms but on detailed questioning the list proves to be based on skin tests done elsewhere and has no connection with the patient's symptoms except in the mind of the patient or parent.

Many parents extrapolate their own food allergies to those of their children, but usually there is no correlation. They are also apt to confuse food dislikes with food allergy. If a child dislikes a food because it causes an uncomfortable sensation in the mouth, there may be a mild urticarial allergic reaction in the mucous membranes of the mouth that indicates allergy to that food. However, a simple dislike with no describable symptoms usually has nothing to do with allergy.

DIETARY RESTRICTION

Dietary restriction is always necessary to confirm a diagnosis of food allergy. If the signs or symptoms do not go away when the suspected food is removed from the diet, the diagnosis is wrong. If the diagnosis is uncertain, it is best to remove the food and return it to the diet on two or three occasions before making a definitive diagnosis. Dietary restriction may be prescribed in several ways: giving all foods in a cooked form (denatured diet), eliminating suspected foods and then reintroducing them, or using various forms of elimination diets. Obviously, the problem is most easily solved by avoiding the offending food or foods, if they can be identified.

Food Diary

A food diary can be useful, particularly when symptoms are thought to be due to foods but occur infrequently. In this case, prolonged use of a strict diet does not seem worthwhile and instead the patient should make an accurate record of all foods eaten even in trace amounts. This record should also include the names of manufacturers of prepared foods so that the physician can find out what ingredients these foods contain if this becomes necessary to identify the common denominator with previous episodes that is responsible for the patient's symptoms. It should be stressed to the patient that the diary is useless unless it is complete.

Infant Diet

In small infants, a soybean substitute plus carrot, squash, beet, pear without farina, banana, applesauce, and lamb is an appropriate restricted diet. Obviously, the number of foods depends on the infant's age. Although all these foods can produce an allergic reaction, they are relatively hypoallergenic. If the signs or symptoms disappear, the responsible foods can be detected by additions to the diet.

Denatured Diet

A striaghtforward denatured diet consists of powdered skim milk reconstituted with water; rice, barley, and oatmeal cereals; well-cooked vegetables; stewed or canned fruits; and well-cooked meats. Some recipes, for example, rice recipes (Appendix 1), should be provided because many people have difficulty making the allowed cereals attractive unless they are given recipes. This diet rigidly excludes ordinary fresh milk, egg, wheat, raw and semiraw foods, peanut, peanut butter, nuts, fish, and shellfish. Frequently it causes all signs and symptoms to disappear, and it is much easier to follow than most other restricted diets.

Elimination Diets

The most useful elimination diets in the author's experience are the Rowe elimination diets (numbers 1, 2, and 3); wheat-free, egg-free, and milk-free diets; and an additive-free diet. The Rowe diets (Appendix 2) are often difficult for the patient to follow, particularly if all meals cannot be eaten at home. However, they are useful in patients with severe symptoms and signs when history and a denatured diet have not identified the cause of the problem and when patients are sufficiently impressed with their symptoms to make the effort required to follow one of these diets for 3 weeks. The wheat-free (Appendix 3), egg-free (Appendix 3), and milk-free (Appendix 3) diets are useful only when one of these foods is strongly suspected and when symptoms are thought to be caused by even trace amounts of the suspected food. These diets are very difficult to follow unless the patient is given exact instructions about what foods must be avoided [2-5].

The additive-free diet (Appendix 4) should be as free as possible from food coloring (especially tartrazine), sulfur dioxide, benzoates, benzoic acid, aspirin, and salicylates. It must also be sufficiently individualized to exclude any food suspected of causing allergic or adverse symptoms in a particular case even if that food is not considered a problem on the basis of additives. For example, if the patient suffers from urticaria, vinegar and cheese must be omitted. This diet is extremely useful in ruling out food additives as a cause of hyperactivity or vague symptoms attributed to food additives by the parent or patient. Often these are not IgE-mediated responses, but the patient believes they are allergic reactions. Of course, the elimination of such foods is just as important to the patient whether the reaction is IgE-mediated or not. It is our practice to prescribe this diet as Special Diet #5 after deleting any suspected foods, without telling the parent that additives are almost entirely absent. Then a report of a good response to the diet is more meaningful.

Restricted Diet Techniques

An appropriately selected elimination diet is a most important means of identifying a food allergy. When a suitable diet is used in conjunction with a good history and correctly performed prick testing, the problem is readily identified in most cases. Unlike dietary manipulation, which may have no beneficial effect even after 2 years, a restricted diet for 3 weeks may prove diagnostic. Selection of which diet is most appropriate is based on the patient's history. If one restricted diet does not relieve the signs and symptoms within a 3-week period and food allergy is still suspected, another completely different diet may be tried for 3 weeks. No restricted diet should be used for longer than 1 month without making sure that it is adequate in calories, carbohydrates, fat, protein, minerals, and vitamins.

Patient compliance is essential for successful use of restricted diets. It is important, therefore, that the patient considers the symptoms severe enough to warrant following the diet. The patient should understand that it is to be tried for a 3-week period, sometimes longer in individual circumstances, but that there is no thought of it being used for continuing treatment. Very explicit instructions must be given, including appropriate recipes. Since wrong information will be obtained if the diet is not used properly, the patient must realize that even a slight deviation can render it useless as a diagnostic tool. The patient must understand the necessity of reading labels on all packaged foods to make sure that they are suitable.

If the patient cannot cope with the diet without additional help, this should be sought from a dietician or a special food store where more expert assistance than the physician feels he or she can provide will be available.

If restricted diets do not solve the problem, the diagnosis of food allergy is very much open to question and other investigations should be considered.

Addition of Foods

Once the signs and symptoms have subsided, additions to the diet must be made in a systematic manner or useful information will not be obtained. Foods should be added singly in pure form, given daily for 5 days, and left in the diet only if signs or symptoms do not recur. In mild food allergies, it is reasonable to go more quickly and add two or three vegetables or two or three fruits at a time. If no signs or symptoms recur, time has been saved. However, if signs or symptoms do return these foods must be tried individually. The first foods to add should be those the child likes that do not appear to have caused a reaction in the past. Eventually, the foods suspected of having caused trouble should be added. Obviously, however, foods that have caused acute reactions should be left out of the diet for at least a year and then cautiously tried again. If a food is tolerated in the cooked form, the same food in its raw form must be regarded as a new food for the purpose of adding to the diet.

SKIN TESTS

Skin tests have been used in diagnosing food allergies for more than 50 years, but they have frequently been criticized as having little value. Of the two methods available, the prick test is much superior to the scratch test. Recent work, largely by May [6] and Bock et al. [7-9], using the prick test correlated with double-blind challenges, has shown that the skin test is a very useful diagnostic tool if one insists on a 3-mm wheal as an indicator of clinical sensitivity and overlooks smaller reactions unless confirmed by history [6-10].

In addition, the correlation of the skin test with the radioallergosorbent test (RAST) supports the validity of the skin test, because the RAST demonstrates specific IgE to the food in the patient's serum [11, 12].

Food skin tests are particularly useful for dermal or respiratory manifestations of food allergy and much less useful for those involving the gastrointestinal tract.

In designing an apppopriate restricted diet, it is reasonable to omit foods implicated by skin test as well as those implicated by history, but one must remember that those foods that give only 1+ (1-mm wheal) and 2+ (2-mm wheal) reactions are frequently not of clinical significance. It is extremely important to impress on the parents that foods are left out of the diet for a prolonged period over and above the restricted diet trial only if they cause symptoms. They are never left out for a prolonged period just because they caused a positive skin test.

PROVOCATION TESTING

Provocation testing is useful when the allergen does not cause severe, life-threatening symptoms. The patient is challenged in a single- or double-blind manner with the quantity of the suspected food that reportedly caused symptoms. The observation of symptoms following such a challenge on two or more occasions is diagnostic. Onset of symptoms may occur from less than 1 hr to several days after testing [13]. Since an unforeseen acute reaction may result from provocation testing, it is necessary to have epinephrine and emergency support equipment available at the time of the test.

If the patient's symptoms have been life threatening in severity, provocation testing should not be done. Usually in such cases the patient's history can be accepted as diagnostic.

Provocative testing by the oral route should be done when the patient is asymptomatic. The suspected food is strictly withheld from the diet for at least 2 weeks prior to the challenge.

Often provocation tests teach both patients and physicians a great deal.

Patients are very adept in deluding themselves about which foods cause symptoms. However, physicians can help their patients only if they are not deluded themselves. Occasionally patients who give a clear history of an allergic or adverse reaction to a food show no symptoms in a laboratory trial of the appropriate amount of food.

The double-blind challenge, in which a suspected food or placebo is given in opaque capsules and the patient is observed for 24 hr, is the most reliable method for diagnosing food intolerance [8, 9, 14]. However, this method has certain disadvantages. It bypasses the upper alimentary tract, which may play a role in the allergic process under investigation. It is not practical for use in the physician's office. The testing is time consuming and involves a large number of capsules filled with dried food or placebo, unless the reaction is brought on by a very small amount of the suspected food. Furthermore, in children who are too young to swallow the capsules, the food must be introduced through a nasogastric tube or masked in another food. For these reasons, the double-blind challenge is more important experimentally than as a clinical tool to confirm the history and correlate with skin tests and RAST.

The suspected food, determined by either history or skin testing, is totally excluded from the diet for at least 2 weeks before challenge. When the patient is symptom-free and medication, if any, has been stabilized, the test foods are administered under double-blind conditions in opaque dye-free capsules or masked in another food for those who cannot swallow capsules. Testing is done at weekly intervals. The initial dose of the dried food varies according to the intensity of the reaction described in the history or obtained by skin testing and ranges between 100 and 2000 mg. If there is no reaction at that dose level, subsequent challenges with 2- to 10-fold dose increments can be carried out at a later date. If 8.0 g of dried food administered in this way does not elicit a reaction, the food is probably not a significant allergen [14].

ADDITIVES

Food Color Challenges

Food color is ubiquitous in our diets. The most commonly used dyes in the United States are FD&C blue #1, brilliant blue FCF; FD&C red #2, amaranth; FD&C red #4, ponceau SX; FD&C yellow #5, tartrazine; FD&C yellow #6, sunset yellow [15]. In Canada, the most commonly used dyes are tartrazine #5, sunset yellow #6, amaranth red #2, erythrosine red #3, brilliant blue #1, and indigotin blue #2 (personal communication from Lauer, Health and Welfare Canada).

The mechanism by which food coloring produces adverse reactions is unknown. There is no conclusive evidence that it is either IgE mediated [16] or related to prostaglandin synthesis [17], and the usual in vivo (skin testing) and in vitro (RAST) tests are not applicable.

Erythrosin B (FD&C red #3) has been shown to inhibit the accumulation of dopamine and other transmitter substances in rat brain homogenates [18]. Thus the adverse effect may occur by another mechanism and may be pharmacological or toxic. One must therefore resort to double-blind oral challenge either with dye-filled capsules or with drinks capable of properly masking the various dyes. When the latter method is used, we have found that reconstituted grape juice concentrate masks the dyes more effectively than other solutions tried.

Except for tartrazine, the dosage of dyes to be used in these challenges has not been established. Tartrazine doses of either 1, 5, 15, 25, and 50 mg [19] or 2.5, 5, 10, and 20 mg [20] appear suitable. These doses can be administered in a double-blind placebo-controlled fashion on separate days.

For asthmatic patients, we give increasing doses of 1, 5, 25, and 50 mg of tartrazine at 30-min intervals followed 48 hr later by an equal number of placebo challenges under double-blind conditions; FEV_1, MMEF changes, the appearance of urticaria, or rhinitis are objective end points.

With regard to other dyes, a reasonable approach would be to challenge the patients with separate mixtures of azo and non-azo dyes and a placebo, correlating the initial test dose with the patient's average intake of these dyes as estimated by a dietician. If any of the mixtures causes a reaction, it can then be broken down and the patient can be challenged with the individual dyes, again starting with a dose that represents the patient's average daily intake.

Metabisulfite Challenge

Several authors have incriminated metabisulfite or sulfur dioxide in foods as a precipitating cause of asthma in susceptible individuals [21-28]. The diagnosis can be suspected from history. For example, the patient may report having had an attack of asthma after ingesting a lettuce salad in a restaurant. (Metabisulfite is commonly used to keep lettuce looking fresh.) However, the diagnosis can only be established by a challenge test.

Stevenson and Simon described a suitable method in which oral testing is conducted under single-blind placebo-controlled conditions [25]. On the first day, the patient receives one placebo capsule every 30 min. FEV_1 values are obtained every 30 min. The next day, under identical conditions, the patient receives in sequential order and at 30-min intervals capsules containing 1, 5, 10, 25, and 50 mg of potassium metabisulfite. FEV_1 values are again obtained every 30 min.

Monosodium Glutamate Challenge

Asthma attacks precipitated by the ingestion of monosodium glutamate have been reported in several patients by Allen and Baker [28-30]. These authors describe a method of challenging such patients but caution that the reaction may appear as late as 11 to 14 hr after the challenge and may be life threatening in severity. They recommend that suspected patients be challenged in the hospital, starting with doses of less than 1 g and increasing the challenges on a daily basis by increments of 0.5 g. However, they do not say how high the doses should go. Initially their method was uncontrolled, but they have subsequently modified it into a single-blind placebo-controlled challenge. Since symptoms may occur late, they recommend giving the challenges in the late evening or early morning so that optimum treatment will be available if required.

ELEMENTAL DIETS

Elemental diets have been reported to have value in severe cases of food intolerance, including food allergy [31]. One such diet is Vivonex (Eaton Laboratories, Norwich, NY), which is described as a nutritionally complete formulation with synthetic essential and nonessential amino acids, glucose, oligosaccharides, oil containing the essential fatty acids, vitamins, and minerals. It is available unflavored and with various flavors. This diet is not indicated for patients with real or suspected food intolerance or food intolerance or food allergy whose problem can be solved from history and more simple elimination diets. However, it is a reasonable approach for patients with a very severe problem that cannot be solved by these simpler methods since it can at least tide them over until they are in a condition to add foods one at a time and find out which they can tolerate.

ROLE OF DRUGS IN DIAGNOSIS AND TREATMENT OF FOOD ALLERGIES

Antihistamines

Antihistamines have been advocated as both diagnostic and therapeutic tools in food allergy. It is the opinion of these authors that they have no value as a diagnostic tool. Therapeutically, they are useful when food allergy causes urticaria, atopic dermatitis, or rhinitis but not for other clinical manifestations, such as gastrointestinal symptoms.

Epinephrine

Epinephrine is the drug of choice for the treatment of anaphylaxis but has no role in diagnosis.

Theophylline and β-Agonists

These drugs are indicated for food-induced bronchospasm.

Steroids

In the opinion of these authors, oral steroids have no place in the diagnosis or treatment of food allergy, except as part of the treatment of anaphylaxis and sometimes in the treatment of very severe gastrointestinal allergies.

Cromolyn Sodium

Cromolyn sodium or Intal may be used as a diagnostic aid in very difficult cases of suspected food allergy to see whether it will relieve symptoms. It may help to avoid the need for extensive tests, such as 5-day stool fat collections, absorption studies, complement studies, and jejunal biopsy. It may be used in difficult cases of chornic urticaria or atopic dermatitis in whom the role of food is very difficult to evaluate. In addition, it may be used in a double-blind study to confirm that a food is actually causing asthma if the FEV_1 does not fall when the food is given with cromolyn sodium but does fall when placebo is given instead. Treatment with cromolyn sodium may be helpful to patients with acute, prolonged symptoms who are unable to tolerate sufficient foods for adequate nutrition. It can be particularly useful in such patients if they often have to eat foods away from home where they cannot follow a very complicated diet.

To be effective, the correct method of administration must be used. The capsule contents are emptied into 1 tsp of hot water, dissolved, and then mixed with some cold water. In infants, the drug must be administered by dropper, with the solution swished around inside the mouth so that it coats the mucous membrane before it is swallowed. The drug is taken four times a day before meals. Although the manufacturer's recommended dose is 100 mg for children and 200 mg for adults, the dose varies greatly from patient to patient and must often be much higher. If the starting dose is too high, the symptoms may be exacerbated during the first few days of treatment. It is therefore advisable to start with a low dose and increase the dose gradually over 10-14 days to the required dose. There is now a vast literature indicating good therapeutic results in properly selected patients [32-41].

ACKNOWLEDGMENT

This chapter was prepared with the assistance of the Medical Publications Department.

REFERENCES

1. Ratner, B., Untracht, S., and Collins–Williams, C. *Ann. Allergy 10*:675, 1952.
2. Sattler, H. R. *The Eggless Cookbook,* A. S. Barnes & Co., Cranbury, New Jersey, 1972.

3. Sainsbury, I. S. *The Milk- and Milk-Free, Egg-Free Cookbook*, Charles C. Thomas, Springfield, Illinois, 1974.
4. Shattuck, R. R. *Creative Cooking Without Wheat, Milk and Eggs*, A. S. Barnes & Co., Cranbury, New Jersey, 1974.
5. Hamrick, B. and Wiesenfeld, S. L. *The Egg-free, Milk-free, Wheat-free Cookbook*, Cygnus Press, Midland, Texas, 1981.
6. May, C. D. *J. Allergy Clin. Immunol. 58*:500, 1976.
7. Bock, S. A., Buckley, J., Holst, A., and May, C. D. *Clin. Allergy 7*:375, 1977.
8. Bock, S. A., Lee, W. Y., Remigio, L., Holst, A., and May, C. D. *Clin. Allergy 8*:559, 1978.
9. Bock, S. A., Lee, W. Y., Remigio, L. K., and May, C. D. *J. Allergy Clin. Immunol. 62*:327, 1978.
10. May, C. D. *N. Engl. J. Med. 302*:1142, 1980.
11. Aas, K., and Johansson, S. G. O. *J. Allergy Clin. Immunol. 48*:134, 1971.
12. Chua, Y. Y., Bremner, K., Llobet, J. L., Kokubu, H. L., and Collins-Williams, C. *J. Allergy Clin. Immunol. 58*:477, 1976.
13. Goldman, A. S., Anderson, Jr., D. W., Sellers, W. A., Saperstein, S., Kniker, W. T., and Halpern, S. R. *Pediatrics 32*:425, 1963.
14. May, C. D. *J. Allergy Clin. Immunol. 58*:500, 1976.
15. Crawford, L. V. In *Allergic Diseases of Infancy, Childhood and Adolescence*, C. W. Bierman and D. S. Pearlman (eds.), Saunders, Philadelphia, 1980, p. 399.
16. Weltman, J. K., Szaro, R. P., and Settipane, G. A. *Allergy 33*:273, 1978.
17. Gerber, J. G., Payne, M. A., Oelz, O., Nies, A. S., and Oates, J. A. *J. Allergy Clin. Immunol. 63*:289, 1979.
18. Logan, W. J., and Swanson, J. M. *Science 206*:363, 1979.
19. Farr, R. S., Spector, S. L., and Wangaard, C. H. *J. Allergy Clin. Immunol. 64*:667, 1979.
20. Weber, R. W., Hoffman, M., Raine, Jr., D. A., and Nelson, H. S. *J. Allergy Clin. Immunol. 64*:32, 1979.
21. Baker, G. J., Collett, P., and Allen, D. H. *Med. J. Aust. 2*:614, 1981.
22. Freedman, B. J. *Clin. Allergy 7*:407, 1977.
23. Freedman, B. J. *Clin. Allergy 9*:423, 1979, Abstract.
24. Freedman, B. J. *Br. J. Dis. Chest 74*:128, 1980.
25. Stevenson, D. D., and Simon, R. A. *J. Allergy Clin. Immunol. 68*:26, 1981.
26. Freedman, B. J. *Clin. Allergy 7*:417, 1977.
27. Snashall, P. D., and Baldwin, C. *Thorax 37*:118, 1982.
28. Allen, D. H., and Baker, G. J. *Med. J. Aust 2*:576, 1981.
29. Allen, D. H., and Baker, G. J. *N. Engl. J. Med. 305*:1154, 1981.
30. Allen, D. H., and Baker, G. J. *N. Engl. J. Med. 306*:1181, 1982.
31. Lessof, M. H. *Q. J. Med.*, N. S. *52*:111, 1983.
32. Freier, S., and Berger, H. *Lancet 1*:913, 1973.
33. Kingsley, P. J. *Lancet 2*:1011, 1974.
34. Kuzemko, J. A., and Simpson, K. R. *Lancet 1*:337, 1975.
35. Shaw, R. F. *Arch. Dermatol. 111*:1537, 1975.

36. Dannaeus, A., Foucard, T., and Johansson, S. G. O. *Clin. Allergy* 7:109, 1977.
37. Dahl, R., and Zetterström, O. *Clin. Allergy* 8:419, 1978.
38. Harries, M. G., O'Brien, I. M., Burge, P. S., and Pepys, J. *Clin. Allergy 8*: 423, 1978.
39. Kocoshis, S., and Gryboski, J. D. *JAMA 242*:1169, 1979.
40. Monro, J., Brostoff, J., Carini, C., and Zilkha, K. *Lancet 2*:1, 1980.
41. Collins–Williams, C. *Sodium Cromoglycate as a Therapeutic and Diagnostic Agent in Food Allergic Disease,* Medmark Communications Inc., Canada, 1982.

APPENDIX 1: RICE RECIPES*

Rice Cookies

3 c rice flour	1 lemon rind, grated
2 tsp baking powder	juice of 1 lemon
1 c sugar	¼ c water
½ c olive oil	

Sift dry ingredients; cream thoroughly with oil. Add grated lemon rind and juice with just enough water to make a stiff dough, and pat into shape. Sprinkle with additional sugar to taste and bake in moderate oven for 5–7 min.

Rice Bread

1 c rice flour	1 tbsp sugar
3 tsp baking powder	½ tsp salt
2 tbsp oil	¾ c water

Sift the dry ingredients. Add the water and oil. Bake in a loaf pan in a moderate oven, 350–375°F, for 45–50 min.

Rice Cupcakes

2/3 c hot water	¼ tsp salt
1½ c rice flour	3 level tsp baking powder
2 level tbsp olive oil	1 tsp vanilla
¼ c sugar	

Pour hot water over half the flour. Cream sugar and oil, and add to the above mixture, beating well. Add the other ingredients, mixing well. Bake in greased muffin pans about 20 min in a fairly hot oven (400°F).

*Appendixes 1 to 4 are reprinted by permission of the publisher from Allergy to Foods other than milk, by C. Collins-Williams and L. Levy, in R. A. Chandra (editor), *Food Intolerance,* Elsevier, New York, 1984.

Rice Biscuits

To make rice biscuits, add 2 tbsp water to 1 c of Nabisco Rice Flakes, blend gently, press out on an oiled cookie sheet, cut with a sharp knife, and bake for 10-12 min at 375°F.

APPENDIX 2: ROWE ELIMINATION DIETS AND RECIPES*

Rowe No. 1 Elimination Diet and Recipes

Foods allowed (not even traces of other foods may be given) are as follows:

Rice	Cane sugar
Tapioca	Sesame oil
Rice biscuit	Olive oil
Rice bread	Salt
Lettuce	Gelatin, plain or flavored with
Chard	lime or lemon
Spinach	Maple syrup or syrup made with
Carrot	cane sugar flavored with
Sweet potato or yam	maple
Lamb	Baking powder
Lemon	Cream of tartar
Grapefruit	Vanilla extract
Pear	Lemon extract
	Baking soda

In addition, the patient should receive Poly-Vi-Sol, 0.3 ml daily, and Calcium-Sandoz Syrup, 1 tbsp twice daily.

Examples of use:

1. Rice or tapioca may be served with the fruit or fruit juice that is allowed or with maple syrup.
2. Homemade jams, preserves, or jellies of the allowed fruits may be used on the bread instead of butter.
3. Fruits may be molded in gelatin.
4. Use olive oil for cooking.
5. The juices of the allowed fruits may be used as beverages.

---

*Rowe diets 1-3 are adapted with the permission of the publisher from A. H. Rowe, *Elimination Diets and the Patient's Allergies.* Copyright 1944 by Lea & Febiger Publishing Co.

Fruit Tapioca

2½ c canned fruit juice and
    water (half and half)
4 tbsp minute tapioca
½ c sugar

¼ tsp salt
1-1½ c chopped or pureed pears
1 tbsp lemon juice

Combine all ingredients in a saucepan, and mix well. Bring mixture to a boil, stirring constantly. Remove from fire. Do not overcook. Cool, stirring occasionally. The mixture thickens as it cools.

Fruit-Free Tapioca

3 c water
1/3 c minute tapioca
1/3 c white sugar or ½ c brown
    sugar

¼ tsp salt
½ tsp maple flavoring or 1 tsp
    vanilla extract or 2 tsp
    carmel flavoring (see below)

(The amount of brown sugar and flavoring may be varied to suit the individual taste.) Combine all ingregiends in a saucepan. Bring mixture quickly to a full boil over direct heat, stirring constantly. Remove from fire. Do not overcook. Stir the mixture occasionally as it cools.

Caramel Flavoring

Cook sugar until it turns golden brown. When cool, add just enough water to dissolve the hard caramel. The resulting liquid may be kept in a jar and used at will for flavoring and coloring.

Lamb Patties

Press ground lamb into small patties. Broil or fry in oil.

Fondant

2 c sugar
¼ tsp cream of tartar
1 c boiling water

¼ tsp salt
½ tsp vanilla

Measure sugar and cream of tartar into a saucepan, and add the boiling water. Stir over a low heat until sugar is dissolved. Do not let the candy boil before the sugar has dissolved and sugar crystals have been wiped down from the sides of the pan with a clean cloth or brush. When the boiling point is reached, cover the saucepan and boil vigorously for 5 min. Remove the cover, wipe crystals from the sides of the pan, and continue cooking without stirring until the medium-ball stage has been reached (240-242°F). When done, pour the candy at once onto a cold, wet platter and let it stand until lukewarm. Sprinkle salt over the surface, add vanilla and beat until white, and knead in the hands until smooth and creamy. Put fondant into a glass jar and cover. It will keep several weeks in a cool place.

Use of Fondant. Put a portion of the fondant into the top part of a double boiler. Melt over hot but not boiling water until fondant softens. Add coloring or flavoring; lemon extract or lemon juice and grated lemon rind may be used. Drop fondant from the tip of a spoon onto waxed paper.

Marshmallows

2 c sugar	¼ tsp salt
¾ c water	1 tsp vanilla extract
2 tbsp gelatin	

Mix sugar and water, and boil until the soft-ball stage has been reached (234–238°F). Remove from the fire. Soften gelatin in ½ c cold water. Pour the hot syrup over the softened gelatin, and stir until dissolved. Let it partly cool, add vanilla and salt, and beat it until the mixture is thick and white and will hold its shape. Pour into straight-sided pans. When firm, cut into squares. Roll in sugar, or, if corn is allowed, powdered corn sugar.

Rice Bread (see Appendix 1)

Rice Fruit Pudding

1½ c cooked rice	½ tsp salt
¼ c sugar	1 c canned pears

Mix all ingredients together, and bake in a moderate oven for 30 min. Serve warm with lemon sauce.

Rice Pudding with Lemon

1½ c cooked rice	1 tbsp lemon juice
¼ c sugar	2 tsp grated lemon rind
½ tsp salt	lemon sauce (see below)

Mix all ingredients together. Serve with additional lemon sauce.

Lemon Sauce

Mix 2 tbsp tapioca flour with ¾ c sugar, flattening all the lumps. Add all at once to 1½ c rapidly boiling water, stirring vigorously. Boil for 2 min. Add 4 tbsp lemon juice and 1 tsp grated rind, with a sprinkle of salt.

Rice Cookies; Rice Cupcakes (see Appendix 1)

Lemon Frosting

1 tbsp grated lemon rind	3 c confectioner's sugar
Dash of salt	2 tbsp lemon juice
2 tbsp sesame oil	1 tbsp water

Mix oil, salt, and lemon rind. Add fruit juice and water alternately with sugar, stirring well after each addition. Place bowl over hot water for a few minutes. Remove and spread over cake. This will cover a two-layer cake or 24 cupcakes.

Lemon Marmalade

Slice six unpeeled lemons very thin and cut crosswise into small pieces. Measure fruit. Add three times as much water. Boil about 1 hr or until tender. Replace liquid boiled away with water. Allow ¾ c sugar to each cup of fruit juice. Cook in 2-c lots to the jelly test (thick, reluctant drops from the spoon, about 10 min). Pour into sterilized jelly glasses. Cover with paraffin. This makes eight 6-oz glasses.

Carrot Marmalade

5 large carrots	Sugar
4 lemons	Water

Squeeze the lemons, removing the seeds, and set the juice aside. Grind lemon rind and pulp and carrots together. Add 8 c of water to the pulp, and boil for 30–45 min. Measure this mixture, and to it add an equal quantity of sugar and the lemon juice. Boil briskly for an hour or until it gels. Pour into sterile glasses, and seal with paraffin.

Pear Butter

Peel and core 1 gal of fresh pears; put into a saucepan, and add 2 c water. Boil slowly, and then when done put through a colander. To every 4 c of pulp, add 2 c of sugar. Place on stove again, and cook slowly until dark and very thick. Stir occasionally. A few minutes before removing, add juice of 1 lemon. Sterilize jars, rubbers, and lids; fill and seal while hot.

Baked Pears

6 medium-sized pears	1 c sugar, white or brown
½ c water	

Wash the pears, and remove blossom ends. Place pears in a baking dish, add sugar and water, cover and bake at 350°F for 1 hr or until pears are tender.

Lemon Ice (Made in the refrigerator)

2/3 c sugar	Pinch of salt
2 c water	1/3 c lemon juice
1½ tsp plain unflavored gelatin soaked in 3 tbsp water	1 tsp grated lemon rind

Boil sugar and water together 3 min. Dissolve soaked gelatin in hot syrup. Add salt, lemon juice, and rind. Turn into the freezer tray, and freeze until solid 1 in. from edge of tray. Scrape from the sides of the tray, and transfer to a chilled bowl. Beat with a chilled rotary beater until fluffy and smooth. Return to tray, and freeze again until firm.

Scotch Broth

2 lb shoulder lamb with bone	½ c diced carrots
2 qt water	salt
¼ c pearl tapioca	

Cut the meat into small pieces, and boil until tender. Cool and strain. Separate the lean meat from the bones, and return it to the broth together with the tapioca and carrots. Simmer gently until tapioca is clear. Salt to taste.

French Dressing

½ c allowed oil	½ tsp salt
¼ c lemon juice	1 tsp sugar

Mix well before using on salads.

Glazed Carrots

6 whole cooked carrots	1 tbsp sugar
2 tbsp sesame oil	½ c water

Dissolve the sugar in the water. Cook carrots in the syrup and oil, turning often to prevent burning.

Rowe No. 2 Elimination Diet and Recipes

Foods allowed (not even traces of other foods may be given) are as follows:

Corn	Apricot
Rye	Prune
Corn pone	Cane or beet sugar
Corn-rye muffin	Mazola oil
Rye bread	Sesame oil
Ry-Krisp	Salt
Beets	Karo corn syrup

Squash

Asparagus

Artichoke

Capon (no hens)

Bacon

Pineapple

Peach

Gelatin, plain or flavored with

pineapple

White vinegar

Baking powder

Baking soda

Cream of tartar

Vanilla extract

In addition, the patient should receive Poly-Vi-Sol, 0.3 ml daily, and Calcium-Sandoz Syrup, 1 tbsp twice daily.

Examples of use:

1. Corn flakes served with fruit or fruit juice that is allowed.
2. Cornmeal served with Karo syrup.
3. Jams, preserves, or jellies of the allowed fruits may be used on the bread instead of butter.
4. Homemade capon broth.
5. Fruits may be molded in gelatin.
6. Use Mazola oil for cooking.
7. The juices of the allowed fruits may be used as beverages.

Corn Pone

1 c cornmeal

½ tsp salt

Boiling water

1 tbsp Mazola oil

Carefully pour enough boiling water onto the cornmeal to make a stiff mixture, stirring constantly. Add the oil, and mix well. Mold into oblong "pones," and fry in hot skillet with enough fat to prevent sticking. When brown on one side, turn and brown on the other side. Serve hot.

Corn-Rye Muffins

1-1/3 c cornmeal

2/3 c rye flour

¼ c sugar

½ tsp salt

2½ tsp baking powder

1 c water

3 tbsp Mazola oil

Sift all the dry ingredients together. Add the water and oil. Pour into well-greased muffin pans. Bake at 400°F for 30 min.

Rye Bread

1½ c rye flour

3 tsp baking powder

½ tsp salt

3 tbsp specified oil

2/3 c water (more if necessary)

Sift dry ingredients, add the oil, and blend with pastry mixer. Add water, and stir until smooth. Put in greased tin and allow to stand for 15 min. Bake 45 min. in a moderate oven (350°F).

Corn Crisps

1 c cornmeal	1 tbsp Mazola oil
1 tsp salt	1 tsp sugar
2 c boiling water	

Mix all together. Pour a very thin layer on a well-greased cookie sheet. Bake 15 min at 350°F. While warm, cut into strips and sprinkle with salt.

Pineapple-Apricot Marmalade

4 c apricot pulp cut in small pieces and packed solidly in the cup	1 c crushed pineapple juice and pulp
	3½ c sugar

Mix fruit and sugar, boil rapidly until thick (approximately 30 min). Seal in hot, sterile glasses.

Capon Croquettes

1½ c cooked capon, chopped fine	1 c capon broth, homemade
½ tsp salt	2 tbsp cornstarch

Cook the cornstarch in the capon broth for 6 min or until thick. Add the capon and salt. Chill, and shape into croquettes. Roll in crushed corn flakes; deep fry in allowed oil, or bake in the oven for 30-45 min at 350°F.

Cornstarch Fruit Blanc Mange

1½ c fruit pulp and juice	4 tbsp cornstarch
1½ c water	3 tbsp sugar

Dissolve cornstarch in a little water. Heat the fruit pulp, water, and sugar. When almost boiling, add the cornstarch mixed in water. Continue cooking for 15-20 min in a double boiler. Pour into molds, and chill. Serve with fruit or pudding sauce.

Clear Pudding Sauce

½ c sugar	1 c boiling water
1 tbsp cornstarch	1 tsp vanilla extract
1/8 tsp salt	

Measure sugar, cornstarch, and salt into a saucepan. Mix well. Add boiling water slowly, stirring carefully to make a smooth sauce. Heat to boiling, stirring constantly until thickened, smooth, and clear. Add vanilla extract, and serve hot.

Rowe No. 3 Elimination Diet and Recipes

Tapioca	Apricot
White potato	Cane sugar
Breads made of any combination	Sesame oil
of soybean, lima bean,	Soybean oil
potato starch and tapioca	Gelatin, plain or flavored with
flours	lime or lemon
Tomato	Salt
Carrot	Maple syrup or syrup made
Lima beans	with cane sugar flavored
String beans	with maple
Peas	Baking powder
Beef	Baking soda
Bacon	Cream of tartar
Lemon	Vanilla extract
Grapefruit	Lemon extract
Peach	

In addition, the patient should receive Poly-Vi-Sol, 0.3 ml daily, and Calcium-Sandoz Syrup, 1 tbsp twice daily.
Examples of use:

1. Tapioca served with fruit or fruit juice that is allowed.
2. Jams, preserves, or jellies made from constituents listed in the diet may be used on the bread instead of butter.
3. Homemade beef broth.
4. Fruits may be molded in gelatin.
5. Use soybean oil or sesame oil for cooking.
6. The juices of the allowed fruits may be used as beverages.

Soy-Potato Muffins or Bread

1 c soybean flour	2 tbsp baking powder
1 c potato starch flour	2 tbsp white sugar
1 tsp salt	¾-1 c water
½ c soybean oil	

Sift the soybean flour once before measuring. Fill the measuring cup lightly, and level off the surface with a knife blade. Sift all the dry ingredients together four times. Add the oil and water, and beat well. Pour the batter into muffin pans that are well greased with soy oil. Bake in a moderate oven (350-375°F) for about 25-30 min. Makes 12 muffins.

For bread, bake in a loaf pan at 350°F for 1¼ hr.
If a moister texture is desired, decrease the potato starch flour to ¾ c.

Soy-Lima-Potato Muffins or Bread

1 c potato starch flour	2 tbsp sugar
¾ c soybean flour	1 c water*
¼ c lima bean flour	6 tsp baking powder
½ c sesame or soybean	½ tsp salt

Sift flour, baking powder, and salt together three times. Blend the oil and sugar
well. Add the sifted flour and the water alternately to the oil and sugar. Beat
well, and pour into muffin pans that have been well greased with sesame or soy
oil. Bake at 375°F for about 25-30 min. Makes 12 muffins. Or, bake in a loaf
pan at 350-375°F for 1¼ hr.

Soy-Potato Pancakes or Waffles

To the recipe for soy-potato muffins, add another ¼ c of water to make a thinner
batter. Bake on a griddle or waffle iron well greased with soybean oil. Serve
with maple syrup or syrup made with brown and white sugar flavored with maple
or caramel.

Lima Bean or Split Pea Soup

1 c split peas or lima beans	1 qt water
2 tbsp bacon fat	salt
diced bacon, crisp	

Cook the split peas or lima beans and salt until they form a smooth puree. Before
serving, add the bacon fat and crisp fried bacon.

Tomato Soup (with Soybean Flour)

1 c strained tomatoes or juice	2 tbsp soybean flour
1 c water	1 tsp salt

Mix the soybean flour thoroughly with some of the water, and add to the hot
tomato juice and water. Boil for ½ hr. This resembles a cream soup in consistency
and flavor. Salt to taste.

*Or 1 c cooked tapioca (2 tsp tapioca cooked in 1 c of water; add water after cooking to
make 1 c).

Soy-Potato Cupcakes or Cake

1 c soybean flour	½ c soybean oil
¾ c potato starch flour	2 tsp vanilla or 1 tsp vanilla and
5 tsp baking powder	1 tsp lemon extract
¾ c sugar	½-2/3 c water
½ tsp salt	

Sift soy flour once before measuring. Sift together all the dry ingredients four times. Mix the oil, sugar, and flavoring, and to this add the flour and water alternately, beginning and ending with flour. Beat well. Pour into muffin or layer cake pans well greased with soy oil, and bake at 375°F for 30 min. Makes 12 cupcakes or two small layers. Or, bake in a loaf pan for 45-50 min.

Variations. Flavor with lemon extract and grated lemon rind or with maple flavoring. Add chopped apricots, and substitute fruit juice for water. Fondant slightly thinned with water or fruit juice may be used for frosting.

Soy-Potato Cookies

Follow the recipe for soy-potato cake. Decrease the water to make a stiff dough. Force through a cookie press onto a cookie sheet well greased with soybean oil. A thinner batter can be dropped from a teaspoon onto a greased cookie sheet. Bake at 375-400°F for 10 or 15 min. A thicker dough can be rolled, kept in the refrigerator, cut in thin slices, and baked as desired. Cookies kept in an airtight container will remain crisp.

Soy Crackers

1 c soybean flour	2 tbsp soybean oil
1 tsp baking powder	1 tsp sugar
¼ tsp salt	1/3 c water

Mix well all ingredients. Dough should be quite thin. Drop from a teaspoon onto a cookie sheet well greased with soy oil. Bake at 350°F until dry and crisp. Sprinkle lightly with salt. These crackers will remain crisp if kept in a tightly covered container.

Soy Cookies

1 c soybean flour	4 tbsp soybean oil
2 tsp baking powder	3-5 tbsp water
¼ tsp salt	¼ tsp vanilla or lemon extract
1/3 c sugar	

Mix oil and sugar, and add the flavoring. Sift soy flour once before measuring, and sift twice more after adding baking powder and salt. Add flour to oil and sugar and sufficient water to make a stiff dough. Form into a roll, and cut into cookies or force through a cookie press. With a softer dough, drop from a teaspoon onto a cookie sheet well greased with soy oil. Bake at 350°F for 15 min. Chopped apricots may be added, or fruit juice may be substituted for water. Cookies will remain crisp if stored in an airtight container.

Soy-Potato Pudding

4 level tbsp soybean flour	¼ tsp salt
1 c water	¼ tsp lemon extract
2 tsp potato starch flour	¼ tsp vanilla extract
3 tbsp sugar	

Cook the soy flour and water for 15 min in the top of a double boiler. Stir potato starch, sugar, and salt into boiling mixture until it thickens. Continue cooking for 20 min. Flavor with lemon and vanilla extracts or with maple or caramel. Serve with fruit sauce, maple, or caramel syrup as desired. More sugar may be desired, or a combination of white and brown sugar may be used.

Caramel Frosting

2/3 c water	3 tbsp soybean oil
2 c brown sugar	1 tsp vanilla extract

Combine sugar and water. Stir slowly while bringing it to a boil. Boil hard, stirring occasionally until the syrup has reached the soft-ball stage (234°F). Remove from the fire, add soy oil and vanilla, and allow to cool undisturbed until lukewarm. Beat the mixture until it is thick and loses its luster. Spread quickly over the cake.

Panocha

2 tbsp sesame or soybean oil	1 c water
2 c brown sugar	1/8 tsp soda
1 c white sugar	

Heat the oil in a saucepan; stir in sugars. Add water and soda, and mix well with sugar. Wipe down sugar from sides of pan. Heat slowly to boiling, stirring until sugar is dissolved. Boil to 240°F, the medium-ball stage (the ball holds its shape when lifted from cold water). Remove from stove, sprinkle a dash of salt over top, and set aside to cool undisturbed until lukewarm. Beat until creamy. Turn into greased pans and cut into squares.

Lemon Frosting

1 tbsp grated lemon rind	3 c confectioner's sugar
dash of salt	2 tbsp lemon juice
2 tbsp sesame or soybean oil	1 tbsp water

Mix oil, salt, and lemon rind. Add fruit juice and water alternately with sugar, stirring well after each addition. Place bowl over hot water a few minutes. Remove, and spread over cake. This will cover a two-layer cake or 24 cupcakes.

Cotlemade

1 qt apricots	Sugar
1 qt lemons	Water

Slice lemons, rind and all, very thin, discarding seeds. Barely cover with water, and cook gently 1 hr. Add the apricots, halved and pitted, and cook another hour, stirring occasionally. Measure the fruit, and add an equal quantity of sugar. Boil rapidly, stirring frequently until the jelly stage is reached. Seal in sterile glasses. This marmalade is rather tart.

Grapefruit Marmalade

3 large grapefruit	Water
Sugar	

Cut the fruit and rind very fine. Measure, and cover with 2½ times as much water. Let it stand overnight, and the next morning boil briskly for 20 min. Remove from the fire, and measure, adding 1 c of sugar to each cup of fruit. Stir well until sugar is dissolved, and let stand several hours. Boil briskly until it jells. Pour into hot sterile glasses, and seal.

Tomato Preserves

Select firm, ripe tomatoes. Remove the skins, cut in slices, and drain an hour or more. For each cup of tomatoes add a cup of sugar, and boil until thick, stirring often. Sliced lemon may be added to the tomatoes while cooking.

Apricot Ice

2/3 c sugar	1½ c apricot nectar or pureed
½ c water	apricots and juice
Pinch of salt	2 tbsp lemon juice
1½ tsp gelatin soaked in 3 tbsp	1 tsp grated lemon rind, if desired
water	

Follow directions for lemon ice.

Lemon Ice (Using a mechanical freezer)

1 c sugar	½ tsp grated lemon rind
3 c water	½ c lemon juice
Rock salt	

Boil sugar and water for 5 min. Remove from stove, and cool. Add lemon juice and rind. Pour into the freezer can and freeze, using 6 or 8 parts of ice to 1 part of rock salt. This makes a little over 1 qt.

Beef Broth

2 c beef stock	Salt to taste
4 tbsp soybean flour	allowed vegetables

Mix the soybean flour with part of the stock, and add to remaining heated stock. Boil for 30 min. Diced carrots, lima beans, peas, or potatoes may be added as desired.

Hamburger-Vegetable Chowder

¾-1 lb ground beef	2 c cubed potatoes
3 tbsp allowed oil	¼ c pearl tapioca
2 c canned tomatoes	2 tsp salt
2 carrots, diced	1½ qt water

Brown the meat in the oil; put all the ingredients in a saucepan, and simmer slowly for an hour.

Tomato Jelly Ring

1 tbsp gelatin	½ tsp salt
½ c tomato juice, cold	1 tsp sugar
1 c tomato juice, hot	1 tbsp lemon juice

Soften gelatin in ½ c cold tomato juice. Add the hot tomato juice, salt, sugar, and lemon juice, and stir until dissolved. Pour into a ring mold. When firm, unmold on a bed of lettuce and fill the center with mixed vegetables that have been marinated in French dressing made with lemon juice and allowed oil. Use only the vegetables allowed in the diet.

Stuffed Tomato Salad

Peel medium-sized tomatoes, scoop out the center, sprinkle with salt, and let them stand upside down until well chilled. Fill the centers with diced cooked carrots and small cooked lima beans.

French Dressing

½ c allowed oil	½ tsp salt
¼ c lemon juice	1 tsp sugar

Mix well before using on salads. Tomato juice may be added for vegetable salads or apricot juice for fruit salads.

Tomato Sauce

2 c strained tomato cooked down to 1 c with the juice of 1 lemon, salt and sugar to taste.

Lima Bean Casserole

1 c dried lima beans	2 c tomatoes
1 tsp salt	3 slices bacon
2 tbsp white sugar	

Soak the lima beans overnight in 1 qt of water. Cook in the same water for 30 min. Drain. Mix lima beans with the other ingredients in a casserole and bake at 250°F until tender (about 2 hr).

Quick Sweet Rolls

2 c flour (½ soybean and ½ potato) ½ c sugar	
6 tsp baking powder	1 tsp salt
½ c sesame oil	½-¾ c water

Mix flour, salt, and baking powder; work in the oil and the water to make a soft dough. Turn out on a floured board; knead lightly for less than 1 min. Roll into an oblong sheet. Sprinkle with the filling (below). Roll up like a jelly roll. Cut into slices ½ in. thick, and bake 15 min. in a hot oven (400°F).

Filling. Mix together ¼ c water, 2 tbsp sesame or soybean oil, and ½ c grapefruit marmalade.

Baked Peach Tapioca Pudding

1/3 c minute tapioca	2½ c water and peach juice (half
4 tbsp sugar	and half)
½ tsp salt	2 c canned sliced peaches,
1 tbsp lemon juice	drained

Combine ingredients in a baking dish. Mix thoroughly. Bake in a moderate oven (375°F) for 30 min, stirring well every 10 min. Serve warm or cold. Apricots may be substituted for peaches.

Golden Turkish Paste

1 c well-drained cooked apricots	2 c sugar
4 tbsp plain gelatin	1 tsp grated lemon rind
½ c apricot juice, cold	2 tbsp lemon juice
½ c apricot juice, hot	

Soften gelatin in cold apricot juice. Mix sugar with the hot juice, and bring to the boil. Add gelatin, lemon juice, and rind, and boil 20 min. Remove from the stove, and add the mashed apricots. Mix well. Pour into a pan lined with waxed paper. After it has set, cut into cubes. Roll in sugar.

APPENDIX 3: OTHER DIETS

Wheat-Free Diet

Wheat and wheat products include white flour, bread flour, cake flour, pastry flour, self-rising flour, whole wheat flour, wheat flour, all-purpose flour, cracked wheat flour, graham flour, enriched flour, entire wheat flour, and phosphated durum flour. They also include wheat, wheat germ, bran, farina, and semolina, as well as malt, bread crumbs, and cracker meal.

In order to remain on a wheat-free diet, it is essential not to use any packaged foods that are not labeled with all their ingredients, and when eating away from home, it is essential to take substitute foods that are known to be free of wheat.

Forbidden Foods

1. Breads, white bread, rolls, biscuits, muffins, whole-wheat bread, graham bread, gluten bread, sweet rolls, doughnuts, johnnycake, pancakes, waffles, pretzels, crackers, zwieback, and popovers. Wheat is also in prepared mixes for waffles, biscuits, doughnuts, breads, rolls, pancakes, and muffins. It may also be in rye, corn, soybean, potato, or rice bread, rolls, or muffins. Therefore, it is not safe to eat any of these unless they are clearly labeled as free of wheat. For example, wheat-free rye bread is readily available, but ordinary rye bread contains some wheat and only reading the label will give confirmation of this. Breaded foods also contain wheat products.

2. Desserts. Doughnuts, dumplings, commercial sherbets, ice creams, ice cream cones, pastry, cakes, cookies, pies, puddings, and custards frequently contain wheat products, as do prepared mixes for cakes, ice creams, puddings, cookies, and pie crusts. Again, it is essential to use only those that have the ingredients listed on the label and exclude wheat.

3. Cereals. Many cereals contain wheat, and it is essential that the label be read carefully in every case.

4. Salad dressings. Many salad dressings are thickened with wheat flour.

5. Soups. Many creamed, vegetable, or meat soups, chowders, and bisbisques contain wheat flour.

6. Candies. Many commercial candies contain wheat products and should not be eaten unless their ingredients are clearly labeled and exclude wheat.

7. Beverages. Some coffee substitutes and similar beverages, malted drinks, beer, and ale contain wheat products.

8. Sauces and gravies. Many sauces and graview are thickened with wheat flour. It is not safe to consume these in restaurants. Prepackaged gravy should be used only if the ingredients are clearly labeled and exclude wheat.
9. Meats, poultry, fish, seafood, and game. Many fish or meat patties contain wheat products. Poultry and game stuffing frequently use wheat products. Swiss steak, chili con carne, and croquettes frequently contain wheat.
10. Vegetables must not be served with sauce thickened with wheat flour.
11. Miscellaneous. Most dumplings, spaghetti, macaroni, mostaccioli, ravioli, soup rings, soup alphabets, vermicelli, and malt products contain wheat.

Milk-Free Diet

The only way to follow the milk-free diet is to eat only foods that are known to be free of milk. The following list includes foods that contain milk in a hidden form in many cases. Foods should be prepared at home or labeled with all their ingredients and explicitly omit milk or milk products.

The only practical way is to buy no packaged foods on which the list of ingredients is not given and, if eating away from home as in restaurants, to order only foods that you are quite sure are free of milk.

Forbidden Foods

1. Milk and milk products that include fresh whole milk, skimmed milk, cultured milk, buttermilk, cream, condensed milk, evaporated milk, dried milk, milk solids, casein, lactalbumin, butter, margarine (unless specifically stated on the label to be free of milk solids), curds, whey, malted milk, and cheese.
2. Beef. Since there is some cross-reaction between beef albumin and milk proteins, a person on a strictly milk-free diet should not eat any beef.
3. Sauces and gravies. Most white or cream sauces contain milk or milk products and should be avoided.
4. Soups. Many canned and dehydrated soups contain milk or milk pro-products and should not be consumed unless their ingredients are labeled and exclude milk.
5. Salad dressings. Many salad dressings contain milk, cream, butter, mar-margarine, or cheese.
6. Desserts. Many cakes, cookies, puddings, and pie crusts contain or are brushed with milk or milk products. These include blanc manges, custard, junket, ice cream, and milk sherbets. These should be homemade

and known to be free of milk or purchased only if they are clearly labeled as free of milk.

7. Meats, poultry, fish, and seafoods. Many commercially prepared meats contain milk products.
8. Candies. Many sweets contain milk or milk products.
9. Vegetables. Creamed and scalloped vegetables often contain milk or milk products.
10. Bread and breaded foods. Pancakes, waffles, crackers, rusks, doughnuts, and foods breaded with bread crumbs or cracker crumbs frequently contain milk products. Most commercial breads and rolls contain some milk and should be eaten only if they are clearly labeled as milk free.
11. Beverages. Many chocolate- or cocoa-containing preparations contain milk or milk products.
12. Miscellaneous. Foods dipped in milk batter, fried in butter or in margarine, creamed and scalloped foods, foods prepared with cheese (au gratin), rarebits, and prepared mixes for cakes, doughnuts, muffins, cookies, biscuits, pie crusts, and waffles frequently contain milk or milk products.

Egg-Free Diet

Following an egg-free diet means eating only foods that are known to be free of egg. The following list includes foods that contain egg in a hidden form in many cases. All foods should be prepared at home or chosen from explicitly labeled egg-free sources.

Buy no packaged foods without a complete list of ingredients, and if eating away from home, eat only foods that you are quite sure are free of egg.

Forbidden Foods

1. Egg dishes, such as those with baked, creamed, deviled, scalloped, fried, scrambled, hard- or soft-cooked eggs, egg drinks, such as eggnog, egg sauces, egg meringue, and egg omelettes.
2. Salad dressings. Many salad dressings include egg; true French dressing is an exception. Unless the salad dressing is clearly labeled with its ingredients, it should not be purchased; a homemade substitute should be used.
3. Breads and breaded foods. Many breads, muffins, waffles, gingerbreads, doughnuts, and griddle cakes contain egg. Many commercial breads and rolls contain egg or have been brushed with egg white, and breads or rolls with a glossy surface must be suspected of having been brushed with egg white. No mixes for these products should be used unless the ingredients are labeled and no forms of egg are present.

4. Baking powder. Many baking powders contain egg white or egg albumen and should not be used unless the ingredients are on the label.
5. Desserts. Custards, Bavarian creams, angel and sponge cakes, macaroons, whips, pie fillings, blanc manges, frostings, ice creams, sherbets, puddings, and cakes frequently contain egg.
6. Beverages. Any prepared drink may contain egg or one of its constituents. Some coffees have been clarified with egg white or egg shell. Some root beers contain egg to make the foam. If you are in doubt about a favorite prepared beverage, a manufacturer will usually let the parent or the physician know whether there is any egg in the beverage.
7. Meats, poultry, fish, seafood, and game. Many sausages, meat loaves, croquettes, or prepared meats contain egg as a binding agent. A patient sensitive to egg should avoid chicken although capon is acceptable.
8. Sauces, such as tartar and hollandaise, frequently contain egg.
9. Candies. Many store-bought sweets contain egg and should not be consumed unless the package is clearly labeled as egg free. Many commercial candies, such as jelly beans, are brushed with egg white to give them a luster and must not be eaten.
10. Soups. Many alphabet, mock turtle, and egg noodle soups, consommes, bouillons, and broths contain egg. No canned soups should be taken unless they are clearly labeled as egg free.
11. Miscellaneous. French toast, fritters, and such products frequently contain egg and should not be consumed unless ingredients are clearly labeled and exclude egg.

APPENDIX 4: SPECIAL DIET NO. 5 (ADDITIVE FREE)

The following foods may be eaten.

Cereals: Wheat, rye, oat, barley, rice, sago, tapioca.

Bread: Homemade bread is preferable. Plain purchased wheat or rye bread will do.

Flour: Wheat, rye, oat, barley, rice, potato.

Pasta: Uncolored spaghetti, macaroni, vermicelli.

Vegetables: Fresh or frozen (not canned or bottled) eggplant, red pepper, lettuce, artichoke, beet, spinach, cabbage, cauliflower, broccoli, Brussels sprouts, turnip, radish, squash, cucumber, asparagus, onion, sweet potato, yam, carrot, celery, mushroom.

Fruits: Fresh (not dried, frozen, canned, or bottled) pineapple, canteloup, muskmelon, honeydew, watermelon, pear, blueberry, grapefruit, lemon, lime.

Eggs: Boiled, or cooked in butter.

Milk products: Whole milk, 2% milk, skim milk, powdered milk, fresh butter, white cheese.

Meats: Fresh, frozen, or salted. Beef, lamb, pork, veal (no sausage or processed meats).

Fish: Fresh, frozen, salted, or pickled (not smoked or canned).

Beverages: Water, weak tea (no black Chinese), lemonade made with fresh lemon, limeade made with fresh lime, fresh grapefruit juice (not canned), fresh pineapple juice (not canned).

Soups: Any homemade using the above ingredients. Not packaged or canned.

Sweets: White sugar, honey, homemade jam, and marmalade.

Condiments: Salt, vinegar, chili, mustard (if prepared at home with pure powder and distilled vinegar).

Cooking oils: Mazola, corn oil.

Chewing gum: None.

Toothpaste: White (not colored) toothpaste.

Note: Under certain circumstances, it may be necessary to avoid vinegar and cheese.

12
Unproven and Unapproved Methods of Diagnosis and Treatment

JOHN A. ANDERSON
Henry Ford Hospital, Detroit, Michigan

Adverse reactions to components of our diet may be quite common. Allergic (immunologically related) reaction and, in particular, hypersensitivity (or IgE-mediated) reactions to foods or food additives are relatively uncommon. Since eating foods is such a necessary and representative part of daily life, it is not unusual that many common complaints — not just those that historically fit the history of allergic reaction, such as anaphylaxis — are unjustly attributed to allergy. The physician who faces the problem of establishing the relationship between a given set of signs and symptoms and the ingestion of a food substance may have an easy or difficult task. In cases in which the signs and symptoms fit the pattern of allergy or immediately related reactions, then those diagnostic procedures and in vitro proven laboratory tests may be helpful in establishing a relationship. An exception may exist when the symptoms and signs encountered are late and/or involve the gastrointestinal tract [1].

In other cases, especially when the signs and symptoms do not fit the pattern common to an allergic or immunologically related reaction, the usual in vivo diagnostic procedures used by an allergist and in vitro immunologically related laboratory tests are not helpful in proving or disproving a relationship with a food ingestant.

The reasons behind this difficulty in diagnosis may be many but include the following.

1. The broad nature of signs and symptoms that the general public as well as select physicians attribute to "allergy." Historically, the term "allergy" refers to an altered response. In this sense, then, almost any

reaction might be identified as an allergy by some, even those reactions that bear little or no resemblance to the classic signs and symptoms of hypersensitivity.

2. The nature of the usual allergen available for study. Most clinical investigators dealing with alleged food reactions have only raw crude allergen mixtures at their disposal. Only a few purified natural food allergens have been well studied, notably cod and peanut [2-5]. The majority of the published scientific articles that deal with the clinical correlation between a set of signs and symptoms and the alleged food reactions are based on studies involving the use of crude food allergens. Even more difficult to critically evaluate are some studies that are based upon chemical food additives used in the test systems.

3. The effect of protein denaturation, as with cooking, as well as with the exact identification of the food allergen in food metabolism, is rarely taken into account. Although the allergenicity of most natural foods decreases with cooking, individual patients can be found to be more sensitive to heat-denatured protein [2, 6]. Enzyme digestion of common raw food allergens may lead to new allergens to which the patient is primarily sensitive, although this concept is debated [7-9].

4. The time sequence involved in many adverse reactions to foods. Those food reactions that result within an immediate period (minutes) are more easily correctly identified. Those alleged reactions, however, that occur hours or even days later become difficult to confirm, especially in cases in which there is a relationship to a modified food allergen [1].

5. The "shock" organ that is usually involved in adverse food reactions. Since the recognition that allergic reactions do exist, it has become common practice among allergists to establish the diagnosis by re-exposing the patient to the suspected substance [10]. Those "true" allergic or hypersensitivity reactions to inhalants, such as pollens and animal danders, or exposure to Hymenoptera insects or drugs, usually involve the skin or the respiratory tract as shock organs. Reactions to foods and food additives, however, frequently involve the gastrointestinal tract as well as the skin as shock organs. Such reactions as hives and atopic dermatitis are more easily studied since the end point to challenge exposure, as with respiratory reactions, are most easily readily identified. Reactions involving the gastrointestinal tract as a shock organ, however, are difficult to study. Symptoms and signs, often late, frequently are confused with other nonimmunologic types of reaction, and because of the nature of the shock organ, offer little opportunity for quantifiable end points. Alleged adverse reactions to foods that involve the nervous system (i.e., migraine headache, fatigue, or hyperkinesis) or the musculoskeletal system (muscle or joint "pains") are even more difficult to study.

6. Lack of defined in vitro or in vivo diagnostic tests to rule in or out immunologic reactions to food or food additives. Although repeated double-blind food challenges may identify patients who truly have adverse reaction to a given food or food additive, such tests do not identify the mechanism of such reactions. No single immunologic test has been shown to be definitive enough to rule in or out all possibilities of an adverse reaction to a given food or food additive. Since the precise diagnosis of a food allergy is difficult, it is not surprising that unconventional methods have surfaced that have been championed by select physicians. As with diagnostic techniques, unconventional treatments that have been alleged to be helpful in patients with a variety of common complaints have also surfaced.

The practice of allergy and clinical immunology has evolved through clinical observations coupled with increasing knowledge of basic immunologic principles. The accepted methods of in vivo and in vitro diagnosis are based upon many laboratory and clinical studies that meet the standards of modern scientific investigation. Significant advances have occurred over the past 15 or 20 years in the recognition of scientific principles and the technical aspects of diagnosing diseases, including hypersensitivity or IgE-mediated reactions, that involve immunologic aspects.

Whenever new concepts, either in diagnosis or treatment, are considered, proper trials should be conducted before the new procedure or therapy is accepted as safe and efficacious. Van Metre has recently outlined those aspects of a trial that should be considered in designing a study of unproven diagnostic procedures or treatment [11]. The same criteria may be used in evaluating published studies concerning unproven techniques.

1. The hypothesis to be tested should be clearly stated and precisely related to established fact and scientific principles.
2. The design of the trial should permit the investigator to separate the effects of the procedure being tested from those effects resulting from other factors.
3. Procedures and reagents should be described in such a way that the work can be repeated by subsequent investigators.
4. The trial should concern a homogeneous group of patients who have the disorder to be studied but who are otherwise well. In some cases, as in the study of adverse reactions to foods, it may be necessary to prove that the patients do indeed have an adverse reaction, regardless of mechanism, before accepting them as suitable study subjects. This may be done with double-blind challenge studies under controlled conditions [12].

5. The subjects under study should be described in sufficient detail that similar patients could be found by a subsequent investigator.
6. Risk factors, such as a study patient sensitive to allergens, should be clearly identified since these factors will modify the response of individual patients to the procedure under study.
7. Test and control study groups should be of appropriate size and number so that statistically significant results can be obtained. (The number of variables to be evaluated will greatly influence the number of patients needed in the study [13].)
8. The study patients should be divided into groups of equal size, each with comparable characteristics and risk factors. By random selection, members of the group should be assigned to either a test or a control procedure.
9. Evaluation of the results of the trial should be as objective as possible and expressed in quantifiable terms. The trial should be conducted in a "double-blind" manner, so that the patient or evaluating physician does not know which patient receives a particular test or control procedure.
10. Appropriate statistical methods for evaluating the significance of the results should be selected at the time of design of the study and used to evaluate the results at the end of the study [13].
11. Patient informed consent should be obtained for all study subjects. The safety and scientific merit of the study should be evaluated and approved by a competent institutional therapeutic trials committee (prior to the start of the study).
12. The results of the trial should be published in a refereed journal.

A critical review of the diagnostic techniques and therapeutic methods considered to be unproven, controversial, and, finally, unapproved will find that proper attention was usually not given to most of the 12 points listed above during trials whose end results promote these unconventional concepts and methods.

SKIN-TEST END-POINT TITRATION (HANSEL-RINKEL TECHNIQUE)

Blackley first noted that, in a sensitive individual, pollen sprinkled upon a scarified portion of skin would result in itching, swelling, and erythema within a few minminutes, localized at the skin site [14]. An immediate-reacting prick, scratch, or puncture as well as intradermal skin test subsequently developed. Prausnitz and Kustner proved that this reaction was due to a transferable serum factor [6]. The antibody class responsible for this skin test reaction has now been recognized as IgE [15].

In common allergy practice, the immediate reacting prick or intradermal skin test is used as a measure of allergen-specific IgE antibody reaction. Although a single concentration of a specific allergen may be selected for testing and the reaction graded for positivity, more information can be obtained if a serial titration series of skin tests can be done using the same allergen [10]. The end point is considered to be that point at which the highest dilution still gives a reaction, generally at a 1+ or 2+ gradation of positivity.

Studies have shown that end-point skin test titration correlates with clinical challenge and with allergen-specific in vitro leukocyte histamine release and levels of allergen IgE-specific antibody as measured by the radio-allergosorbent test (RAST) under optimal conditions [16]. In a study by Sweet and colleagues, clinical sensitivity was found more likely to be associated with a positive skin test reaction than a positive allergen-specific RAST [17]. Only those patients who were very sensitive to allergens, as demonstrated clinically and by high dilutional skin test end-point reaction, were likely to have positive allergen-specific IgE reaction in the serum. Skin test end-point titration also has been used to follow the course of allergen immunotherapy [18].

Skin-Test End-Point Titration to Determine the Optimal Dose for Immunotherapy

Allergy skin testing, as well as skin test titration, has deep roots within the science of this specialty. Where the use of this latter technique differs from conventional doctrine is the concept of determining the therapeutic allergen dose to be used in immunotherapy (such as in the treatment of pollen hypersensitivity) by end-point skin test titration. Phillips first introduced the concept in 1926 [19]. Hansel renewed the concept in 1941 [20]. Rinkel introduced the fivefold serial titration method and the currently used terminology [21]. An excellent review of the technique was published by Willoughby [22]. According to the technique, a safe starting dose for allergen immunotherapy is 0.01–0.15 ml of the skin test endpoint dilution; the optimal therapeutic dose was close to 0.5 ml of the skin test end-point dilution; the specific safe starting dose rarely, if ever, caused untoward reaction; and the specific optimal therapeutic dose rarely, if ever, caused untoward reaction and, in many cases, promptly relieved the symptoms [11]. A review of how this works in clinical practice as well as the reasons for failure of the technique in the eyes of the proponents of the titration technique can be seen in Goldberg's publication [23].

The concept of end-point titration relative to optimal dose is not compatible with the accepted published data. In recent years, a series of properly controlled trials has clearly demonstrated that low-dose allergen therapy is no more effective clinically than placebo [24]. Furthermore, only high-dose therapy has been demonstrated to produce measurable immunologic changes.

During high-dose therapy, cutaneous reactions have been shown to decline gradually over years – not in days as claimed by Rinkel [18, 21, 23]. Low-dose therapy does not change skin test reactivity [18]. Skin test reactions do not correlate with the maximal dose of allergen tolerated [18].

The recent controlled studies comparing allergen immunotherapy utilizing doses on the basis of the Rinkel technique versus placebo or versus conventional high-dose therapy in the treatment of allergic rhinitis due to ragweed pollen have not shown the Rinkel technique to be of benefit [25-27]. These control studies provided no support for Rinkel's claim that the usual optimal dose for providing relief of allergy symptoms is 0.5 ml of the skin test end-point titration. Following the Rinkel technique, only low-dose therapy was achieved. In the studies comparing the Rinkel technique with conventional therapy, the median accumulative dose of allergen achieved for the conventionally treated patient was 1000-fold higher than those patients treated on the basis of the Rinkel concept [26]. When patients who had been obtaining low-dose therapy on the basis of the Rinkel concept and had fared no better than placebo-treated patients clinically, and immunologically were then given conventional therapy, they then improved clinically and immunologically [28].

The process of skin test end-point titration is time consuming and labor intensive. The cost of doing this procedure for each allergen to which the patient is sensitive is much greater than using single skin tests based upon a standard allergen concentration. These costs are usually passed on to the patient.

In addition, conventional allergen immunotherapy is usually based upon one battery of skin tests. This frequently is not the case when practitioners follow the Hansel-Rinkel concept. When treatment failures occur, it is usually assumed that the treatment dose is less than optimal because the patient's sensitivity may have changed. Retitration is then advocated in order to readjust (usually upward) the allergen immunotherapy dose [23]. Again, these costs are usually passed on to the patient.

Although the technique of skin test end-point titration may be useful in experimental situations as a method for quantifying skin sensitivity to allergenic extract and for obtaining information about the sensitization of patients to allergy, it is not a practical clinical diagnostic procedure. Proper trials have not confirmed the Rinkel hypothesis concerning the value of the technique in establishing either the proper starting dose or the optimal therapeutic treatment allergen immunotherapy dose. Finally, the increased cost of this technique may be unjustifiably passed on to the patient without offering that patient increased benefits. The American Academy of Allergy and Immunology has labeled the use of the technique as controversial and reserved for experimental use [29].

Although ordinary conventional immunotherapy is not recommended for the treatment of food hypersensitivity, it should be understood that the Hansel-Rinkel technique has been advocated by some in the diagnosis of adverse reactions to foods. Furthermore, the provocative testing and neutralizing therapy techniques are based upon end points obtained by the same technique of skin test end-point titrations [23].

PROVOCATIVE FOOD TESTING AND NEUTRALIZATION

The intracutaneous provocation test for diagnosing food "allergy" and the subsequent neutralization therapy was introduced in the early 1960s by Lee [30]. The technique was based upon attempts at food desensitization, which, in turn, was based upon end points obtained by skin test titration [31, 32]. The principle of the diagnostic test was the induction of symptoms by intracutaneous injection of food allergen, followed by alleviation of the symptoms with subsequent injection of a more dilute food allergen solution than the one that produced an end point on titration. Generally, 0.01 ml of a number 2 dilution (Rinkel 1:500 w/v) [22] of a food extract is injected intracutaneously. The size of the whealing response is then noted at 10 min. The clinical response of the patient is also observed, particularly for signs and symptoms that the patient may relate to a food ingestion.

Subjective symptoms, which are believed important to observe, include a wide variety of common complaints, including feelings of nausea, headache, dizziness, fatigue, pain in any part of the body, dry mouth, thirst, mental confusion, visual disturbances, pressure in the chest, dyspnea, irritability, chilliness, depression, and intoxication [31]. Objective symptoms included by Lee include, in addition to the more classic allergy signs and symptoms, the signs of hiccup, sweating, crying, tachycardia, irritability, flushing, and such eye signs as rubbing of the eyes, circles around the eyes, "a far-away look," and "vagueness" [31].

If no symptoms are produced upon initial screening, the size of the skin-test test wheal governs the next dose. If the wheal is small, the next dose is larger. If the wheal is large, the next dose is smaller. Should symptoms be provoked on any test dilution, one is again guided by the size of the skin test wheal. Stronger food allergen solutions are injected when the wheal size is small, and vice versa. When any provoked symptoms are relieved by one of the injected food allergen solutions, this dose is considered to be the neutralization dilution [23].

An extension of the diagnostic or clinical testing technique is to recommend that the patient continue to eat the food in the same quantities that he or she did prior to testing and to use the neutralization food allergen dilution injections frequently. If the injections later fail to relieve the patient's symptoms, the patient must be retested so that a new neutralizing dilution may be established [33].

The clinical symptom provocative aspect of the procedure was adapted to use the same food allergen dilutions, introduced now as drops under the tongue (instead of intracutaneous injections) by Dickey and Pfeiffer [34]. After observing the patient for 10-20 min, if no symptoms develop, a stronger solution is used or another food is tested. If a food allergen provokes a reaction, a more dilute solution of the same food extract is applied sublingually in an attempt to neutralize the symptoms. "Neutralization drops" (of the same dilution of food extract that neutralized the provoked symptoms) are then prescribed for the patient to take regularly before meals that contain the offending food [23, 35].

The rationale for the use of the sublingual route is that rapid absorption of the allergen is achieved through access to the systemic venous circulation, which bypasses the portal circulation. Food allergens thus avoid change due to gastrointestinal tract digestion. The method by which the neutralization may work is not explained in current immunologic terms [23, 35].

CONTROLLED TRIALS EVALUATING THE EFFICACY OF PROVOCATIVE TESTING AND NEUTRALIZATION TREATMENT PROCEDURES

A number of anecdotal reports of the clinical application of both the intracutaneous and the sublingual methods of provocative testing and neutralization therapy for alleged adverse reactions to foods have emerged over the past 20 years [23, 33-36]. In recent years, reports on "double-blind testing" of these techniques have given rise to the claim of successful control of a wide variety of usual allergy allergy, as well as other unusual complaints (headache, fatigue, myalgia, arthritis, hyperkinesis, and mental confusion) [37-41].

The reports of these latter studies usually do not fulfill the 12 aspects of an adequate trial of a new diagnostic or therapeutic technique as outlined by Van Metre, to convince the general medical community of the validity of the reported conclusions of the studies [11].

Studies evaluating either the intracutaneous or sublingual methods of provocative testing and neutralization therapy have not been successful in demonstrating the efficacy of these techniques [42-48]. Based upon this published information, the American Academy of Allergy and Immunology and the National Center for Health Care Technology have stated that these techniques should be reserved for experimental use only in well-controlled trials [29, 36, 49].

In spite of this evaluation of the published studies on provocation-neutralization techniques, reports continue to be submitted allegedly "proving" the validity of the technique [50, 51]. In one report, in which a wide variety of somatic complaints were allegedly provoked and then neutralized by food allergens, bizzare changes in several immune factors (total hemolytic complement-CH_{50}, C3, "total RAST," and "immune complex levels", as well as "serotonin levels" plus fluctuation of the erythrocyte sedimentation rate) are claimed. These reports do not satisfy the criteria of an adequate trial [11].

One study, however, rates consideration [52]. This study concerns the effect of neutralization therapy upon animal dander antigen-induced bronchospasm and reports significant benefit from this form of treatment. As reported, the study is well designed. The response with neutralization therapy is similar to that reported by other authors using conventional immunotherapy in cat-induced asthma [53, 54]. The significance of the results of the study reported by Boris and colleagues, if confirmed, in the relationship to the diagnosis or therapy of adverse reactions to foods is not clear at this time.

RADIOALLERGOSORBENT TEST (RAST) AND OTHER IN VITRO TESTS TO MEASURE IgE–SPECIFIC ANTIBODY TO FOOD ALLERGENS

Since the radioallergosorbent in vitro test (RAST) was introduced in 1967 to measure allergen-specific antibodies of the IgE type, hope has been given that many of the fundamental problems relating to the diagnosis and treatment of allergy-related problems may be solved [55]. This new assay has been a true technological advance and has been a boon to allergy research. The value of in vitro measurement of IgE allergens, however, has been largely limited to the laboratory. Generally, there is a good correlation between the various tests available for studying IgE-mediated allergen disease, such as prick skin testing, the IgE-RAST, the leukocyte histamine release, and clinical challenge [56]. The IgE-RAST uses the same allergens that can be used with the prick skin test. In clinical use, the prick skin test is more sensitive than the in vitro IgE measurement [17]. In situations where food allergen prick skin test has been critically studied, in relationship to double-blind food challenge under controlled conditions, such as with atopic dermatitis, a negative challenge follows a negative prick skin test [12]. It is generally felt that measurement of a food allergen IgE RAST would not be of any more value than a simple prick skin test using the same allergen. However, it is recognized that food allergen IgE RAST can correlate well with clinical pictures, especially when documented food anaphylaxis is involved. This is especially true when very purified allergens are used in the test system [4, 5, 57].

Problems Concerning the Use of In Vitro IgE-Specific Allergen Assays in Food Allergy Diagnosis

Measurement of IgE-specific food allergens is a valuable laboratory tool. Clinically, however, it has been abused in a variety of ways [58]. For this reason, guidelines have been put forth by the American Academy of Allergy and Immunology [59]. The problems concerning the clinical use of these techniques in the diagnosis of food allergy falls into the following categories.

1. Sole reliance upon any in vitro IgE allergen-specific assay as an indicator of the diagnosis of allergy or no allergy.

2. Use of the IgE RAST for diagnosis of food allergy in cases where the skin test is negative. If the skin test is negative, so should be the IgE allergen-specific RAST [12, 59].

3. Use of the IgE RAST test without proper controls and standardization. Evans and his colleagues of the American Academy of Allergy and Immunology, in a collaborative study, have shown the importance of this problem in the day-to-day and laboartory-to-laboartory variance of RAST results that are possible [60].

4. Use of a "modified" RAST system to allegedly increase "sensitivity." Nalebuff and his colleagues have modified the technique of the IgE RAST to allegedly increase the sensitivity of the test [61]. With the modification that he and his colleagues advocate, the RAST test is capable of detecting IgE antibody to a sensitivity of 0.2 Phadebas RAST units (PRU) in contrast to the lower limit of 0.35 PRU with the Phadebas conventional RAST system [62]. Santrach and colleagues critically evaluated this new method and compared this test with the conventional IgE RAST technique in 40 patients with allergic rhinitis, using clinical nasal challenge as an end point. The modified RAST technique was able to identify clinical sensitivity in 8 of 13 (62%) patients who had a positive nasal challenge test and a negative conventional RAST (<0.35 PRU). However, with the extended cutoff range, the modified RAST classified 5 of the 8 patients who had negative nasal challenge in the class I (equivocally positive) range (63%). In addition, using a human serum albumin negative control with the modified RAST system, 7 of 21 assays (33%) were classified positive. Thus, the high number of false-positive tests far outshadow the false-negative results that the use of this modified RAST technique presents. This factor is especially true when evaluating the test as one to diagnose "allergy" in situations where the clinical factors are unknown (indiscriminate laboratory screening), unclear (clinical evaluation and interpretation by untrained observer), or equivocal (clinical signs and symptoms not clear-cut as to the mechanism of reaction).

5. Use of a "modified" IgE RAST system as a titration in a similar fashion as used for the skin test wheal size in the Hansel-Rinkel technique, and to base the initial immunotherapy dose upon this method. The modified RAST system has been linked to the use of the "titration endpoint technique" in order to allegedly improve the efficiency of allergen immunotherapy [63]. When this system was critically evaluated by Santrach and colleagues, several conclusions could be made [62]. In 15 instances out of 50 trials (30%), highly skin test sensitive patients were identified in whom there was a wide distribution in regard to the modified IgE RAST score. If the RAST score were to be used to calculate a starting point for immunotherapy, the potential exists for an

adverse treatment reaction. In highly sensitive patients, therefore, this technique could be dangerous. In these 15 highly sensitive patients (to ragweed pollen), the allergen-specific modified RAST score changed over time (without immunotherapy), whereas the skin test remained fairly stable. Using the modified RAST schedule, some patients were begun on allergen doses more dilute or weaker than would be usually thought necessary using conventional techniques, thus promoting the tendency for "low-dose" (and ineffectual) therapy [59, 62]. Other workers have concluded that although determination of the usual immunotherapy dose in allergen-induced rhinitis based upon the modified RAST technique may be safe, it is not precise enough considering the variability of allergenic extract potency and does not offer any advantages, currently, over conventional methods [36, 62, 64].

6. Promotion of the IgE RAST as an in vitro laboratory technique for commercial purposes without regard to the techniques limited its specific value in the diagnosis of allergy, especially food allergy. Abuse of the technique may mislead the public. This may be a misdirection of the health care dollar resources. Since the in vitro allergen-specific assay offers only limited use in a clinical sense, it seems unjustified to overpromote its use, especially by individuals not skilled in the clinical evaluation of allergic disease [58, 59]. The commercial overuse of this technique seems particularly unjustified in the field of adverse reaction to food clinical diagnosis and treatment, since measurement of IgE antibodies to food allergens is only occasionally helpful in a clinical situation.

LEUKOCYTOTOXIC TESTS (BRYAN AND BRYAN, INCLUDING THE LEUKOPENIC INDEX, BLACK)

The leukopenic index was introduced in 1934 [65]. In this clinical test, the total white cell count was believed to fall following oral challenge of a specific food and, with this end point, clinical "allergen sensitivity" could allegedly be established. This test is not thought to be of value by most investigators [11, 23, 36].

In 1947, Squire and Lee reported their studies in which whole blood from ragweed hay fever allergic patients was incubated in vitro with ragweed allergens [66]. In the report of their studies, white cells were lysed and a reduction of the white cell numbers occurred. Black introduced the leukocytotoxic test for the in vitro diagnosis of food allergy in 1956 based upon observations by Squire and Lee [67]. In 1960, Bryan and Bryan refined the test that now frequently bears their name [68, 69].

In this test system, the blood buffy coat plus 1 drop of water and 4 drops of autologous plasma are placed in suspension, then applied to siliconized slides with exposure to dried food allergen within a ring of petrolatum jelly [36, 69, 70]. The food allergen-plasma cell suspension preparation is compared to a control preparation consisting of physiologic saline and the plasma cell suspension. Neutrophil changes are read from 10 min to 2 hr and graded as follows: negative, no change; slight, half leukocytes round and half active; moderate, all leukocytes round and few disintegrated; marked, majority of leukocytes are disintegrated [36].

The rationale for the test is based upon the observations noted by Black, Squire and Lee, and the Bryans. No mechanism, immunologic or otherwise, has been determined that explains the results of the test [49].

Since the test became popular, several studies have allegedly shown that the test is of value as an accurate diagnosis of food "allergy." This contention is, at best, questionable [11, 23, 29, 36, 49]. In well-done, controlled, blinded clinical trials of the leukocytotoxic test, using the Bryan and Bryan methodology, the test has not been found to be an accurate measure of the diagnosis of atopic reactions to foods [70]. Lieberman and colleagues studied 45 patients from the ages of 4 through 45 years for 50 food allergens. A total of 15 patients with well-documented allergic reactions to foods were compared with 10 patients with other somatic complaints, allegedly as a result of food allergen ingestion (headache, fatigue, dyspnea, maculopapular rash, nasal congestion, and diarrhea) and with 20 other patients who had no history of adverse food reaction. Interpretation of the test was found by Lieberman and his colleagues to be highly subjective. There was little concordance between examiners when the same slide was examined by two people. When five patients were tested upon successive days, entirely random sets of "positive" food reactions were seen. Positive tests were found to be at least one food allergen in all but one patient, regardless of the clinical response to food ingestion. False-positive reactions (positive leukocytotoxic test to food, which failed to provoke symptoms clinically) occurred equally in patients who were clinically allergic to one food; to controls who were not allergic at all; as well as in the group of patients who had other alleged clinical reactions to food. The test had little sensitivity evaluating the allergic group (73% false-negative test reactions) or in evaluating the nonallergic group (80% false-positive test reactions). The test also lacked specificity. In all 15 atopic patients, who were usually allergic only to one food, false-positive reactions averaged 5.5 foods (range, 1–11 food allergens per patient) [70]. In another study by Benson and Arkins, nine atopic patients and five controls were studied in a double-blind fashion using Bryan's technique [71]. Each patient was studied six times with 10 food allergens. The tests were found to be reproducible. However, the incidence of false-positive results in the atopic group was 70% and in the controls was 57%.

According to the position statement of the American Academy of Allergy and Immunology and the Center for Health Care Technology, the leukocytotoxic test lacks specificity and sensitivity. There is no proof that the test is efficacious in the diagnosis of immunologic reactions to foods – "food allergy." Finally, the test should be considered only for experimental use in well-controlled trials [29, 49].

Unfortunately, within recent years, this test has been the subject of unwarranted commercial promotion as a valid test of food allergy. This seems to be a shameful deception of the public and a waste of the health care dollar resource.

AUTOLOGOUS URINE IMMUNIZATIONS

In 1947, Plesch reported upon the results, in 12 patients, allegedly allergic, with a treatment consisting of injecting urine intramuscularly. According to the report, fresh urine from each patient was sterilized by filtration, boiling, or both and then injected into the patient in volumes of 0.25-5 ml [72]. This anecdotal report concerned relief of symptoms and signs, such as eczema, asthma, hay fever, urticaria, and food allergy, as well as jaundice, weakness, abdominal pain, constipation, migraine, and such conditions as rheumatic heart disease and pulmonary disease.

Urine injections were associated with significant local and occasional systemic reactions [11]. A suggestion, based on experimental animal information that such a treatment could be dangerous in that anti-glomerular basement membrane antibody might be produced and subsequently produce chronic human diseases, such as Goodpasture's syndrome, has been entertained [29]. This treatment has been condemmed by the American Academy of Allergy and Immunology, as well as other scientific organizations, as a practice that is not acceptable in the treatment of allergic disease [29, 73].

DEFINED DIETS AND BEHAVIORAL PROBLEMS

Tension–Fatigue Syndrome

Shannon noted in 1922 the symptoms of restlessness, irritability, and constant crying in children with food allergy [74]. Rowe in 1930 first described a syndrome that was usually attributed to food but sometimes as a result of sensitivity to inhalant allergens. This syndrome was characterized by fatigue, weakness, sleeplessness, and inability to think clearly [75]. The condition was associated with gastrointestinal disturbances, headaches, and aching of the muscles and joints. According to Rowe, when the offending food was eliminated from the diet, the somatic symptoms cleared. Speer, in 1954, enlarged on the syndrome and emphasized that the behavior of affected children had two contributing facets, which were termed "allergic tension" and "allergic fatigue"; hence, the name of the syndrome [76].

The reports concerning this syndrome are based upon anecdotal experience [77]. No double-blind studies done under strict control conditions have convincingly demonstrated that primary changes in the nervous system may be consistently provoked by exposure to food allergens. The subjective symptoms of irritability and tiredness may be simply a manifestation of chronic disease rather than specific allergen sensitivity.

Attention Deficit Disorder (with Hyperactivity)

The attention deficit disorder was first described by Hoffman in 1845 [78]. This syndrome usually describes children who are difficult to discipline or who receive poor grades in school. Hyperactivity is a component of this syndrome in some cases, as is impulsivity, distractibility, and excitability [79]. This syndrome may involve an estimate of 5-10% of American school children.

The cluster of symptoms does not represent a single disease. Rather than having a single etiology, the syndrome may be secondary to (1) organic factors, such as trauma, infection, lead intoxication, and significant birth hypoxia, (2) genetically defined predisposing factors, as well as (3) psychosocial factors, such as anxiety, maternal depression, and environmental stress [80]. In some, the etiology is unclear [79].

The possible relationship between this disorder and the presence of natural salicylates or other food additives was presented by Feingold in 1973 [81]. Later, a diet commonly bearing Feingold's name became popularized [82]. This diet was devoid of color, particularly tartrazine, as well as the known natural salicylates and the preservative sodium benzoate and BHA/BHT (butylated hydroxyanisole/butylated hydroxytoluene). Feingold claimed that 50% of the children who are hyperactive would be improved if they adhered to this defined diet [81, 82].

The exact mechanism by which the diet might work was not clear, except that Feingold suggested that a "toxicity" reaction occurred of some sort. Others linked the alleged hyperkinesis reaction to type I food reactions and the attention-fatigue syndrome [83].

Several well-controlled studies have challenged the Feingold hypothesis [78]. In an elaborate study done by Harley and his associates, reported in 1978, evaluating 36 school-aged children, no support for the beneficial effect of the diet in the hyperkinetic children was found as a consensus of parent and teacher ratings, classroom observations, and neuropsychiatric tests [84]. In a smaller study, involving 10 preschool boys, however, parents rated the majority improved on the Feingold diet [84]. A specific double-blind challenge with 27 mg of a mixture of artificial dyes to nine hyperactive boys failed to elicit a change in behavior [85]. In another challenge study, 35 mg of a color blend, disguised in a soda pop, demonstrated that 2 of 22 (9%) of the hyperactive children showed a significant deterioration in behavior [86].

Swanson and his colleagues challenged 20 hyperactive children with 100–150 mg of artificial dye mixture under controlled conditions in a laboratory situation. Using a special learning test, the children demonstrated progressively more errors when given the dye mixture than the placebo mix (and progressively less errors when given the placebo mix). This adverse effect appeared at ½ hr after ingestion and lasted approximately 3½ hr.

In the opinion of many, little if any value is given for the use of the Feingold diet in children with hyperkinesis [36, 78]. However, the NIH Consensus Conference on the subject, held in January 1982, came to the following conclusions [80].

1. The defined diet of the Feingold type may be helpful in a small number of young children with hyperkinesis. Changes, however, have not been consistent in nature.
2. Challenge with a very high dose of food colors in susceptible children might produce a pharmacological (drug) effect to depress learning in specific test situations.
3. Other factors in the diet are not well studied as to their affect on behavior (preservatives, natural components of the diet, metabolic effects, and sugars).
4. Allergic (hypersensitivity), as well as other immunologic reactions to foods or food additives, probably has nothing to do with any observed effects of the diet upon behavior.

The Consensus Conference was of the opinion that, though controversial and inconvenient, the Feingold type of defined diet has not been shown to cause clinical harm. It was further recommended that the diet may be tried once the child has been thoroughly investigated concerning other reasons for abnormal behavior [80].

The sugar content of the diet has been alleged to adversely affect behavior in young children. In an epidemiological study by Prinz and colleagues, he noted that hyperactive children tend to become more aggressive and restless and that normal children become more active on high-sugar diets [87]. Rappaport, however, recently used a double-blind sugar challenge in children reported by parents to be adversely behaviorly affected by sugar ingestion [88]. These children were challenged with either glucose or sucrose or a placebo (saccharin) in the amount equivalent to the sugar content of two candy bars. The sugar challenge was associated with a calming effect upon behavior.

Frequently, hyperactive behavior in children has been attributed to or associated with the atopic state [77, 83]. Often these children are accused of having "sugar" allergy (allegedly sensitive by specific source – corn, beet, or cane). In other cases, specific atopic IgE-mediated reactions to different foods are implicated. Usually, the exact mechanism of adverse reaction, however, has not been defined.

Recently, "double-blind" studies claim that adverse behavioral effects can be provoked by small amounts of allergen exposure and then neutralized [37–40]. These reports were based upon techniques described by Lee et al. and adapted by Dickey and Pfeiffer to the sublingual method (see Provocative Food Testing and Neutralization) [30, 34].

These studies do not establish the relationship between atopic disorder in children and hyperactive behavior. They do not represent adequate trials of the provocative-neutralization technique of diagnosis and treatment [11].

These techniques must still be considered unproven at this time and used only in well-controlled research situations [29]. Furthermore, diet manipulations in the management of the attention deficit syndrome with hyperkinesis should only be done under physician management once other possible causes of the syndrome have been investigated [80].

Though children with hyperkinesis may also be atopic, allergy per se has not been shown to be directly related, so that allergy-related diagnostic techniques and treatments are usually not indicated [78].

CONCLUSION

The diagnosis and treatment of adverse reactions to foods, in 1986, has not often reached the level of an exact science. Much must be learned before this level of perfection can be achieved. The emergence of those diagnostic and therapeutic techniques as well as their continued popularity is largely based upon our ignorance. It is hoped that the future will bring new resources to bear so that the many questions that exist in the field of diagnosis and treatment of adverse food reaction can be answered. Only then will diagnostic tests and treatment of dubious value fade from the medical scene and be of historical interest only.

REFERENCES

1. Ford, R. P. K., Hill, D. J., and Hosking, C. S. Cow's milk sensitivity: Immediate and delayed clinical patterns. *Arch. Dis. Child. 58*:856, 1983.
2. Galant, S. Common food allergens. In *Allergic Diseases of Infancy, Childhood and Adolescence*, C. W. Bierman and D. S. Pearlman (ed.), W. B. Saunders, Philadelphia, 1980, pp. 211–218.
3. Moroy, L. A., and Yung, W. H. Kunitz soybean trypsin inhibitor. *N. Engl. J. Med. 302*:1126, 1980.
4. Sachs, M. I., Jones, R. T., and Yunginger, J. W. Isolation and partial characterization of a major peanut allergen. *J. Allergy Clin. Immunol. 67*:27, 1981.
5. Hoffman, D. R., Day, E. D., and Miller, J. S. The major heat stable allergen of shrimp. *Ann. Allergy 47*:17, 1981.
6. Prausnitz, C., and Kustner, H. Studien uber neberempfindlichkeit. *Zentralbl. Bakteriol. 86*:160, 1921.

7. Spies, J. R., STevan, M. A., Stein, W. J., and Coulson, E. J. The chemistry of allergens. XX. New antigens generated by pepsin hydrolysis of bovine milk protein. *J. Allergy 45*:208, 1970.
8. Haddad, Z., Kaba, V., and Verma, S. IgE antibodies to peptic and peptic-tryptic digests of beta-lactoglobulin: Significance in food hypersensitivity. *Ann. Allergy 42*:368, 1979.
9. Schwartz, H. R., Nerurkon, L. S., Spies, J. R., Scanlon, R. T., and Bellanti, J. A. Milk hypersensitivity: RAST studies using new antigens generated by pepsin hydrolysis of beta-lactoglobulin. *Ann. Allergy 45*:242, 1980.
10. Norman, P. In vivo methods of the study of allergy. In *Allergy – Principles and Practice,* E. Middleton, C. Reed, and E. Ellis (eds.), C. V. Mosby, St. Louis, 1978, pp. 256–264.
11. Van Metre, T. Critique of controversial and unproven procedures for diagnosis and therapy of allergic disorders. *Pediatr. Clin. North Am. 30*:807, 1983.
12. Sampson, H. Role of immediate food hypersensitivity with pathogenesis of atopic dermatitis. *J. Allergy Clin. Immunol. 71*:473, 1983.
13. Siegel, S. *Non-parametric Statistics for the Behavior Sciences.* McGraw-Hill, New York, 1956.
14. Blackly, C. H. *Hay Fever: Its Courses, Treatment and Effective Prevention; Experimental Research.* Balliere, Tindall and Cox, London, 1880.
15. Ishizaka, K., and Ishizaka, T. Human reagenic antibodies and immunoglobulin E. *J. Allergy 42*:330, 1968.
16. Arbesman, C. E. In vitro and in vivo measurement of ragweed sensitivity. *J. Allergy Clin. Immunol. 53*:81, 1974.
17. Sweet, L., Yanari, S., Ringwald, U., Anderson, J., and Callies, Q. Comparison of radioallergosorbent test (RAST) with standard allergy diagnostic procedures in 100 unselected patients. *J. Allergy Clin. Immunol. 53*:82, 1974.
18. Sprecase, G. A., Pomper, G. G., Sherman, W. B., Lemlich, A., and Ziffer, H. The effect of antigen injections on skin reactivity to antigens. *J. Allergy 38*: 9, 1966.
19. Phillips, E. W. Relief of hayfever by intradermal injections of pollen extract. *JAMA 86*:182, 1926.
20. Hansel, F. K. Co-seasonal intracutaneous treatment of hay fever. *J. Allergy 12*:457, 1941.
21. Rinkel, H. J. Inhalant allergy. *Ann. Allergy 7*(I):625; (II):631; (III):639, 1949.
22. Willoughby, J. W. Serial dilution titration skin tests in inhalant allergy. *Otolaryngol. Clin. North Am. 7*:579, 1974.
23. Golbert, T. M. A review of controversial diagnostic and therapeutic techniques employed in allergy. *J. Allergy Clin. Immunol. 56*:170, 1975.
24. Norman, P. S. An overview of immunotherapy. *J. Allergy Clin. Immunol. 65*:87, 1980.
25. Van Metre, T., Adkinson, N., Lichtenstein, L., et al. A controlled study of the effectiveness of the Rinkel method of immunology for ragweed pollen hay fever. *J. Allergy Clin. Immunol. 65*:288, 1980.

26. Van Metre, T., Adkinson, N., Amodio, F., et al. A comparative study of the effectiveness of the Rinkel method and the current method of immunotherapy for ragweed pollen hay fever. *J. Allergy Clin. Immunol. 66*:500, 1980.

27. Hirsch, S., Kalbfleisch, J., Golbert, T., et al. Rinkel injection therapy: A multicenter controlled study. *J. Allergy Clin. Immunol. 68*:133, 1981.

28. Van Metre, T., Adkinson, N., Amodid, F., et al. A comparison of immunotherapy schedules for injection treatment of ragweed pollen hayfever. *J. Allergy Clin. Immunol. 69*:181, 1982.

29. American Academy of Allergy, Position Statement — controversial techniques. *J. Allergy Clin. Immunol. 67*:333, 1981.

30. Lee, C. H. A new test for diagnosis and treatment for food allergies. *Buchannon Co. Med. Bull. 25*:9 (Jan.), 1961.

31. Lee, C., Williams, R., and Buckley, E. Provocative testing and treatment for foods.

32. Rinkel, H. The managementof clinical allergy. IV. Food and mold allergy. *Arch. Otolaryngol. 77*:302, 1963.

33. Miller, J. *Food Allergy: Provocative Testing and Injection Therapy.* Charles C. Thomas, Springfield, Illinois, 1972.

34. Dicky, L. D., and Pfeiffer, G. Sublingual therapy in allergy. *Trans. Am. Soc. Ophthalmol. Otolaryngol. Allergy 5*:37, 1964.

35. Morris, D. L. Use of sublingual antigen in diagnosis and treatment of food allergy. *Ann. Allergy 27*:289, 1969.

36. Grieco, M. Controversial practices in allergy. *JAMA 247*:3106–3111, 1982.

37. Miller, J. A double-blind study of food extract injection therapy: A preliminary report. *Ann. Allergy 38*:185, 1977.

38. Rapp, D. Double-blind confirmation and treatment of milk sensitivity. *Med. J. Aust. 1*:571, 1978.

39. Rapp, D. Food allergy treatment for hyperkinesis. *J. Learning Disabilities 12*:42, 1979.

40. O'Shea, J., and Porter, S. Double-blind study of children with hyperkinetic syndrome treated with multi-allergen extract. *J. Learning Disabilities 14*: 189, 1981.

41. King, D. Can allergic exposure provoke psychological symptoms? A double-blind test. *Biol. Psych. 16*:3, 1981.

42. Kallin, E., and Collier, R. Relieving therapy for antigen exposure. *JAMA 217*:78, 1971.

43. Bronsky, E., Buckley, D., and Ellis, E. Evaluation of the provocation skin test technique. *J. Allergy 47*:104, 1971 (abstract).

44. Draper, L. Food testing in allergy: Intradermal, provocative or deliberate feeding. *Arch. Otolaryngol. 95*:169, 1972.

45. Breneman, J., Crook, W., Deamer, W., et al. Report of the Food Allergy Committee on sublingual method of provocative testing for food allergy. *Ann. Allergy 31*:382, 1973.

46. Breneman, J., Hurst, A., Heiner, D., et al. College of Allergists on the clinical evaluation of sublingual provocation testing method for diagnosis of food allergy. *Ann. Allergy 33*:164, 1974.

47. Crawford, L., Lieberman, P., Harfi, H., et al. A double-blind study of sub-cutaneous food testing sponsored by the Food Committee of the American Academy of Allergy (abstract). *J. Allergy Clin. Immunol. 57*:236, 1976.
48. Lehman, C. A double-blind study of sublingual provocative food testing: A study of its efficacy. *Ann. Allergy 45*:144, 1980.
49. *Federal Register,* vol. 48, no. 162, Friday, August 19, 1983, pp. 37716–37722.
50. McGovern, J., Rapp, D., Gardner, R., et al. Reliability of provocative-neutralization procedure. *Arch. Otolaryngol.* (submitted).
51. Rea, W., Podell, R., William, M., et al. Intracutaneous neutralization of food food sensitivity: A double-blind evaluation. *Arch. Otolaryngol.* (submitted).
52. Boris, M., Schiff, M., Weindorf, S., and Inselman, L. Bronchoprovocation blocked by neutralization therapy (abstract). *J. Allergy Clin. Immunol. 71*(2):92, 1983.
53. Taylor, W., Ohman, J., and Lowell, F. Immunotherapy in cat-induced asthma. *J. Allergy Clin. Immunol. 61*:283, 1978.
54. Ohman, J. Double-blind trial of immunotherapy in cat-induced asthma: In vitro responses (abstract). *J. Allergy Clin. Immunol. 71*(2), 1983.
55. Wide, L., Bennich, H., and Johansson, S. G. O. Diagnosis of allergy by an in vitro test for allergen antibodies. *Lancet 2*:1105, 1967.
56. Tipton, W. R. Evaluation of skin testing in the diagnosis of IgE-mediated diseases. *Pediatr. Clin. North Am. 30*:785, 1983.
57. Aas, K., and Lundkvish, U. The radioallergosorbent test with a purified allergen from codfish. *Clin. Allergy 3*:255, 1973.
58. Adkinson, N. F. Editorial. The radioallergosorbent test: Uses and abuses. *J. Allergy Clin. Immunol. 65*:1, 1980.
59. Position statement of the American Academy of Allergy and Immunology: Skin testing versus RAST. *NER Allergy Proc. 4*:224, 1983.
60. Evans, R. Variance in the measurement of serum-specific IgE antibody using the radioallergosorbent test (RAST) procedure (abstract). *J. Allergy Clin. Immunol. 65*:197, 1978.
61. Nalebuff, D., Fadal, R., and Ali, M. IgE in investigation and management of atopic disorders: Recent advances. *J. Cont. Educ. Otolaryngol. Allergy 40*:47, 1978.
62. Santrach, P., Parker, J., Jones, R., and Yunginger, J. Diagnostic and thera-peutic applications of a modified radioallergosorbent test and comparison with the conventional radioallergosorbent test. *J. Allergy Clin. Immunol. 67*:97, 1981.
63. Nalebuff, D. J., Fadal, R. G., and Ali, M. The study of IgE in the diagnosis of allergic disorders in an otolaryngology practice. *Otolaryngol. Head Neck Surg. 87*:351, 1979.
64. Kane, J., Wypych, J., Reisman, R., et al. Evaluation of serum RAST titers to determine initial doses of ragweed immunotherapy (abstract). *J. Allergy Clin. Immunol. 65*:33 (Suppl.), 1980.

65. Vaughan, W. Further studies on the leucopenic index in food allergy. *J. Allergy 6*:78, 1934.

66. Squire, T., and Lee, H. Lysis in vitro of sensitized leukocytes by ragweed antigen. *J. Allergy 18*:156, 1947.

67. Black, A. A new diagnostic method in allergic disease. *Pediatrics 17*:716, 1956.

68. Bryan, W. T. K., and Bryan, M. P. The application of in vitro cytotoxic reaction to clinical diagnosis of food allergy. *Laryngoscope 70*:810, 1960.

69. Bryan, W. T. K., and Bryan, M. P. Allergy in otolaryngology. In *Otolaryngology*, M. M. Paparella and D. A. Shumrick (eds.), W. B. Saunders, Philadelphia, 1973, Vol. 3, pp. 69–94.

70. Lieberman, P., Crawford, L., Bjelland, J., et al. Controlled study of the study of the cytotoxic food test. *JAMA 231*:728, 1975.

71. Benson, T., and Arkin, J. Cytotoxic testing for food allergy: Evaluation of reproducibility and correlation.

72. Plesch, J. Urine therapy. *Med. Press 218*:128, 1947.

73. Report from National Center for Health Care Technology. *JAMA 246*:1499, 1981.

74. Shannon, W. R. Neuropathic manifestation in infants and children as a result of anaphylactic reactions to foods contained in their dietary. *Am. J. Dis. Child. 24*:89, 1922.

75. Rowe, A. H. Allergic toxemia and fatigue. *Ann. Allergy 8*:72, 1950.

76. Speer, F. Allergic tension fatigue in children. *Ann. Allergy 12*:168, 1954.

77. Crook, W. G. Can what a child eats make him dull, stupid or hyperactive. *J. Learning Disabilities 13*:281, 1980.

78. Ribon, A., and Joshi, S. Is there any relationship between food additives and hyperkinesis? *Ann. Allergy 48*:275, 1982.

79. American Psychiatric Association, Committee on Nomenclature and Statistics. *Diagnostic and Statistical Manual of Mental Disorders (DSM-III)*, Third Edition. Washington, D. C., Am. Psychiatric Assoc., 1978.

80. NIH Consensus *Development Panel: Defined Diets in Childhood Hyperactivity*. Office for Medical Applications of Research, NIH Bldg. #1, Washington, D. C., 1982.

81. Feingold, B. F. Editorial: Food additives and child development. *Hosp. Pract. 8*:11, 1973.

82. Feingold, B. F. *Why your child is hyperactive*. Random House, New York, 1975.

83. Rapp, D. J. Does diet affect hyperactivity? *J. Learning Disabilities 11*:383, 1978.

84. Harley, J. P., Ray, R. S., Tomasi, L., et al. Hyperkinesis and food additives: Testing the Feingold hypothesis. *Pediatrics 61*:818, 1978.

85. Harley, J. P., Mathews, C. G., and Eichenman, P. Synthetic food colors and hyperactivity in children: A double-blind challenge experiment. *Pediatrics 62*:975, 1978.

86. Weiss, B., William, J. H., Margen, S., et al. Behavioral responses to artificial food colors. *Science 207*:1487, 1980.
87. Prinz, R. J., Roberts, W. A., and Hartman, E. Dietary correlates of hyper-active behavior in children. *J. Consult. Clin. Psychol. 48*:760, 1980.
88. Rapoport, J. L. Effects of dietary substances in children. *J. Psychiatr. Res. 17*:187, 1983.

13
Maintaining Patient Compliance During an Elimination Diet

EILEEN RHUDE YODER
Medical Diet Systems, Inc., Orland Park, Illinois

Many patients are willing to comply with the restrictive nature of an elimination diet during the diagnostic phase because they know it is a temporary measure to be enforced only until the offending food allergens are detected. However, once the food allergens are detected and identified and the patient must adhere to a diet based upon avoidance of the offending food allergens for an extended period of time, for 1-12 months, the patient soon finds the diet overwhelming and impractical [1-3].

Once the doctor has discovered which foods must be eliminated from the diet, the responsibility for complying with an elimination or avoidance diet falls to the patient. Unfortunately, it is not an easy responsibility and the patient soon encounters many difficulties in complying with the new diet.

PATIENT DIFFICULTIES WITH COMPLIANCE

Additional Time Necessary for Meal Management

Finding the time necessary for proper meal management is one major problem inherent in an elimination diet. The patient, or in the case of a child, the parent, must take extra time to read labels, to locate substitute ingredients, to seek out practical information on food allergies from professional sources, to prepare all meals using natural ingredients, to avoid processed or convenience foods, and, in some cases, to prepare separate hypoallergenic meals for different members of the family.

Inability to Identify Original Sources of an Ingredient

Seeking out practical information on food allergies involves determining which foods to substitute for those that produce food allergies. This involves reading labels very carefully. Eggs, for instance, might not appear on the label but a portion of the egg may be used in preparing the processed food, and the ingredient may be listed as "albumen." The same is true for milk. Even if milk is not listed on the label or the food product is listed as "non-dairy", it may still contain casein, a milk protein [4].

Sometimes food manufacturers label a specific food product in general terms. Modified food starch, for instance, is the general name applied to a substance that could be made from soybean, wheat, tapioca, or even potato. Another common problem involving ingredients is the nonspecific label. For example, a label may say, "May contain one or more of the following ingredients: soybean, cottonseed or corn oil." This means the food manufacturer has used the less costly or most available food ingredient for the product.

Sometimes the substitute ingredient is a by-product of the original ingredient. In the case of corn, for instance, the label may list "dextrose" or "fructose" or even "carmel flavoring," all of which may be derived from corn. To make matters worse, the patient may be wise enough to avoid all these ingredients and select a diet soft drink as a beverage, not knowing that the carbonation in the soda is part of the fermentation process of corn [5].

Even beyond food preparation, one must be careful. Some manufacturers of English muffins routinely dust the baking pan with corn meal and then fail to list it on the label because it is really not a true ingredient. This results in an unsuspecting consumer and a mysterious allergic food reaction.

Difficulties in Locating Hypoallergenic Ingredients

Of course, the more exotic the substitute ingredient, the more difficult it is to find a store that sells the ingredient. Many supermarkets sell the common grains, but only health food stores deal with the more unusual substitute ingredients, such as tapioca starch and potato starch. Health food stores also offer a wider selection of specialty foods – unusual foodstuffs like 100% rice flour bread – so people with food allergies should make a determined effort to locate as many health food stores as possible within a convenient radius of the home [6].

If the supermarket or the health food store fails to carry a wide enough selection of appetizing substitute ingredients, the food manufacturer can be contacted directly. Information on which stores in the local community carry a line of foods will be provided, or a bulk order can be sent directly from the factory to the customer. All of this depends on the distance to the nearest retail food outlet and the volume of ingredients or specialty foods needed.

Lack of Information on How to Cook with Substitute Ingredients

Many people fail to realize that when one ingredient is substituted for another, the proportions need to be changed. For example, when cooking without wheat, the gluten that helps hold together the bread is also eliminated. Other substitutes, including such grains as barley, rye, or rice, do not have the same consistency as wheat, so if formerly a cup of wheat was used in the recipe, a cup and a third of oat flour must now be used to compensate for the lack of consistency. Because of a change from one grain to another, the food must also be cooked at a different temperature. The easiest solution to preparing allergy-free meals is to use recipes from specially written allergy-free cookbooks.

Difficulties in Eating Out

Dealing with food allergies is difficult enough for an adult but it is especially painful for a child. Children are very sensitive to the psychological trauma of being identified as "different." Those who cannot share in the simple joys of milk and cookies can be labeled odd and strange by their young peers.

The child thus is faced with an awkward and potentially dangerous dilemma: eat the allergen and remove the stigma, or pass up the illness-producing foods and risk the stares and murmurs of all those around the child. It is not an easy choice. And with a little understanding and advance preparation on the part of parents and children alike, it is a choice that does not have to be made. For instance, if a child in the group is allergic to cookies and cookies are planned for the entire group, prepare a simple snack the child can eat and still enjoy the company of friends. The same applies for milk. Give the child juice, or give all the children the the choice of milk or juice. That way they can each select the beverage of choice and this removes the onus of singling out one child for "different" treatment.

Although this approach will work in a social environment, it is impractical for everyday use in school. In this instance, it is wise for the parent to meet with the principal, the secretarial staff, the cafeteria staff, and the child's teacher or teachers. The secretarial staff is important because often the child's medicine is kept in the school office and the secretarial staff will have more contact with the child when he or she needs the medicine than anyone else. It is also important to engage the secretarial staff as an ally in the event the child suffers a food allergy attack when a substitute teacher is conducting class. The secretarial staff will assure the substitute teacher that the child's medical needs are genuine at a time when every minute is critical [7].

Dealing with the child's noontime meal is easy if the school supplies a menu in advance. The parent or child decides which meals the child can eat and prepares a lunch for those days when an inappropriate meal is to be served. Or, if the menu is not sufficiently detailed, the parent can resolve the problem by preparing all the child's lunches at home.

Problems with allergy-producing ingredients sometimes arise when traveling, especially if one is in a situation where the menu presented is limited. Airlines, for instance, offer a limited choice or no choice at all. To avoid this situation entirely, call the airline before a trip and order a special meal or bring a home-prepared meal.

At dinner parties, one can do approximately the same thing. Simply contact the hostess as soon as the invitation is received and explain the problem. Politely inquire about the menu and identify any foods that might trigger an allergic reaction. The hostess will probably respond by changing the menu or preparing alternate dishes from which to select. One can also offer to bring allergy-free dishes for all the guests.

For situations in which one meal is served to a large group of people, just eat the foods that are safe. It is generally wise to snack a little before the meal, if possible, or certainly after the dinner if still hungry.

Developing New Food Allergies

Another common problem experienced by food allergy sufferers is the emergence of new allergies. Often when an ingredient is removed from the diet and another is substituted, the patient will eat large amounts of the substitute ingredient. Since the body has already reacted to the original ingredient in a negative way, it can react the same way to the substitute ingredient after repeated or prolonged exposure. Thus, in time, the body can reject both the original and the substitute ingredients. One way to avoid this is to vary the diet. Discover many substitutes, if possible, and vary one's diet so there is no dependence on any one ingredient to the exclusion of other suitable ingredients [8].

DIETARY ORGANIZATION

Faced with difficulty in deciding which ingredients to use in place of those that bring on allergic reactions, and then where to find the ingredients, how to prepare them, and, of course, whether the family will like them at all, many people simply give up and run the risk of bringing on the the original food allergy by reverting to the original ingredient. These are usually patients who suffer milder reactions. They might argue that the hassles of finding new ingredients, preparing them, and then suffering through a less-than-wonderful meal simply do not outweigh the enjoyment and light-to-moderate suffering that goes with eating the offending ingredient. So they do. Others, however, especially those who experience severe or disabling, perhaps even life-threatening allergic reactions, will usually opt for a very bland but safe diet that is easy to prepare but boring to eat. It is all a value judgment, and it depends on how difficult it is to find and prepare the substitute meals versus the possible harm that can come from eating the offending ingredient.

One of the first steps in overcoming the difficulties of a dietary change is to prepare and maintain a dietary notebook. This helps the patient overcome the many frustrations of learning an entirely new way of life. It serves as an educational manual and cookbook. It also serves as an education manual to other family members who are not familiar with allergy-free cooking.

The notebook should be hardcovered, two- or three-ringed, and have dividers with folders or pockets. The dividers should be labeled into different sections, for example,

1. List of acceptable allergy-free foods
2. List of allergenic foods to avoid
3. Master grocery list
4. List of acceptable name brands and food sources
5. Recipes
6. Menus
7. Practical tips and suggestions
8. Miscellaneous

On the inside front cover, the notebook should contain the following information:

Physician's name, address, and phone number
Hospital's name, address, and phone number
Pharmacy's name, address, and phone number
Emergency phone numbers of anyone else
List of any medications patient is taking along with directions for
    administration
Any other pertinent information

The first section (list of acceptable allergy-free foods) should emphasize all the many different foods allowed and include the various ways the food can be obtained. For example, apples can be served as apples, applesauce, or apple juice, or rice can be served as brown rice, rice flour, cream of rice, rice vinegar, puffed rice cereal, rice cakes, rice syrup, or rice noodles.

The next section should include the list of allergenic foods to avoid and should also include the many different ways a food can be processed and where the offending food might be found. For example, if milk is to be eliminated from the diet, all the different dairy products should be listed plus a list of the other names for milk, like casein or whey.

Creating a master grocery list saves many hours in trying to remember what foods are allowed and what needs to be bought. If a master copy is typed up, photocopies can be made and kept in the folder. Keep a copy of the list attached to the bulletin board or refrigerator. As foods are needed, they can be checked off or circled immediately and the list can be brought to the grocery store or health food store. If there are many stores to go to each week, the master list can be divided into sections listing each store's name and what foods can be obtained at that particular store.

People with restrictive diets are usually looking for new foods to try. Sometimes, after a particular food was bought, the location, name of the store or brand name of the food might not be remembered. By keeping a systemized list of the new foods that are bought along with where the store is located, and the brand name and food manufacturer's address, it will be easier to obtain the same brand of food again.

In the next section, an individualized collection of good-tasting recipes can be kept. Any variations in the recipe or comments about the recipe should be included.

After one has created a well-balanced, appetizing meal, it would be helpful to write down the menu. Menus can be divided into sections, such as lunch, dinner, holiday meal, summer picnic, or parties. Again, this list is primarily a time saver when one is unable to think of what to eat.

As one begins to adhere to the restrictive diet, new facts are discovered that will help in adjusting to the diet. These practical tips and suggestions should be written down so they may be shared with other allergy sufferers or recalled at a later time. For example, tapioca starch or arrowroot starch makes a good substitute for wheat flour.

Any additional information, such as articles and newsletters related to food allergies or a daily food diary, can be kept in the miscellaneous section.

Obviously, this notebook will take additional effort in the beginning to assemble and to maintain, but over a period of time, it will serve as both a time saver and as an educational source of information for everyone who must deal with the patient's allergies.

MEAL MANAGEMENT

As the elimination diet is undertaken, much time will be spent reading labels to determine if there are any hidden food allergens in the packaged, processed foods. The most common allergens are milk, eggs, and wheat, and these are the most difficult to remove from the diet. Corn, because of its many uses, is another common allergen that is almost impossible to avoid in all its forms. Instructions for milk-, egg-, wheat-, and corn-free cooking are given. If the patient has other food allergens, information on how to cook without the allergen can be collected and included in the patient's individualized notebook.

Wheat-Free Cooking

Wheat and other grain members (corn, rice, oats, rye, and barley) are the staples of the human diet. Because most Americans eat wheat on a daily basis, avoidance becomes difficult.

Special recipes are needed to prepare acceptable foods. Breads, cakes, cookies, and pastries made without wheat do not always have the same taste, texture, appearance, and aroma as the baked products one is used to.

Wheat flour contains gluten, which gives a good structural framework to breads and cakes. Other flours contain little or no gluten and therefore are generally used in combination with wheat flour. Read the labels carefully; even the soybean-based baked goods and rye or potato bread may contain some gluten or wheat to help it rise.

Baked products made without wheat flour tend to be heavier and more crumbly than those made with wheat flour. This difference is most noticeable in breads and cakes.

Flours

Flours and starches suitable for use in baked products are milled from cereal grains and other starchy portions of plants, such as roots.

Oats, barley, corn, rice, and rye are all from the grass family. Oat flour tends to produce a somewhat sticky feel in the mouth. Rice flour gives a distinct graininess to baked goods and is bland in flavor. It is used most successfully when mixed with potato flour and in recipes in which eggs and milk are used. Rye flour has a dark color and distinctive flavor. Rye baked goods are more compact and heavier than wheat products because of the low amount of gluten. Corn flour produces a heavy, crumbly baked good since it is gluten free. Barley has a mild flavor and contains a slight amount of gluten, making a nice substitute for wheat.

Barley, oats, rye, and wheat must all be eliminated by those individuals who are gluten intolerant.

Potato flour is made from cooked potatoes and is useful as a thickener in sauces. When mixed with soybean flour, potato flour makes acceptable baked goods. Soy flour is generally milled from the whole bean and therefore has a high fat content. Tapioca flour is the starch made from the fleshy root of the bitter manioc or cassava plant. It is best used as a thickener or for small cookies. Arrowroot starch can be derived from the arrowroot plants, although there are eight different biologic families of arrowroot.

Buckwheat flour is not a grain but a member of the rhubarb family. It makes acceptable pancakes and breads or can be mixed with another grain.

Newly rediscovered amaranth is in a different family from the grains. Used by the Aztecs some 3000 years ago, it was their primary source of food. In order to control the Aztec population, Cortez ordered all the amaranth destroyed. It was recently discovered growing wild in Central America and was brought to the United States. It is high in protein and, when mixed with a grain, contains 100% of the essential amino acids [9]. Recipes have been developed for hypoallergenic individuals.

Substitutions

Various flours can be substituted for 1 c of wheat:

> 1 c corn flour
> ¾ c coarse cornmeal
> ¾ c cornstarch
> 5/8 c potato flour
> 7/8 c buckwheat
> 7/8 c rice flour
> 1-1/3 c ground rolled oats
> 1-1/8 c oat flour
> ¾ c soybean flour
> 1 c barley
> 1 c millet
> 1¼ c rye flour
> 1 c tapioca flour

> *Flour Combinations Equaling 1 c of Wheat.*

> ½ c rye flour + 1/3 c potato flour
> 1/3 c rye flour + 5/8 c rice flour
> 1 c soy flour + ¾ c potato flour
> 5/8 c rice + 1/3 c potato flour
> ½ c cornstarch + ½ c rye flour
> ½ c cornstarch + ½ c potato flour

> *Spaghetti and Noodle Substitutes.*

> Chinese bean threads (mung beans)
> Rice
> Rice noodles
> Corn noodles

Thickeners. To replace 1 tbsp of wheat flour in soups, sauces, gravies, and puddings, use one of the following:

½ tbsp cornstarch
½ tbsp potato starch
½ tbsp rice flour
½ tbsp arrowroot
2 tsp quick-cooking tapioca
2 tbsp uncooked rice
½ tbsp lima bean flour
½ tbsp gelatin
1 tbsp tapioca flour
1 egg

Many processed foods contain wheat as an ingredient; therefore it is important to know the names of ingredients that indicate the presence of wheat [10]:

All-purpose flour
Bran
Bread crumbs
Bread flour
Bulgar
Cake flour
Cracked wheat flour
Cracker meal and crumbs
Durum
Enriched flour
Farina flour
Gluten flour
Graham crackers and crumbs
Graham flour
Hydrolyzed vegetable protein (HVP)*
Malt†
Malt syrup†
Monosodium glutamate (MSG)*
Pastry flour
Phosphated flour
Semolina
Wheat
Wheat flour
Wheat germ

*Gluten and/or wheat is often present, but not always.
† Although gluten is not present in these products, the protein of malted barley may bring about a reaction to those sensitive to gluten. This is thought to happen when glutenlike proteins are created within the body when combined with other proteins in the body [4].

Wheat starch
White flour
Whole wheat flour

Cooking Suggestions

Wheat-free products should be baked at a lower temperature and for a longer period of time.

Substitute flours have a higher fat content than wheat; therefore, decrease the amount of shortening in each recipe.

When combining flours, sift several times to make sure the flours are well mixed.

To help improve the texture of baked goods, an extra amount of baking powder (½ tsp per c of flour) should be added..

Refrigerating dough a half-hour before baking helps improve the texture and flavor.

Foods tend to stick to baking pans; therefore, grease pans well or use paper liners. Because of the tendency to crumble, it is better to make cupcakes instead of cakes.

It is best to use small-sized loaf pans for quick breads; do not pour the dough higher than 2–4 in. because the bottom will not be cooked thoroughly.

A faster and easier way to prepare baked goods is to buy wheat-free ready mixes.

Substitute crushed corn flakes or Rice Krispies for breading foods.

Corn-Free Cooking

Corn is one of the most widely used ingredients in America because it is easily and cheaply grown. Corn can be found in practically all processed foods and therefore is one of the most difficult foods to avoid. Learning how to identify corn in its many forms is the first step in developing a corn-free diet [11].

Corn can be made into corn syrup, corn meal, corn oil, and corn starch. It can be further processed into

Modified food starch*
Dextrin
Fructose
Maltodextrins
Dextrose
Lactic acid

*Modified food starch can also be derived from other ingredients, such as tapioca, potatoes, or wheat.

Sorbitol
Mannitol
Caramel color
Alcohol

Corn is used in the preparation of more foods than any other edible food. Below is only a partial list of some of the many foods in which corn may be used [12].

Baby foods	Gelatin desserts
Bacon	Glucose and fructose products
Baking mixes	Graham crackers
Baking powders	Grape juice
Batters for frying	Gravies
Beers	Grits
Bleached wheat flours	Gums, chewing
Bourbon and other whiskeys	Gin
Breads and pastries	Ginger ale
Cakes	Hams, cured
Candies	Harvard beets
Carbonated beverages	Ices
Catsups	Ice cream
Cereals	Jams and jellies
Cheeses	Leavening agents and yeasts
Chili	Liquors
Chop suey	Margarines and shortenings
Chow mein	Meats, processed and cold cuts
Coffee, instant	Milk, in paper cartons
Colas	Monosodium glutamate
Cookies	Peanut butter and canned peanuts
Confectioner's sugar	Pickles
Cream pies	Powdered sugar
Dextrose	Puddings and custards
Eggnog	Salad dressings
Fish, prepared and processed	Salt
Foods, fried	Sandwich spreads
French dressing	Sauces for sundaes, meats, fish, etc.
Frostings	Sausages
Fruits, canned and frozen	Sherbets
Fruit juices	Soft drinks
Fruit pies	Spaghetti
Frying fats	Soups, creamed, thickened, and vegetable

Soybean milk
Syrups, corn
Teas, instant
Tortillas
Vanillin
Vegetables, canned creamed and frozen
Vinegar, distilled
Waffles
Wines

Remember, read the labels since some of the products may be corn free.

Nonfood Uses

Corn can also be used in other ways. Plastic food wrappers, waxed paper cartons for milk and some juices, paper cups, and waxed coated paper plates are dusted with cornstarch to prevent sticking. Cornstarch is even in body powders, cosmetics, toothpastes, and soaps. Corn is used in many medicines and vitamins. Corn may also be used as an adhesive for postage stamps and envelopes.

Because of the widespread use of corn, the only way to avoid corn is through home preparation of all foods. Corn-free cooking is still the easiest part of staying on a corn-free diet. Simply substitute another starch for thickening foods. Buy corn-free baking powder and use maple syrup, honey, or sugar in place of corn syrup. Use corn-free oil, such as safflower oil [8].

Egg-Free Cooking

Egg is probably the second most common food allergy in infants and young children, with egg whites causing the most problems.

Eggs are found in most processed foods. Sometimes the presence of eggs is not indicated on the label. For example, egg whites may be brushed on breads, rolls, pretzels, and other baked goods to give a glazed effect. Wine, beer, real root beer, coffee, bouillon, and consomme may be clarified with egg. Some cholesterol-free "egg replacers" may have egg whites as an ingredient [13].

Egg is present if the label indicates any of the following:

Albumen
Ovalbumen
Globulin
Ovomucin
Ovomucoid
Powdered or dried egg
Silicoalbuminate
Vitellin

Ovovitellin
Yolk
Livetin

Cooking Suggestions

For cake mixes, use 1 tsp of vinegar for each egg called for in the recipe.

Since egg is a binder, baked goods without eggs will crumble easily. It is best to make cupcakes instead of a cake.

Use 1 tsp of xanthan gum in each recipe to help hold the baked good together (available through Gluten Intolerance Group, Seattle, WA).

Add an extra half-teaspoon of egg-free baking powder for each egg called for in a recipe.

For thickening cream dishes and sauces, add extra flour or cornstarch.

A good egg replacer mix for 1 egg [8] is:

2 tbsp allowed starch	½ tsp baking powder
½ tbsp allowed shortening	2 tbsp liquid

Grease and lightly flour the cookie sheet to prevent cookies from spreading.

Add extra ingredients, like raisins, nuts, coconut, seeds, or spices to disguise the flavor of egg-free cookies and cakes.

Substitute mashed bananas, apricot puree, or pureed vegetables in place of eggs (2 tbsp for each egg replaced).

Use unflavored gelatin (1 tsp dry gelatin or mixed with 2 tbsp liquid) to replace an egg.

Since homemade egg-free mayonnaise generally tastes more like flour and vinegar mixed together, it is best to avoid recipes calling for mayonnaise, or try Hain's imitation mayonnaise. (Alwasy read the label first to see if ingredients may have changed.)

Milk-Free Cooking

Milk allergy is the most common allergy among infants and children under the age of 3 [4]. This is because of the immature or inefficient gastrointestinal system [14-17]. Milk allergy can cause a variety of symptoms throughout life. For example, after a period of avoidance and freedom from symptoms, the symptoms may change if milk is once again ingested. An infant may suffer from diarrhea, but when older, the young child may suffer from rhinitis.

Milk has many different protein fractions, but casein and whey are the most allergy causing.

The whey fraction, which contains lactalbumin and β-lactoglobulin, causes the most reactions. Individuals who are allergic only to the whey (not the casein) may be able to tolerate goat's milk since the whey fraction differs from cow's milk, or they may tolerate powdered, boiled, or evaporated cow's milk, since the whey protein is changed by the heating process. Those allergic to just the whey (lactose intolerant) will have to avoid cottage cheese and other soft processed cheeses but may be able to tolerate hard cheeses, such as Swiss, Edam, Parmesan, Cheddar, Gruyere, and Romano.

Casein remains stable during the heating process, so powdered, evaporated, or boiled milk cannot be consumed. The casein is similar both in goat's milk and cow's milk, so both must be avoided. Even "nondairy" creamers, imitation processed cheeses, imitation cream cheese, imitation sour cream, and soybean-based ice cream may contain casein. Read all labels carefully.

Labels may have one of the following names if a product contains milk or milk protein:

Lactose
Caseinate
Potassium caseinate
Casein
Lactalbumen
Lactoglobulin
Curds
Wheys
Milk solids

Substitutions

An equal amount of any liquid can be substituted for milk.

Goat's milk, fresh, powdered, or evaporated
Soybean milk; add 1 tsp vanilla or lime juice to improve the flavor
Banana, nut, or oat milk (see recipes)
Vegetable water, that is, water used to cook vegetables (add 1 tbsp extra shortening to recipe)
Fruit juices or vegetable juices (add 1 tbsp extra shortening or oil to recipe)

For sour cream, mix ½ c allowed starch with ¾ c water, soybean milk, or goat's milk; stir in ¼ c vinegar.

Cooking Suggestions

Try fruits or fruit juices in place of milk on hot cereal.
Chill soybean milk first and add flavoring.
Freeze fresh goat's milk first, then thaw; this eliminates some of the strong flavor and odor.

Use kosher margarine, bread, and processed meats.
Use fruit juice in place of milk when making quick breads.
Use pure broth as a substitute for milk in sauces and gravies.
Fry foods in safflower oil or allowed oil instead of butter or margarine.

REFERENCES

1. Crawford, L. V. Allergic diets. In *Allergic Diseases of Infants, Childhood and Adolescence*, C. W. Bierman and D. S. Pearlman (eds.), W. B. Saunders, Philadelphia, 1980.
2. Saarineu, U., and Kajosaari, M. Does dietary elimination in infancy prevent or only postpone a food allergy? *Lancet 1*:166–167, 1980.
3. Gerrard, J. W. *Food Allergy: New Perspectives*. Charles C. Thomas, Springfield, Illinois, 1980.
4. Frazier, C. *Coping with Food Allergies*. Quadringle/The New York Times Book Co., New York, 1974.
5. Yoder, E. *Corn-Free Cooking*. Healthful Living Co., New York, 1982.
6. Greer, R. New foods for special diets. *Nutr. Food Sci. 3*:23–24, 1978.
7. Yoder, E. *Allergy-Free Cooking, A Guide to an Allergen-Free Elimination Diet*. Healthful Living Co., New York, 1982.
8. Stevens, L. *The Complete Book of Allergy Control*. Macmillan, New York, 1983.
9. Cole, J. A. *From the Past, for the Future*. Rodale Press, Emmaus, Pennsylvania, 1982.
10. Allergy Foundation of Canada, *A Guide to Living with Wheat Allergy*, Allergy Coundation of Canada, Sask., Canada, 1978
11. Randolph, T., and Yeager, L. B. Corn sugar as an allergen. *Ann. Allergy*, Sept.–Oct., 1949.
12. Breneman, J. *Basics of Food Allergies*. Charles C. Thomas, Springfield, Illinois, 1978.
13. Allergy Foundation of Canada, *A Guide to Living with Egg Allergy*, Sask., Canada, 1978.
14. Grogan, F. T. Food allergy in children after infancy. *Pediatr. Clin. North Am. 16*:217–225, 1969.
15. Shiner, M., Ballard, J., and Smith, M. E. The small-intestine mucosa in cow's milk allergy. *Lancet 1*:136–140, 1975.
16. Deamer, W. C., Gerrard, J. W., and Speer, F. Cow's milk allergy, a critical review. *J. Family Pract. 2*:223–232, 1979.
17. Halpern, S. R., Sellers, W. A., Johnson, R. B., Anderson, D. W., Saperstein, S., and Reisch, J. Development of childhood allergy in infants fed breast, soy or cow's milk. *J. Allergy Clin. Immunol. 3*:139–151, 1972.

APPENDIX 1: FOOD MANUFACTURERS

AFTER THE FALL PRODUCTS, INC.
Box B, Newfane, VT 05345
> Apple-raspberry juice
> Apple-apricot juice
> Apple-pineapple juice
> Apple-cherry juice
> Purepear juice

AMERICAN MAPLE PRODUCTS, CORP.
Newport, VT 05855
> Old Colony Pure Maple Sugar Candy (100% pure maple syrup)
> Old Colony Pure Maple Butter Spread (100% pure maple syrup whipped until creamy)
> Old Colony Pure Maple Syrup (100% pure)
> Old Colony Granulated Maple Sugar (100% pure; comes in a shaker dispenser or hard slabs)

ARDEN ORGANICS, INC.
99 Pond Road, Asheville, NC 28806
> Arden Plain Rice Cakes (organic, whole brown rice and sea salt)
> Arden Rice Cakes (with sesame)
> Arden Plain Rice Cakes (no salt added)

ARROWHEAD MILLS, INC.
110 South Lawton, Hereford, TX 79045
> Arrowhead Mills Oils (no preservatives, unrefined; sunflower, safflower, soybean, peanut, and sesame)
> Deaf Smith Peanut Butter (100% peanuts)
> Arrowhead Mills Organic Grains, Seeds, and Nuts

CALIFORNIA GOAT DAIRYMEN'S ASSOC., INC.
P.O. Box 934, Turlock, CA 95380
> Miracle Brand Evaporated Goat Milk
> Miracle Brand Powdered Goat Milk

CHICAGO DIETETIC SUPPLY, INC.
405 East Shamut, La Grange, IL 60525
> Feather River Rice Cakes (whole brown rice, sesame seeds, and water)
> Featherweight Cereal-Free Baking Powder
> Featherweight Tapioca Starch Flour
> Featherweight Potato Starch

Featherweight Oat Flour
Featherweight Rice Flour
Featherweight Full Fat Soybean Flour
Featherweight water packed fruits and vegetables
Mail orders accepted.

CHICO-SANS, INC.
P.O. Box 810, Chico, CA 95926
Rice Crackers (whole brown rice, sesame seeds, and salt)
Yinnie's Taffy
Yinnie's Rice Syrup (rice, water, and barley malt)
Yinnie's Caramel [oat powder, raisins, almonds, sesame oil, coconut, lecithin
    lecithin (from sesame seeds), natural vanilla, and agar]
Miso (soybeans)
Seaweeds

CZIMER FOOD, INC.
Box 285, Lockport, IL 60441
Organic foods, exotic meats and fish
Mail orders accepted.

EL MOLINO MILLS
Box 2250, City of Industry, CA 91746
Sunflower and sesame seeds (no preservatives or additives)
Cara Coa Carob Powder (100% carob)
Brown rice (natural, unpolished, 100% pure)
Rolled oats, puffed rice cereal (100% whole grain, no sugar or additives)

ELAM'S
2625 Gardner Road, Broadview, IL 60153
Elam Brown Rice Flour
Elam Soy Flour
Elam Steel Cut Oatmeal

ENER-G FOODS, INC.
Box 24723, Seattle, WA 98124
Arrowroot Starch
Unsweetened Coconut
Ener-G Rice Mix
Ener-G Oat Mix
Ener-G Egg Replacer
Jolly Joan Pure Soyquik

Nut Milk
Many other low-allergen foods
Mail orders accepted.

HAIN'S PURE FOOD CO., INC.
P.O. Box 54841, Terminal Annex, Los Angeles, CA 90054
Hain Natural Potato Chips (safflower oil)
Hain Eggless Mayonnaise (soy, water, honey, cider, vinegar, lemon juice,
natural spices, algin, and onion oil)
Hain Safflower Margarine (safflower, soybean, water, salt, and lecithin,
colored with carotene)
Hain Soy Oil Shortening (solid soy and vitamin E)
Hain Nut Butters: Almond, Cashew, Peanut, and Sesame
Hain Preserves: Apple, Apricot, Grape, Orange Marmalade, Red Raspberry,
Seedless Blackberry, and Strawberry
Hain Cider Vinegar
Hain Sea Salt
Hain Natural Imitation Catsup

INTERSALES, INC.
55 Virginia Avenue, West Nyack, NY 10994
Ka-Me Plain Rice Crunch
Ka-Me Saifun Bean Threads (cellophane noodles containing mung bean
starch and water)

SHEDD'S FOOD PRODUCTS
Detroit, MI 48238
Willow Run Margarine

VERMONT COUNTRY MAPLE, INC.
P.O. Box 53, Jerico Center, VT 05465
Pure Maple Syrup
Pure Maple Sugar Granules

APPENDIX 2: RECIPES

Beverages

Apricot–Apple Shake

1 can (16 oz) water-packed apricots, drained	½ c milk or allowed substitute 6-10 ice cubes
½ c applesauce	

Combine all ingredients in blender, and liquefy. Makes 2¾ c.

Banana Ade

2 ripe bananas, cut into pieces	5-6 pineapple chunks
2 c pineapple juice	

Put pineapple juice into blender container, and process at high speed, adding small chunks of fruit a few at a time. Blend until smooth and frothy.

Tropical Shake

1 frozen banana	2½ c milk or allowed substitute
½ c flaked, unsweetened coconut	½ tsp pure vanilla
2 tbsp peanut butter or nut butter	

Puree banana, coconut, peanut butter, and 1 c milk or allowed substitute. Blend until creamy, then add remaining milk or allowed substitute and vanilla. Makes 4 c.

Nut, Banana, or Oat Milk

1/3 c nuts or seeds (cashews, walnuts, sliced almonds, sunflower seeds, or sesame seeds	*or* 2 tsp rolled oats *or* ½ small banana 1 c water

Combine nuts, seeds, oats, or banana and water in blender on highest speed until smooth. Use instead of cow's milk for baking and on cereals. Banana milk is good on cereal but must be used immediately.

Coconut Milk

meat of 1 coconut, cut into pieces	liquid from 1 fresh coconut 2 c hot water

Whirl all ingredients in blender at high speed until liquefied. Let cool to luke-warm. Strain in a sieve, pressing out liquid. The milk can be used in recipes and freezes well. (Use grated coconut left in sieve for baking.)

Bread, Muffins, Pancakes, and Cereals

Corn Bread

1 c cornmeal	2 eggs or egg substitute
2 tbsp sugar	½ c milk or allowed substitute
¼ tsp salt	2 tbsp allowed margarine
2 tsp baking powder	

Mix dry ingredients. Melt margarine. Add margarine, eggs, and milk all at once
to dry ingredients, and blend well. Pour into greased 8-in. square pan. Bake at
425°F for 20-25 min.

Barley Bread

1 tsp sugar	¼ tsp salt
1 c barley flour	2 tbsp milk or allowed substitute
¼ c rice flour	2 tbsp allowed oil
1 tbsp baking powder	1 c water
¼ tsp baking soda	

Put all dry ingredients in bowl unsifted. Put all wet ingredients in at once. Mix
until blended. Bake at 350°F for about 45 min.
Bread will keep for a week in the refrigerator.

Oatmeal Bread

1 c rolled oats	2 eggs or egg substitute
1 c hot water	¼ tsp baking soda
¼ c maple syrup or honey	3 tsp baking powder
¼ tsp salt	

Mix rolled oats and hot water. Let stand 5 min. Stir in honey, eggs, and salt.
Add flour, soda, and baking powder, and stir until all ingredients are well mixed.
Turn into greased 9 X 5 in. loaf pan, and let stand 20 min in a warm place. Bake
at 350°F for 45 min.
Bread is about 1½-2 in.

   Variations.   You may substitute 1 mashed banana for eggs.

Cornmeal Potato Starch Muffins

2/3 c cornmeal, white	½ tsp sugar
1/3 c potato flour	1 egg or egg substitute
2 tsp baking powder	½ c milk or allowed substitute
½ tsp salt	1 tsp allowed margarine, melted

Sift dry ingredients together. Beat egg slightly, add milk, and stir gently into dry
ingredients. Add melted margarine, and stir only enough to combine. Fill greased
muffin tins two-thirds full. Bake at 400°F for about 30 min.

Cream of Rye Muffins

½ c Cream of Rye cereal	4 tsp baking powder
1 c rice flour	½ tsp salt
2 tbsp brown sugar, firmly packed	2 tbsp allowed oil

Blend dry ingredients, add oil and 1 c water, and mix well. Batter will seem too thin but will thicken if left to stand only a couple of minutes. Spoon into oiled muffin tins. Bake in preheated 400°F oven for 15 min.

Potato Pancakes

1 c mashed potatoes, seasoned	½ tsp salt
1 c finely grated uncooked	½ tsp baking powder
potatoes	2 tbsp allowed margarine

Combine all ingredients, and shape into pancakes. A little oat flour may be added, if necessary, to hold pancakes together. Sprinkle both sides of cakes with oat flour. Heat oil over medium heat. Place pancakes in oil, and allow raw potatoes to cook.
Serve with maple syrup.

Rice Waffles

2 c rice flour	2 c water
4 tsp baking powder	3 tbsp allowed oil
1 tbsp sugar	

Sift dry ingredients together. Add water and oil, gradually stirring mixture constantly until smooth. Bake on a hot waffle iron greased with allowed oil.

Granola

¼ c unsweetened applesauce	¾ tsp salt
¼–½ c honey	2¼ c rolled oats
1 tbsp allowed oil	½ c sliced almonds or cashews
1 tsp pure vanilla	¼ c grated unsweetened coconut

Mix applesauce, honey, oil, vanilla, and salt in a large mixing bowl. Add oats, nuts, and coconut. Stir enough to coat dry ingredients. Spread in a 13 X 9 in. pan, and toast at 375°F for 20–25 min, stirring occasionally. Cool, and add ¼ c raisins, if desired.
Store in an airtight container.
Eat within 2 weeks.

Casseroles and Meat Dishes

Baked Chicken with Tomato Rice Stuffing

2 lb cut-up chicken	1 c cooked tomatoes
1/3 c chopped celery	½ c water
¼ c chopped green pepper	¾ tsp salt
1/3 c chopped onion	dash pepper
2/3 c uncooked rice	¼ tsp powdered sage

Brown chicken in oil in heavy skillet. Preheat oven to 350°F. While chicken browns, combine remaining ingredients in mixing bowl. Turn rice mixture into 11 X 7 in. baking dish. Arrange chicken on rice. Sprinkle with additional salt, pepper, and paprika. Cover. Bake 1 hr, or until chicken is tender.

Baked Fish in Chips

4 fish fillets	1 tsp onion powder or garlic powder
2 tbsp allowed oil	1 tsp dried parsley
1 tbsp lemon juice (optional)	1½ c crushed potato chips

Dip fish in blended oil, lemon juice, onion powder, and parsley. Roll in crushed chips, and lay on rack in shallow pan. Bake in 425°F oven for 20 min. or until fish flakes easily.

Beef Stew

2 lb boneless beef chuck in 2 in. pieces	2 small bay leaves
	2 tsp salt
4 c water	¼ tsp pepper
pinch of allspice	6 carrots, scraped
1 tsp lemon or pineapple juice	4 small onions
1 tsp sugar	2-4 potatoes, pared and cubed
1 clove minced garlic	1 slices medium onion

Brown beef in oil in heavy saucepan. Add water, spices, juice, sugar, garlic, and onion. Cover tightly and simmer 1¾ hr. Add carrots, small onions, and potatoes. Cook 30 min. more or until vegetables are done.

Easy Meat Loaf

1 lb lean ground beef	1¼ tsp salt
3 tbsp minute tapioca	¾ c natural tomato juice
2 tbsp minced onion	

Combine ingredients. Place in small loaf pan. Bake at 350°F for 1 hr.

Lamb Stew

½ lb lamb, cut for stew	1¼ c hot water
1 tbsp rice flour	1½ c sweet potatoes, diced and pared
¾ tsp salt	
1 tbsp lamb drippings	1 tbsp rice flour

Broil lamb in mixture of flour and salt. Brown in hot drippings. Add water. Cover and simmer 1 hr. Add potatoes, cover and cook 25 min. longer, or until tender.
Make gravy with liquid and 1 tbsp rice flour.
Makes 3 servings.

Lamb with Rice

3 tbsp rice flour	½ tsp salt
2 tbsp lamb drippings	1 c diced lamb
1 c hot water	1½ c hot cooked rice

Brown rice flour in drippings. Add water and salt. Cook and stir until thick and smooth. Add lamb, and heat thoroughly. Serve over rice.
Makes 3 servings.

Rabbit

1 rabbit, cut into serving pieces	½ c rice flour
¼ c allowed oil	½ tsp salt
3 tbsp potato flour	

Blend flours and salt in clean paper bag. Drop in pieces of rabbit, and shake to coat. Brown over high heat in allowed oil, reduce heat, cover, and cook for 30-45 min. Uncover to crisp coating.
Serves 4.

Condiments

Cream of Rice White Sauce

2 c milk or allowed substitute	3 tbsp Cream of Rice for medium
½ tsp salt	sauce; 2 tbsp for thin; ¼ c for thick

Combine ingredients, and bring to boil, stirring constantly. Reduce heat, and continue stirring; simmer 1 min. Cover, and set aside 4 min. Puree in blender until smooth, taking care not to splash hot mixture. Repeat as needed.
Makes 2 c.

Variations.

1. For seasoned white sauce, add 1 tbsp chopped parsley and 1 tbsp chopped chives after blending.
2. Saute ½ c chopped onion and 1 c chopped celery in 2 tbsp allowed margarine. Add to white sauce.

Minute Tapioca White Sauce

2 c milk or allowed substitute	3 tsp Minute Tapioca for thin sauce;
½ tsp salt	5 tsp for medium; 7 tsp for thick

Mix all ingredients, and let stand 5 min. Bring to boil, stirring constantly. Remove from heat, cover, and let stand 5 min. Reheat. If desired, puree in blender for smoother sauce.

Potato Flour Mayonnaise

1½ tbsp potato flour	¾ c boiling water
¼ tsp dry mustard	2 tbsp lemon juice
½ tsp salt	1 tbsp white vinegar
2 tsp sugar	½ c allowed oil
¼ c cold water	

Mix dry ingredients in saucepan, then stir in cold water and mix well. Add hot water, and cook just until mixture is clear. Cool to lukewarm, then gradually add remaining ingredients, beating constantly.

Corn-Free Baking Powder

¼ c baking soda	¼ c potato starch
¼ c cream of tartar	

Sift each ingredient before measuring. Mix together thoroughly. Sift again. Keep baking powder dry in a tightly covered jar. To check if baking powder is still active, add several drops of water to a little baking powder. If it bubbles vigorously, it is still good. Use as you would any commercial double-acting baking powder.
Makes ¾ c.

Egg Substitute

1 c soy flour	2 tbsp allowed oil
2 c water	¼ tsp salt

Thoroughly blend flour and water in a blender at high speed. Pour into the top of a double boiler, and cook over boiling water, covered, for about 1 hr. Beat in oil and salt with an electric mixer. Refrigerate. Will thicken when cooled.

Use about ¼ c of the substitute for each egg. A half extra teaspoon baking powder per egg can be added to make batter rise.

Blueberry Jam*

4 c fresh blueberries	1 package Knox gelatin
2 c sugar	1 tsp lemon extract

In a large saucepan, slightly crush half the berries. Add remaining berries, sugar, and gelatin. Heat to boiling, stirring constantly. Boil hard for 2 min, stirring constantly. Stir in lemon extract. Pour into clean jelly glasses or jars; seal.
Makes 3 half-pints.
May be frozen.

*From *How To Improve Your Child's Behavior Through Diet*, Laura Stevens.

Catsup*

½ c apple cider vinegar	¼ c water
½ tsp whole cloves	2 tbsp dried minced onion or ½
1 2-in. stick cinnamon	onion, finely chopped
½ tsp celery seed	1/8 tsp black pepper
4 lb (about 12 medium tomatoes,	¼ c honey
washed and quartered)	2 tsp salt

Combine vinegar, cloves, cinnamon, and celery seed in a small covered saucepan. Bring to a boil. Remove from heat. Let stand.

In a large kettle or Dutch oven cook tomatoes, water, onion, and pepper over medium heat until tomatoes are quite soft. Put tomato mixture through sieve or food mill. Return juice to stove. Add honey and salt. Bring to a boil. Reduce heat and simmer until volume has been reduced by half. Stir in vinegar. Strain tomato mixture, discarding spices. Continue simmering until desired consistency is reached, stirring frequently. Pour into sterilized canning jars, leaving a ½-in. headspace. Seal. Process in boiling water bath for 5 min.

Or, cool and refrigerate in a covered container.
Makes 2 cups.

Chicken Stock

4 lb (about) chicken bones or	1 carrot, diced
whole carcass, broken up	Several stalks celery, diced
1 medium onion, diced, or ¼ c	Salt and pepper to taste
instant minced onion	4 qts cold water

Cover chicken bones with cold water in a Dutch oven. Add onion, carrot, and celery, and bring slowly to a boil. Simmer for 2-3 hr. Strain, season, and cool. Refrigerate. Skim off layer of fat on top when ready to use stock.
Makes 2 qts.

Desserts

Carob Balls

1 c peanut butter	1 c unsweetened coconut
½ c carob powder	¼ c banana flakes (or soy flour)
½-¾ c honey	

Mix all ingredients. Form into balls. Wrap in wax paper, and refrigerate.

---

*From *How To Improve Your Child's Behavior Through Diet,* Laura Stevens.

These balls can also be baked for 15 min, if preferred, at 350°F.

Variation.   Add nuts or raisins.

Almond Cookies

2 c finely ground almonds	¼ c water
½ c honey	3 tbsp carob powder (optional)
½ tsp salt	

Grind nuts in blender. Mix with remaining ingredients. Drop by teaspoonful onto a greased cookie sheet. Bake at 350°F for 10-12 min. Place whole almonds on top of each cookie for decoration.
Makes 2 dozen cookies.

Blender Broiled Frosting

1 c honey	1 tsp vanilla
½ c allowed oil	2 c unsweetened shredded coconut

Mix first three ingredients in blender. Pour liquid into a mixing bowl, and add coconut. Stir until well mixed. Spread on cake, and broil until bubbly.

Note: Chopped mixed nutmeats and/or seeds may be substituted for some or all of the coconut.

Barley Drop Cookies

1/3 c allowed margarine	2 c barley flour
¾ c sugar	1 tbsp baking powder
1½ tsp pure vanilla	½ tsp salt

Cream margarine and sugar, and stir in vanilla. Add dry ingredients alternately with ½ c water. Blend well. Drop from teaspoon onto greased cookie sheet and bake in preheated 350°F oven for 12-14 min.
Makes about 4½ dozen cookies.

Vegetables, Salads, and Side Dishes

Banana Honey Salad

1 banana	2 tbsp shredded coconut
¼ c peanut butter	2 tsp lemon juice
¼ c honey	

Put lettuce leaves on two salad plates. Slice whole banana in half, then slice lengthwise. Place bananas on top of lettuce leaves. Sprinkle lemon juice over banana to keep from browning. Mix peanut butter and honey. Pour over bananas and sprinkle with coconut.
Serves 2.

Green Beans with Almonds

2 lb green beans	¼ c almonds, blanched and
½ c boiling water	slivered
½ tsp salt	2 tbsp allowed oil
2 tsp finely chopped onion	¼ c chopped parsley

Wash and trim beans and cut into 1 in. pieces. Add salt, onion, and beans to boiling water. Quickly return to boil. Reduce heat to low, and steam until tender (7–10 min). Stir in almonds, oil, and parsley.

Hash Brown Potatoes

4 c shredded cooked potatoes	Dash pepper
1-2 tbsp grated onion	1/3 c allowed margarine
1 tsp salt	

Chill cooked-in-jacket potatoes, peel, and shred to make 4 c. Add onion, salt, and pepper. Melt margarine in skillet. Pat potatoes into pan, leaving ½-in. space around edge. Cover, and brown for 10-12 min. Check potatoes, reduce heat if necessary, and cook 8-10 min longer until golden. Place platter over pan, and invert potatoes onto platter.

Potato Salad

6 c (6 medium) potatoes, cooked, peeled, and cubed	1 tsp salt
	¼ tsp pepper
¼ c chopped onion	3 hard-boiled eggs
¾ c chopped celery (1 large stalk)	¼ c sunflower seeds
1½ c sliced fresh mushrooms	1/3 c allowed mayonnaise

In a large bowl combine all ingredients except sunflower seeds. Toss gently until well mixed. Refrigerate. Just before serving, toss with sunflower seeds. Serves 6.

Something Special Sweet Potatoes

2 c cooked sweet potatoes, cubed	½ c raisins
	¼ tsp salt
½ c maple syrup	2 tbsp allowed margarine
½ c well-drained unsweetened crushed pineapple	¼-½ c almonds, slivered

Combine syrup, pineapple, raisins, and salt. Arrange potatoes in 1 qt dish. Spread fruit mixture over top. Dot with margarine, and sprinkle with almonds. Bake at 350°F for 40-45 min. Serves 6-8.

Stuffed Mushrooms

32 fresh, whole mushrooms	4 green onions, finely chopped
½ c allowed margarine	2½ tbsp chopped fresh parsley
2 tbsp chopped walnuts	Salt and pepper to taste

Wash and dry mushrooms. Remove stems. Lay caps upside down in well-greased baking dish. In small skillet, melt 2 tbsp margarine. Add mushroom stems. Saute lightly. In small bowl, combine stems, remaining margarine, onions, parsley, salt, and pepper. Mix thoroughly. Fill each cap with a rounded teaspoon of mixture. Heat under broiler and broil mushrooms for 3-5 min until bubbly. Serve immediately.

Sunflower Salad

2 c coarsely shredded carrots	2 tbsp unsweetened pineapple
1 c thinly sliced celery	juice
2 firm bananas, sliced	¼ tsp salt
½ c sunflower seeds	¼ tsp pepper
¼ c allowed oil	Crisp lettuce cups

Combine carrots, celery, bananas, and sunflower seeds. Stir oil, juice, salt, and pepper together. Pour over salad mixture, and toss lightly. Serve in lettuce cup. Makes 4 servings.

14
Prophylaxis of Food Allergy

DOUGLAS E. JOHNSTONE
University of Rochester School of Medicine and Dentistry, Rochester, New York

Efforts at prophylaxis of allergic disease require a familiarity with dietary factors that may affect the development of atopy once the genetic die is cast. It is well known that heredity plays a key factor in the development of atopy, but it has been shown that not all identical twin offspring of two asthmatic parents develop frank atopic disease. This finding suggests that environmental factors, such as diet, among other forces, play a role in the determination of which child will develop allergic disease.

Atopic diseases associated with food allergy may be prevented [1] at four states in their pathogenesis: (1) avoidance of an antigen to which the patient is sensitized, (2) prevention of entry of the antigen, (3) modification of a damaging state of sensitization, and (4) avoidance of damaging sensitization. Some of these stages occur prenatally and some occur after birth.

PRENATAL FACTORS

In 1927, Ratner et al. [2] demonstrated in guinea pigs that it is possible to sensitize the fetus in utero, both passively and actively. They postulated that human fetuses might similarly be able to be sensitized to a food in a mother's diet. Matsamura et al. [3] reported that they were able to demonstrate the presence of egg white antigen in human cord blood, amniotic fluid, meconium, and first voided urine specimens. They implied this finding supported the thesis that prenatal in utero food sensitization could take place. Ratner and Greenburgh [4] reported a case of a mother who ate peanuts in large quantities during her pregnancy. Her child was not breast fed. Within a short time after birth the child gave marked skin reactions when touched with peanut. These authors speculated that this child had been atopically sensitized to peanut protein in utero. Michael et al. [5] have provided the most convincing evidence that in utero sensitization occurs in humans. They reported three newborns who had in their cord blood IgE-type antibodies to cow's milk as measured by the radioallergosorbent test (RAST) technique. None of their mothers had IgE antibodies to cow's milk in their sera. This finding strongly suggests the likelihood that sensitization of these three infants to cow's milk protein had taken place prenatally.

POSTNATAL FACTORS

Once a child of an allergic family is born, what are the physiologic and immuno-logic factors that seem important in "turning on" the allergic process? First, it has been shown that the infant's gut is very leaky. Wilson and Walzer [6] presented convincing evidence that unaltered food protein molecules cross the intestinal wall into the circulation in infants. Walzer [7] also demonstrated the rapidity with which antigens gain access to the circulation after ingestion. He did this in an experiment in which he injected human serum containing anti-egg white antibodies into the skin of the arm of an infant. He then fed the infant a bottle of milk containing a minute amount of egg white protein. Before the infant had finished the bottle, the serum-injected site on his forearm revealed a positive Prausnitz–Kustner reaction, indicating that some molecules of egg white protein in the infant's bottle had passed through his gut and had reached the skin test site and reacted with the anti-egg white antibodies at the intradermal site. Despite the absorption of food proteins intact across the intestinal mucosa in normal children in sufficient amounts to be immunogenic, only a few individuals seem to become atopically sensitized to these antigens. Paganelli et al. [8] demonstrated that, after challenge with foods a patient was suspected to be allergic to, abnormally high levels of immune complexex containing the suspected food were detected. In normal individuals these complexes rapidly cleared. These same investigators showed that the same atopic individuals with food sensitivities, if pretreated with sodium cromoglycate, had less antigen entry into their circula-tion, diminished immune complex formation, and no atopic symptoms. They studied a patient who developed itching atopic eczema and asthma after eating egg. When he was pretreated with oral sodium cromoglycate, the patient could eat egg without bronchospasm or skin itching.

Buckley and Dees [9] demonstrated that abnormal leakiness of the gut occurs when it is not coated with sufficient IgA immunoglobulin. They examined the sera of a large number of children with low serum IgA concentrations. These sera contained high titers of IgG-precipitating antibodies to cow's milk proteins. These children did not exhibit milk allergies; they simply made a greater than normal IgG immunologic response to milk proteins, suggesting that their gastrointestinal tracts were unusually "leaky." Similarly, Soothill et al. [10] observed that immunodeficient children often have allergic diseases, so he speculated that atopic individuals and other patients with common immunopathological diseases might also have common minor immunodeficiencies. He believed that persistent overactivity of an ordinary protective mechanism may occur as a result of failure of effective antigen handling by another mechanism. Kaufman and Hobbs [11] reported an increased proportion of abnormally low serum immunoglobulins, especially of serum IgA, in atopic subjects. Also, Sloper et al. [12] reported that atopic eczematous infants have significantly lower IgA plasma cell counts in their jejunal mucosa than do age-matched infants without eczema or a family history of atopy. They interpreted these findings as suggesting an immune response deficiency that allows antigenic sensitization through the jejunum at a time when neonate IgA production should be taking over from persisting maternal IgM. A prospective study by Taylor et al. [13] of newborn offspring of atopic parents showed that, before symptoms had developed, those who later became clinically atopic, that is, developed eczema, had lower serum IgA levels than did those who did not develop atopic symptoms. By 1 year of age, the difference between the two subgroups had disappeared. They interpreted their findings as an argument for withholding commonly allergenic foods from the diets of infants of allergic families until their guts became coated with IgA of their own making and thus less "leaky." They theorized that if one withheld certain allergenic foods until that had happened, these children might be less likely to "turn on" the IgE system, which sets the stage for clinical atopic disease.

Rossi et al. [14] reported a case of a child whose history revealed an interesting example of how food avoidance can influence a variety of immunologic mechanisms. They described a girl who at 2 months of age developed severe generalized atopic eczema. Eating egg induced angioedema. After receiving oral polio vaccine, she developed fever and severe diarrhea. At 12 months of age she began to suffer from recurrent middle ear infections, furunculosis, bronchospasm, mucocutaneous candidiasis, aphthous stomatitis, and herpetic keratitis, which led to blindness in one eye. Numerous hospitalizations, steroids, antibiotics, and antifungal treatments were of little help. At age 5 she was found to have negative delayed hypersensitivity skin test reactions, low level of circulating T lymphocytes, and grossly elevated blood eosinophil counts and serum IgE, as well as positive RAST serum tests to milk, egg, and *Staphlococcus aureus.* After being placed on a diet free of cow's milk and egg, in only 1 day she improved markedly clinically. Her severe atopic dermatitis and pruritus disappeared. She gained weight. Her oral candidiasis and recurrent infections subsided. Fascinatingly, her blood eosinophil count and total and specific IgE levels gradually fell. Her T-lymphocyte counts and the motile response of neutrophils increased. These observations suggest that severe allergy can induce an immunologic dysfunction of many proportions that may be treated and perhaps even be prevented with dietary prophylaxis.

Papageorgiou et al. [15] have reported that neutrophil chemotactic activity may also play a significant role in food allergy. They reported four patients with milk-induced asthma in whom skin tests, RAST (IgE and IgG$_4$), basophil histamine release, and serum precipitins, all using appropirate milk extracts, were negative. After drinking milk, all subjects developed a reproducible and dose-dependent increase in airflow limitation. In three of the four subjects who gave an early reaction to drinking milk, wheezing was accompanied by an elevation in circulating neutrophil chemotactic activity. In each of these cases, the immediate asthmatic response in peak expiratory flow rate and the elevation in neutrophil chemotactic activity were inhibited by prior oral administration of either disodium cromoglycate or oral beclomethasone.

Although Soothill has theorized that atopic disease is a consequence of overstimulation of the IgE-forming cells in children at a time when their serum IgA is relatively low, Juto [16] has presented an alternative theory to explain the clinical findings in children of allergic families. He asks the question, "Could atopic allergy represent an example of disturbed cell-mediated immunity?" He based his question on observations of others. Hamburger [17] suggested that in children of atopic parents, 60–80% of the control of serum IgE synthesis is genetically determined. Thus, less than 20–40% of the marked variation in serum IgE levels is likely to be due to environment, diet, and other forces. Buckley and Becker [18] reported that many children with immunodeficiencies have an impaired cell-mediated immunity in addition to elevated serum IgE levels. Canonica et al. [19] found that subpopulations of T-cell lymphocytes are diminished in atopic individuals. Bousquet et al. [20] found that serum IgA deficiency is often associated with T-cell lymphopenia. Hovmark [21] reported that eczema patients have hyporeactivity to tuberculin. Tada [22] has shown that T-suppressor cells in human atopic disease, by both mitogen assays [23] and monoclonal antibodies [24], support the view that such systems may be relevant. With these reports of suggestions of defects in cellular immunity, Juto [16] studied serum IgE levels at various ages during the first year of life. He found that these levels appeared to be related to the number of T-cells measured at the age of 1 month and to the type of feeding the infant had received. Babies fed cow's milk and having low T-cell counts had higher serum IgE levels at 3 and 6 months of age than did breast-fed babies with low T-cell counts. Of the babies fed cow's milk, those with low T-cell counts had higher serum IgE levels than those with normal T-cell counts. He found that initiation of cow's milk feeding before 3 months of age in babies with low T-cell counts was associated with continuously elevated serum IgE levels during the first year of life compared with the levels in babies with normal T-cell counts. Juto concluded that in T-cell-deficient infants there might exist a crucial time period during which the onset of cow's milk feeding can be associated with a subsequent increase in IgE synthesis and, presumably, the subsequent development of atopic disease.

ROLE OF BREAST-FEEDING IN THE PROPHYLAXIS OF ALLERGIC DISEASE

It has been suggested that the way to human immunocompetence is through the infant's stomach. Examination of a drop of breast milk or colostrum under the microscope reveals rather startling findings. Whereas 2% of adult serum leukocytes are monocytes, nearly 90% of leukocytes in breast milk are monocytes. These monocytes have anti-infection qualities by secreting complement components, lysozyme, and the iron-binding protein, lactoferrin. Breast-feeding can pass on to the infant delayed-type sensitivity to such antigens as tuberculin from the mother. Breast milk facilitates the coating of the infant's gut with IgA immuno-globulin. Walker and Isselbacher [25] demonstrated that IgA antibodies can prevent the transport of foreign proteins, including sensitizing food allergens, across the gut wall. They suggested that this mechanism may explain the lessening of sensitization of breast-fed babies to cow's milk and other foods. Studies of Eastham and Walker [26] have shown that human milk contains a factor that stimulates the development of intestinal mucosa.

Clinical Reports of the Benefit of Breast-Feeding

Kaufman and Frick [27] reported that babies who were breast-fed for 6 weeks were less likely to develop bronchial asthma than those given cow's milk formulas. They prospectively followed 94 full-term infants of 92 allergic mothers for 2 years. Only 2 of 38 breast-fed infants developed asthma, but 10 of 56 infants who received cow's milk became asthmatic during the 2-year study. In separate studies, Chandra [28] and Saarinsen et al. [29] reported that prolonged breast-feeding significantly protects children from developing atopic disease. Stevenson et al. [30] demonstrated that IgE antibodies to cow's milk appeared earlier in babies who had been fed cow's milk than in breast-fed infants.

Potential for Atopic Sensitization of Infants by Breast Milk

It is important to remember that, although breast-feeding for potentially allergic newborns is strongly advocated, certain potential allergens may gain entrance to the infant's relatively leaky gut via the mother's breast milk.

Bjorksten and Saarinen [31] demonstrated cow's milk-specific IgE antibodies in exclusively breast-fed infants by positive prick tests and RAST tests on infants' sera. These authors pointed out that the feeding of cow's milk on the first night in the nursery to infants who will then be exclusively breast fed might cause allergy to cow's milk. Kaplan and Solli [32] compared the feeding habits of 18 young atopic infants with IgE antibodies to cow's milk proteins in their serum with those of 18 symptomatic infants whose serum did not contain IgE antibody to cow's milk. They found that the incidence of breast-feeding was significantly higher than in the control group of the age-matched patients without IgE antibodies to milk. Warner [33] reported infants with eczema whose rash exacerbated when their breast-feeding mothers ate egg. The eczema cleared when the mothers stopped eating egg and recurred when they ate it again. Jakobsson and Lindberg [34] studied 19 breast-fed infants with "colic." When their mothers were put on a diet free of cow's milk, the colic disappeared in 13 of the 19 infants. The colic recurred in 12 of the 13 infants when their mothers again drank milk. They demonstrated by Ouchterlany technique the presence of cow's milk proteins in the breast milk of mothers who drank milk. When the mothers were off milk for 1 or 2 days, their breast milk no longer contained cow's milk proteins. These findings suggest that perhaps mothers of potentially allergic infants should be on a diet free of cow's milk while breast-feeding.

CLINICAL EXPERIENCE WITH DIETARY PROPHYLAXIS

In the 1920s, allergists and pediatricians noted that infants who were fed egg yolk to prevent the development of iron-deficiency anemia and lessen hunger and crying of infants who were exclusively breast fed frequently developed classic atopic eczema. Similarly, Grulee and Sanford [35] noted that seven times as many infants fed whole cow's milk developed atopic eczema as did those who had been exclusively breast fed. Ratner et al. [36] observed that 60–80% of those eczematous children went on to develop major respiratory allergies. With this in mind, it was a natural development in this field that pioneer pediatric allergists, such as Hill and Galser, began to popularize the recommendation that one should deliberately withhold egg, wheat, chicken, and cow products from the diets of children of allergic families from the time of birth until 9 months of age. Glaser also suggested that these foods should be restricted or withheld from the mothers' diets during their pregnancies, on the assumption that the fetus might develop intrauterine sensitization to these foods.

In 1953, Glaser and Johnstone [37] reported that, in infants fed a diet free of egg, wheat, and milk for the first 9 months of life, the incidence of atopic eczema was significantly less than their siblings as well as another retrospectively picked control group of offspring of atopic mothers. Also, of those children on the special diet who did develop eczema, only 15% went on to develop asthma, pollenosis, or perennial allergic rhinitis. By contrast, 60% of their eczematous siblings not on this diet developed major respiratory allergies.

Johnstone and Dutton [38] repeated the Glaser and Johnstone study as a prospective controlled trial of the effectiveness of withholding cow's milk, chicken egg, and milk products from the time of birth in children of allergic families. They randomly placed newborns of allergic families either on the diet free of milk, egg, and wheat or on normal pediatric diets that permitted these foods. They then carefully followed the clinical courses of these children up to

12 years. Their data revealed that significantly fewer children placed on this diet developed bronchial asthma (9 of 115) compared with infants of allergic parents not on such a diet (28 of 120). They found that 12 of 115 of the diet group developed hay fever compared with 22 of 120 of the control group. Also, 8 of 115 of those on the special diet developed perennial allergic rhinitis compared with 40 of 120 of the controls (p < 0.001). Interestingly, not only did fewer of those on the diet develop these major respiratory allergies, but by the end of the 13-year study period, differences in persistence of these conditions persisted in the two groups. At the end of the study, hay fever persisted in 11 of 115 of the diet group and in 23 of 120 of the controls. Asthma persisted in 7 of 115 of the diet group and in 18 of 120 of the controls. Perennial allergic rhinitis persisted in 8 of 115 of the diet group and in 41 of the 120 of the control group. Thus, it appeared that for those on the diet free of milk, wheat, and egg, some prophylactic benefit persisted through midchildhood. Halpern et al. [39] using a somewhat different protocol, were unable to confirm these findings. Detailed critiques of the comparison of the studies of Johnstone and Dutton with that of Halpern et al. have appeared elsewhere [40, 41]. Several independent clinical studies [28–30] have demonstrated the prophylactic value of exclusive breast-feeding. Matthew et al. [42] carried on a prospective study of a group of infants of allergic parents to evaluate the value of a program designed to prevent allergic disease. In that study, infants of allergic parents were either placed on an allergen-avoidance program or managed conventionally. Those on the regimen were encouraged to continue breast-feeding for at least 6 months. They were to be given no cow's milk, fish, or egg. They were to avoid contact with pets, horse hair mattresses, and feather quilts. An anti-house mite measure was instituted during the 6-month period. The group on the allergen-avoidance regimen had less eczema and lower serum IgE levels than the control group. The authors theorized that food allergen sensitization requires antigen entry with adjuvantizing *Escherichia coli* endotoxin [43]. They also observed that Hanson [44] has demonstrated that maternal or infant IgA prevents attachment of *E. coli* to mucosal cells.

Orgel et al. [45] followed the serum IgE levels from birth to 12 months of age in 34 atopic and nonatopic families. They found that elevation of serum IgE levels at or before 1 year of age was highly correlated with atopic disease in the first 2 years of life. The elevation of serum IgE preceded the manifestation of allergic disease.

One of the concerns of workers in the field of animal immunology has been that delaying introduction of cow's milk into the diets of newborn humans might actually increase rather than decrease sensitization to milk. They based this postulation on findings that young animals fed large quantities of food allergens develop tolerance to these same allergens on later immunization. Mellon et al. [46] examined this hypothesis during a prospective allergy prevention study com-

composed of offspring of immunologically documented atopic (65% bilateral) parents. Their hypoallergenic regimen entailed breast-feeding for at least 3 months, a casein hydrolysate formula, solid food ingestion only after 6 months of age (excluding cow's milk, egg, wheat, and fish), and maternal avoidance of cow's milk and egg during the third trimester of pregnancy and while breast-feeding. Only 5% of the first 100 infnats at 2 months of age had cow's milk-specific IgE antibodies in their serum compared with the finding of 15% reported by Juto and Bjorksten [47] in prospectively studied infants who ingested cow's milk in their first 6 months. Mellon fed cow's milk to a group of infants with negative skin tests to milk at 12 months of age. Total serum IgE and cow's milk-specific IgE by RAST did not significantly increase in 24 of 25 such infants by age 24 months. Cow's milk-specific IgE remained negative in all 25 infants after beginning cow's milk at 12 months. Consequently, these authors concluded that delayed milk feeding does not increase the risk of developing IgE sensitization to milk in potentially atopic infants and may even reduce it.

Thus, it seems that prevention of atopic disease may be influenced by advocating avoidance of commonly sensitizing foods in the first 6-9 months of life, efforts at prevention of allergen entry perhaps with the help of sodium cromoglycate in some instances, and encouraging breast-feeding while suggesting that the mother avoid certain common offending food allergens during the third trimester of pregnancy and while nursing her infant in the first 3-6 months of life.

REFERENCES

1. Soothill, J. Prevention of atopic allergic disease. *Ann. Allergy 51*:229, 1983.
2. Ratner, B., Jackson, H., and Gruehl, H. Transmission of protein sensitiveness from mother to offspring. I. Critique of placental permeability. *J. Immunol. 14*:269, 1927.
3. Matsamura, T., Kurome, T., Iwasaki, I., and Oguri, M. Congenital sensitization to food of humans. *J. Allergy 18*:858, 1957.
4. Ratner, B., and Greenburgh, J. Congenital protein hypersensitiveness transmitted from other to child. *J. Allergy 3*:149, 1931.
5. Michel, F., Bousquet, J., Yves, C., Coulomb, Y., Gauci, L., Greillier, P., and Robinet-Levy, M. Comparison of clinical and immunological parameters for the prediction of infant allergy. *J. Allergy Clin. Immunol. 65*:167, 1980.
6. Wilson, S., and Walzer, M. Absorption of undigested proteins in human beings. IV. Absorption of unaltered egg protein in infants and children. *Am. J. Dis. Child. 50*:49, 1935.
7. Walzer, M. Transfer of skin sensitizing antibody. *J. Allergy 2*:282, 1931.
8. Paganelli, R., Levinsky, R., Brostoff, J., and Wraith, D. Immune complexes containing food proteins in normal and atopic subjects after oral challenge, and effect of sodium cromoglycate on antigen absorption. *Lancet 1*:1270, 1979.

9. Buckley, R., and Dees, S. Correlation of milk precipitins with IgA deficiency *N. Engl. J. Med. 281*:456, 1969.
10. Soothill, J., Stokes, C., Turner, M., Norman, A., and Taylor, B. Predisposing factors in the development of reaginic allergy in infancy. *Clin. Allergy 6*: 305, 1976.
11. Kaufman, H., and Hobbs, J. Immunoglobulin deficiencies in an atopic population. *Lancet 2*:1061, 1970.
12. Sloper, K., Brook, C., Kingston, D., Pearson, J., and Shiner, M. Eczema and atopy in early childhood: Low IgA plasma cell counts in the jejunal mucosa. *Arch. Dis. Child. 56*:939, 1981.
13. Taylor, B., Norman, A., Orgel, H., Stokes, C., Turner, M., and Soothill, J. Transient IgA deficiency and pathogenesis of infantile atopy. *Lancet 2*:111, 1973.
14. Rossi, P., Galli, M., Cantani, A., Perlin, R., Dellitto, F., and Businco, L. A case of hyperimmunoglobulinemia E treated with cow's milk and egg-free diet. *Ann. Allergy 49*:159, 1982.
15. Papageorgiou, N., Lee, R., Nagakura, T., Cromwell, O., Wraith, D., and Kay, A. Neutrophil chemotactic activity in milk-induced asthma. *J. Allergy Clin. Immunol. 72*:75, 1983.
16. Juto, P. Elevated serum immunoglobulin E in T cell-deficient infants fed cow's milk. *J. Allergy Clin. Immunol. 66*:402, 1980.
17. Hamburger, R. Allergies in infants – perhaps they can be prevented. *Consultant 19*:23, 1979.
18. Buckley, R., and Becker, W. Abnormalities in the regulation of human IgE synthesis. *Immunol. Red. 41*:18, 1978.
19. Canonica, C., Mingari, M., Melioli, D., Colombatti, M., and Moretta, L. Imbalances of T cell subpopulations in patients with atopic diseases and effect of specific immunotherapy. *J. Immunol. 123*:2669, 1979.
20. Bousquet, J., Clot, J., Dardenne, M., Robinet-Levy, M., and Michel, F. Lymphocyte markers, serum thymic factor, and IgE in IgA deficiency. *Ann. Allergy 43*:174, 1979.
21. Hovmark, A. An in vitro and in vivo study of cell mediated immunity in atopic dermatitis. *Acta Derm. Venereol. 55*:181, 1975.
22. Tada, T. Regulation of reaginic antibody formation in animals. *Prog. Allerg. 19*:122, 1975.
23. Jensen, J., Cramers, M., and Threstrup-Pedersen, K. Subpopulations of T lymphocytes and non-specific suppressor cell activity in patients with atopic dermatitis. *Clin. Exp. Immunol. 45*:118, 1981.
24. Butler, M., Atherton, D., and Levinsky, R. Quantitative and functional deficit of suppressor T cells in children with atopic dermatitis. *Clin. Exp. Immunol. 50*:92, 1982.
25. Walker, W., and Isselbacher, K. Uptake and transport of macromolecules by the intestine. *Gastroenterology 67*:531, 1974.
26. Eastham, E., and Walker, W. Effect of cow's milk on the gastrointestinal tract: A persistent dilemma for the pediatrician. *Pediatrics 60*:477, 1977.

27. Kaufman, H., and Frick, O. Prevention of asthma. *Clin. Allergy II.* 549, 1981.
28. Chandra, R. Prospective studies of the effect of breast feeding on the incidence of infection and allergy. *Acta Paediatr. Scan. 68*:691, 1981.
29. Saarinen, U., Kajosaar, M., Bakcman, A., and Sumes, M. Prolonged breast feeding as a prophylaxis for allergic disease. *Lancet 2*:163, 1979.
30. Stevenson, D., Orgel, A., Hamburger, R., and Reid, R. Development of IgE in newborn human infants. *J. Allergy Clin. Immunol. 48*:61, 1971.
31. Bjorksten, F., and Saarinen, V. IgE antibodies to cow's milk in infants fed breast milk and milk formulae. *Lancet 2*:624, 1978.
32. Kaplan, M., and Solli, N. Immunoglobulin E to cow's milk protein in breast fed atopic children. *J. Allergy Clin. Immunol. 64*:122, 1979.
33. Warner, J. Food allergy in fully breast fed infants. *Clin. Allergy 10*:133, 1980.
34. Jakobsson, I., and Lindberg, R. Cow's milk as a cause of infantile colic in breastfed infants. *Lancet 1*:437, 1978.
35. Grulee, C., and Sanford, H. The influence of breast and artificial feedings on infantile eczema. *J. Pediatr. 9*:273, 1936.
36. Ratner, B., Collins-Williams, C., and Untracht, S. Allergic dermal respiratory syndrome in children. *Am. J. Dis. Child. 82*:666, 1951.
37. Glaser, J., and Johnstone, D. Prophylaxis of allergic disease in children. *JAMA 253*:620, 1953.
38. Johnstone, D., and Dutton, A. Dietary prophylaxis of allergic disease in children. *N. Engl. J. Med. 274*:715, 1966.
39. Halpern, S., Sellars, W., Johnson, R., et al. Development of childhood allergy in infants breast, soy, or cow's milk fed. *J. Allergy Clin. Immunol. 51*:139, 1973.
40. Johnstone, D. In *Yearbook of Pediatrics,* S. Gellis (ed.), Year Book Medical Publishers, Chicago, pp. 82–83, 1974.
41. Johnstone, D. Letters to the editor. *Ann. Allergy 48*:246, 1982.
42. Matthew, E., Taylor, D., Norman, A., Turner, M., and Soothill, J. Prevention of eczema. *Lancet 1*:321, 1977.
43. Buller, C. Resistance of breast fed infant to gastroenteritis. *Br. Med. J. 3*: 338, 1971.
44. Hanson, L. *E. coli* infections in childhood. Significance of bacterial virulence and immune defense. *Arch. Dis. Child. 51*:727, 1976.
45. Orgel, H., Hamburger, R., Barazol, M., Gorrin, H., Groshong, T., Lenoir, M., Miller, J., and Wallace, W. Development of IgE allergy in infancy. *J. Allergy Clin. Immunol. 56*:296, 1975.
46. Mellon, M., Heller, S., O'Connor, R., Hamburger, R., and Zieger, R. No increase in cow's milk sensitization after delayed cow's milk ingestion in infancy. *J. Allergy Clin. Immunol. 71*:98, 1983.
47. Juto, P., and Bjorksten, B. Serum IgE in infants and influence of the type of feeding. *Clin. Allergy 10*:953, 1980.

15
New and Promising Treatments

ROBERT N. HAMBURGER and GARY A. COHEN
University of California – San Diego, La Jolla, California

The phenotypic expression of IgE-mediated disease appears to be regulated by multiple genetic factors [1-5] and modulated by environmental exposures [6, 7]. Food sensitivity usually appears early in life partly due to the increased permeability of the immature neonatal gastrointestinal tract to macro-molecular food antigens [8, 9]. Allergic manifestation may then develop locally in the gastrointestinal tract and/or systemically in the respiratory tract, skin, or in almost any organ system in the body.

The ultimate treatment goal is prevention for any disease process in the susceptible individual rather than treatment of the acute process or chronic symptoms. Prevention of allergic disease may have to begin while the infant is still in utero [10], especially in the highly susceptible infant with bilateral familial atopy. Providing the pregnant mother with a modified, nutritional, hypoallergenic diet and a hypoallergenic environment and continuing this regimen during lactation and throughout the infant's first year of life may be the most successful preventive measure [6]. Breast-feeding associated with the delaying of introduction of cow's milk protein and solid foods is the cornerstone for any allergy prevention program in infancy [7, 11-15]. Breast milk not only minimizes the susceptible infant's exposure to large quantities of potentially sensitizing antigens (cow's milk proteins) but also supplies the infant with factors of humoral and cellular protective immunity. The maternal diet must also be hypoallergenic since food antigens may pass to the infant via breast milk [16-18]. Other environmental factors, such as dust and dander exposures, also must be minimized.

The optimal mode of treatment for the patient who is already food sensitized is avoidance of the offending food(s). However, if severe, multiple food sensitivities exist or if basic or essential foods are incriminated whose total elimination may lead to malnutrition, then pharmacological intervention becomes a reasonable addition. Acute reactions to ingested allergens are treated the same as any other allergen-induced anaphylactic reaction, that is, with epinephrine, antihistamines, bronchodilators, and, if necessary, corticosteroids. For chronic food-provoked symptoms, a safe drug used with a high degree of success is oral cromolyn sodium. Newer agents, such as a nonsteroidal anti-inflammatory drugs, cromolynlike variants, IgE-blocking peptides, and regulatory molecules, are at present under investigation. Hyposensitization in atopy due to foods is currently experimental. New treatments of food allergies appear to be promising, especially as the use of genetic engineering and altered regulation, such as turning off IgE production, becomes a reality in the not-to-distant future.

AVOIDANCE

Avoidance, as mentioned earlier, is the ideal management for food sensitivity. This is usually simple when only a few foods are involved. Apparently, "simple avoidance" can be confounding to the physician and disappointing to the conscientious patient when unlisted ingredients are included in the prepared foods. Common examples of "hidden food allergens" are corn proteins in certain sweeteners or cereal fillers in some meat products. However, in patients in whom multiple sensitivities exist or the potential for malnutrition occurs with the elimination of specific foods, then pharmacological intervention needs to be considered.

ANTIHISTAMINES

The classic antihistamines act by binding to H_1 histamine receptors and therefore blocking the action of histamine on target organs. Thus, to be effective, antihistamines should be taken regularly in the case of multiple food sensitivity. Some patients may be able to tolerate limited quantities of allergenic foods by taking an antihistamine 30 min prior to the anticipated food exposure [10, 19]. Unfortunately, there have been no controlled clinical trials to date to document that these drugs are efficacious in the management of food sensitivity [20]. Combination of H_1 and H_2 antihistamines have been used recently with good results in patients with chronic urticaria, which, in some cases, is secondary to food sensitivity [21, 22].

Oral Cromolyn

Oral cromolyn sodium has been used with favorable results [23–28] for many years in Europe to treat patients with multiple or intractable food hypersensitivity.

Theoretically, cromolyn given orally is poorly absorbed and therefore is effective by inhibiting local gastrointestinal mast cell degranulation, thereby preventing gastrointestinal symptoms and secondarily limiting systemic reactions by reducing allergen entry into the circulation [29, 30]. Both antihistamines and cromolyn sodium given orally, prior to challenge, in rats sensitized with ovalbumin, will reduce the subsequent gut wall edema [31]. A recent article by Businco et al. attests to the protective effect of 30 mg/kg per day of oral cromolyn sodium in preventing symptoms in children with cow's milk and/or egg allergy. Cromolyn may also be useful for food additive sensitivity [32, 33] and in nursing mothers to prevent reactions in infants with severe food hypersensitivity [34].

CROMOLYNLIKE VARIANTS

Since the advent of cromolyn sodium, experts have begun to synthesize drugs with greater potencies and absorptive properties than those of cromolyn. Some of these drugs are structurally related to cromolyn (doxantrazole), whereas others, though structurally dissimilar, have pharmacological activity thought to be related to that of cromolyn (cinnarizine, ketotifen, and ladoxamide) [35]. A number of these drugs have other activities in addition to inhibiting mediator release and antigen-induced bronchoconstriction. For example, ketotifen also has a strong anti-anaphylactic and anti-histaminic effect and has been used to protect from oral provocation in aspirin-induced asthma and in some cases of chronic urticaria [21]. Cinnarizine, which has anti-seritonin and anti-kinin effects as well as the capacity to inhibit complement activation, has been used with some success in patients with chronic urticaria [36]. However, properly controlled clinical studies have yet to be performed to confirm the appropriate use of these drugs in food sensitivity.

NONSTEROIDAL ANTI-INFLAMMATORY AGENTS

Nonsteroidal anti-inflammatory drugs inhibit the synthesis of prostaglandins via inhibition of the cyclo-oxygenase system and have been reported to be useful in some patients in preventing food-induced gastrointestinal symptoms [37]. In 1978, Buisseret et al. reported that the prophylactic use of aspirin, indomethacin, and ibuprofen could prevent symptoms of food intolerance in patients unable or unwilling to avoid the specific food. In experimental studies of rat intestinal anaphylaxis, these agents significantly suppress [^{125}I] bovine serum albumin extravasation from the blood into the intestinal tissue [38]. These drugs have not yet been studied in detail, and their chronic use may produce detrimental gastrointestinal side effects as well as adverse effects on other atopic disease (e.g., asthma and aspirin).

CORTICOSTEROIDS

Adrenal corticosteroids have been shown to be useful for eosinophilic gastroenteritis [39], which may be associated with food allergies, as well as in some infants with intractable diarrhea [40]. However, because of the well-known complications associated with chronic corticosteroid use, it would be wise to reserve them for specific indications serious enough to warrant their use.

IgE BLOCKING PEPTIDES

Small peptides derived from the F_c portion (third constant domain) of the IgE heavy chain (ϵ) are currently being studied. In a recent double-blind placebo-controlled clinical trial, human IgE pentapeptide (HEPP) was evaluated in 12 patients with IgE-mediated atopic disease. Statistically significant differences were observed in allergy symptoms scores, medication use, and skin test suppression between the treatment and control groups [41]. This study also confirmed previous results concerning the safety of HEPP and its ability to suppress IgE-mediated skin test responses. A larger multicenter clinical study has recently been completed utilizing this new medication s.c. for the treatment of allergic diseases, and preliminary analysis suggests confirmation of the clinical effectiveness and safety of this unique modality [42, 43]. Nasal spray and opthalmalogic drops of this pentapeptide are presently undergoing clinical trials.

IMMUNOTHERAPY AND HYPOSENSITIZATION

Immunotherapy or hyposensitization is a form of treatment used to modify the immunologic response of an atopic allergic individual to specific allergens. Immunotherapy by subcutaneous injection of one or more antigens has been proven efficacious for inhalant allergy (pollens, dust, danders, mites, and mold spores) [44–48] and in insect venom hypersensitivity [49]. The treatment involves injecting increasing doses of specific allergens subcutaneously into the sensitive individual. This may lead to an increase in the serum blocking antibody (IgG), a decrease in specific allergen antibody (IgE), and a decrease in specific-allergen induced mast cell histamine release [50]. Desensitization procedures have also been used for patients with drug hypersensitivities (pencillin [51, 52], insulin [53, 54], and aspirin [55]) and vaccine sensitivities due to egg-grown viruses, such as measles [56].

Although different routes have been attempted for hyposensitization in individuals with food allergies, none have yet been proven to be uniformly successful [57]. With regard to sublingual testing and/or therapy, both Breneman et al. [58] and Grieco [58a] found it to be "not proven to be useful" when appropriate controlled studies have been performed. Most studies of subcutaneous injections of food antigen extracts have produced poor results and frequent severe side effects [59–62]. Oral hyposensitization methods have also produced poor results in humans. In several different species of animals, tolerance has been induced by feeding the antigen as well as inducing a decrease in antigen absorption by the gut [63, 64]. This has not been possible in humans. Unsuccessful attempts to produce an allergen-specific antibody (such as secretory IgA) in the gut have been made in an effort to provide a protective barrier at the mucosal level. Unsatisfactory results have also been observed in double-blind studies utilizing sublingual food antigens [58, 58a] for treatment or desensitization.

It is obvious that further studies are necessary to delineate the role of hyposensitization for food allergy patients. Results with current methods have been disappointing. New studies must take into account the different allergic manifestations and mechanisms of food sensitivity, the age and immunologic state of the individual, and the nature of the specific antigen in question. One major unsolved problem is that each foodstuff contains numerous covert antigens that may be altered by digestive enzymes to produce new antigens while traversing the gastrointestinal tract, and thus the specific antigen responsible for an allergic reaction may not be recognizable or discoverable. Furthermore, there appear to be significant differences in the results obtained in various mammalian species compared with similar studies in humans.

REFERENCES

1. Orgel, H. A., Hamburger, R. N., Bazaral, M., Gorrin, H., Groshong, T., Lenoir, M., Miller, J. R., and Wallace, W. W. Development of IgE and allergy in infancy. *J. Allergy Clin. Immunol. 56*:296, 1975.
2. Kaufman, H. S., and Frick, O. L. The development of allergy in infants of allergic parents: A prospective study concerning the role of heredity. *Ann. Allergy 37*:410, 1976.
3. Bazaral, M., Orgel, H. A., and Hamburger, R. N. Genetics of IgE and allergy serum IgE levels in twins. *J. Allergy Clin. Immunol. 54*:288, 1974.
4. Bazaral, M., Orgel, H. A., and Hamburger, R. N. IgE levels in normal infants and mothers and an inheritance hypothesis. *J. Immunol. 107*:794, 1971.
5. Gerrard, J. W., Horne, S., Vickers, P., Mackenzie, J. W. A., Galuboff, N., Garson, J. Z., and Maningas, C. S. Serum IgE levels in parents and children. *J. Pediatr. 85*:660, 1974.
6. Hamburger, R. N., Heller, S., Mellon, M. H., O'Connor, R. D., and Zieger, R. S. Current status of the clinical and immunological consequences of a prototype allergic disease prevention program. *Ann. Allergy 51*(2):281, 1983.
7. Businco, L., Marchetti, F., Pellegrini, G., Cantani, A., and Perlini, R. Prevention of atopic disease in "at risk newborns" by prolonged breast-feeding. *Ann. Allergy 51*:(2):296, 1983.
8. Udall, J. N., Pang, K., Fritze, L., Kleinmen, R., and Walker, W. A. Development of gastrointestinal mucosal barrier. I. Effect of age on intestinal permeability to macromolecules. *Pediatr. Res. 15*:241, 1981.

9. Eastham, E. J., Lichauco, T., Grady, M. I., and Walker, W. A. Antigenicity of infant formulas: Role of immature intestine in protein permeability. *J. Pediatr. 93*:561, 1978.

10. Bahna, S. L., and Gandhi, M. D. Milk hypersensitivity. II. Practical aspects of diagnosis, treatment and prevention. *Ann. Allergy 50*:(5):295, 1983.

11. Chandra, R. Prospective studies of the effect of breast feeding on incidence of infection and allergy. *Acta Paediatr. Scand. 68*:691, 1979.

12. Grulee, C. G., and Sanford, H. N. The influence of breast and artificial feeding on infantile eczema. *J. Pediatr. 9*:223, 1936.

13. Johnstone, D. E., and Dutton, A. M. Dietary prophylaxis of allergic disease in children. *N. Engl. J. Med. 274*:415, 1966.

14. Matthew, D. J., Taylor, B., Norman, P. A., Turner, M. W., and Soothill, J. F. Prevention of eczema. *Lancet 1*:321, 1977.

15. Saarinen, U. M., Kajosaari, M., Backman, A., and Siimes, M. A. Prolonged breast feeding as prophylaxis for atopic disease. *Lancet 2*:163, 1979.

16. Gerrard, J. W., and Shenassa, M. Sensitization to substances in breast milk: Recognition, management and significance. *Ann. Allergy 51*:(2):300, 1983.

17. Cogswell, J. J., and Alexander, J. Breast feeding and eczema-asthma (letter). *Lancet 1*:910, 1982.

18. Shacks, S. J., and Heiner, D. C. Allergy to breast milk. *Clin. Immunol. Allergy 2*:(1):121, 1982.

19. Goldman, A. S., and Heiner, D. C. Clinical aspects of food sensitivity: Diagnosis and management of cow's milk sensitivity. *Pediatr. Clin. North Am. 24*:(1):133, 1977.

20. Bock, S. A. Food sensitivity: A critical review and practical approach. *Am. J. Dis. Child. 134*:973, 1980.

21. Zanussi, C., Ortoloni, C., and Pastorello, E. Dietary and pharmacologic management of food intolerance in adults. *Ann. Allergy 51*:(2):307, 1983.

22. Phanuphak, P., Schocket, A., and Kohler, P. F. Treatment of chronic idiopathic urticaria with combined H_1 and H_2 blockers. *Clin. Allergy 8*:429, 1978.

23. Freier, S., and Berger, H. Disodium cromoglycate in gastrointestinal protein intolerance. *Lancet 1*:913, 1973.

24. Kuzemko, P. J., and Simpson, K. R. Treatment of allergy to cow's milk. *Lancet 1*:337, 1975.

25. Esteban, M. M., Casas, J. A. O., Borrego, M. T. L., and Marcos, C. P. Oral disodium cromoglycate in food allergy. *Acta Allergol. 32*:413, 1977.

26. Dahl, R., and Zetterstrom, O. The effect of orally administered sodium cromoglycate on allergic reactions caused by food allergens. *Clin. Allergy 8*:419, 1978.

27. Gerrard, J. W. Oral cromoglycate: Its value in the treatment of adverse reactions to foods. *Ann. Allergy 42*:135, 1979.

28. Danneus, A., Foucard, T., and Johansson, S. G. O. The effect of orally administered cromoglycate on symptoms of food allergy. *Clin. Allergy 7*:109, 1977.

29. Brostoff, J., Carini, C., Wraith, D. G., and Johns, P. Production of IgE

complexes by antigen challenge in atopic patients and the effect of sodium cromoglycate. *Lancet 2*:1268, 1979.

30. Paganelli, R., Levinsky, R. J., and Brostoff, J. Immune complexes containing food proteins in normal and atopic subjects after oral challenge and effect of sodium cromoglycate on antigen absorption. *Lancet 1*:1270, 1979.

31. Byars, N. E., and Ferraresi, R. W. Intestinal anaphylaxis in the rat as a model of food allergy. *Clin. Exp. Immunol. 24*:352, 1976.

32. Businco, L., Cantini, A., Benincori, N., Perlini, R., Infussi, R., DeAngelis, M., and Businco, E. Effectiveness of oral sodium cromoglycate in preventing food allergy in children. *Ann. Allergy 51*:(1):47, 1983.

33. Ortolani, C., Pastorello, E., and Zanussi, C. Prophylaxis of adverse reactions to foods. A double-blind study of oral sodium cromoglycate for the prophylaxis of adverse reactions to foods and additives. *Ann. Allergy 50*:105, 1983.

34. Soothill, J. F. Prevention of food allergy. *Clin. Immunol. Allergy 2*:(1): 243, 1982.

35. Bernstein, I. L. Cromolyn sodium in the treatment of asthma: Changing concepts. *J. Allergy Clin. Immunol. 68*:(4):247, 1981.

36. Kalino, K., and Jansen, C. T. Treatment of chronic urticaria with an inhibitor of complement activation. *Ann. Allergy 44*:34, 1980.

37. Byars, N. E., and Ferraresi, R. W. Inhibition of rat intestinal anaphylaxis by various antiinflammatory agents. *Agents Action 10*:252, 1980.

38. Buisseret, P. D., Youlten, J. F., Heinzelmann, D. I., and Lessof, M. H. Prostaglandin-synthesis inhibitors in prophylaxis of food intolerance. *Lancet 1*:906, 1978.

39. Katz, A. J., Falchuk, Z. M., Garovoy, M., Zeiger, R. S., and Twarog, F. J. Eosinophilic gastroenteritis in childhood: Basis for allergic etiology (abstract). *J. Allergy Clin. Immunol. 61*:157, 1978.

40. Lloyd-Still, J. D., Schwachman, H., and Filler, R. M. Protracted diarrhea of infancy treated with intravenous alimentation. I. Clinical studies of 16 infants. *Am. J. Dis. Child. 125*:358, 1973.

41. Cohen, G. A., Hamburger, R. N., and O'Connor, R. D. Dose response to human IgE pentapeptide (HEPP). *Ann. Allergy 50*:351, 1983.

42. Dennis, S., Haddad, Z., Kniker, W., Mansmann, H., Meltzer, E., Mendelson, L., Prenner, B., Rosenthal, R., Segall, N., Tinkelman, D., Wold, R., and Ziering, R. HEPP (IgE Pentapeptide) in Allergic Rhinitis. *J. Allergy Clin. Immunol. 77*:213, 1986.

43. Prenner, B., Rohr, A., Cohen, G., and Sainz, C. Preliminary results of a multicenter study of the antiallergy pentapeptide "HEPP" (abstract). *Ann. Allergy 52*:240, 1984.

44. Lichtenstein, L. M. An evaluation of immunotherapy in asthma. *Am. Rev. Respir. Dis. 117*:191, 1978.

45. Norman, P. S. An overview of immunotherapy: Implications for the future. *Allergy Clin. Immunol. 65*:87, 1980.

46. Warner, J. O., Price, J. F., Soothill, J. F., and Hey, E..N. Controlled trial of hyposensitization to dermatophagoides pteronyssinus in children with asthma. *Lancet 2*:912, 1978.

47. Taylor, W. W., Ohman, J. L., and Lowell, F. C. Immunotherapy in cat-induced asthma. Double-blind trial with evaluation of bronchial responses to cat allergens and histamine. *J. Allergy Clin. Immunol.* *61*:(5):283, 1978.

48. Warner, J. O. Hyposensitization in asthma: A review. *J. R. Soc. Med.* *74*: 60, 1981.

49. Lichtenstein, L. M., Valentine, M. D., and Sobotka, A. K. Insect allergy: The state of the art. *J. Allergy Clin. Immunol.* *64*:5, 1979.

50. Patterson, R., Lieberman, P., Irons, J. S., Pruzansky, J. J., Metzger, W. J., and Zeiss, C. R. Immunotherapy. In *Allergy: Principles and Practice*, E. Middleton, C. R. Reed and E. F. Ellis (eds.), Vol. II, 2nd ed., C. V. Mosby, St. Louis, pp. 1119–1142, 1983.

51. Sullivan, T. J., Yecies, L. D., Shatz, G. S., Parker, C. W., and Wedner, H. J. Desensitization of patients allergic to penicillin using orally administered beta-lactam antibiotics. *J. Allergy Clin. Immunol.* *69*:275, 1982.

52. Brown, L. A., Goldberg, N. D., and Shearer, W. T. Long term ticarcillin desensitization by the continuous oral administration of penicillin. *J. Allergy Clin. Immunol.* *69*:51, 1982.

53. Davidson, J. A., Galloway, J. A., Peterson, B. H., Wentworth, S. Y., and C Crabtree, R. E. Use of purified insulin in insulin allergy. *Diabetes 23*(Suppl. 1):352, 1974.

54. Grammer, L. C., Chen, P. Y., and Patterson, R. Evaluation and management of insulin allergy. *J. Allergy Clin. Immunol.* *71*:(2):250, 1983.

55. Pleskow, W. W., Stevenson, D. D., Mathison, D. A., Simon, R. A., Schatz, M., and Zeiger, R. S. Aspirin desensitization in aspirin-sensitive asthmatic patients: Clinical manifestations and characterization of the refractory period. *J. Allergy Clin. Immunol.* *69*:11, 1982.

56. Herman, J. J., Radin, R., and Schneiderman, R. Allergic reactions to measles (rubeola) vaccine in patients hypersensitive to egg protein. *J. Allergy Clin. Immunol.* *69*:51, 1982.

57. American Academy of Allergy, Position statements — Controversial techniques. *J. Allergy Clin. Immunol.* *67*:333, 1981.

58. Breneman, J. C., et al. Final report of food allergy committee — Sublingual testing. *Ann. Allergy 33*:164, 1974.

58a. Grieco, M. Controversial practices in allergy. *JAMA 247*:3106, 1982.

59. Rowe, A. H. In *Food Allergy: Its Manifestation and Control and the Elimination Diets*. Charles C. Thomas, Springfield, Illinois, pp. 431, 1972.

60. Tuft, L., and Blumstein, G. I. Studies in food allergy. *J. Allergy 17*:329, 1946.

61. Speer, F., and Dockhorn, R. In *Allergy and Immunology in Children*. Charles C. Thomas, Springfield, Illinois, p. 363, 1972.

62. Samter, M. In *Immunologic Diseases*. Brown, Boston, Massachusetts, p. 1384, 1978.

63. Thomas, H. C., and Parrott, D. M. V. The induction of tolerance to a soluble protein antigen by oral administration. *Immunology 27*:631, 1974.

64. Hanson, D. G., Vaz, N. M., Maia, L. C. S., Lynch, J. M., and Simon, K. M. Tolerance to protein induced by feeding (abstract). *Ann. Allergy 881*:386, 1977.

Index

A

Acetanilid, 71
  adult food toxicity and, 71
  pneumonopathy and, 71
  rapeseed oil and, 71
ACTH (adrenocorticotrophic
    hormone), 14
Additives
  adverse reactions to, 126
  asthma and 141, 187
  chronic urticaria and, 139
  dyes, 130
  eczema and, 85, 86
  Feingold and, 224
  food color, 186
  free diet, 183, 209
  hyperactivity and, 224
  metabisulfite, 187
  monosodium glutamate, 187
  treatment, 146, 182
  triggers of reactions, 130
    aspirin, 130
    bisulfites, 130
    dyes, 130
    flavorings, 130
    preservative, 130
  salicylates, 130
Adult food allergy, 71
  anaphylaxis and, 77
  arthritis, 76, 77, 139
  central nervous system, 76, 77,
    139
  epilepsy, 76
  migraine, 76
  psychiatric, 77
  controversial tests, 80
  cromoglycate, 75
  diagnosis, 77
  ELISA (enzyme-linked immuno-
    assay), 73
  double-blind food challenge, 81
  gastrointestinal, 74
  immune complexes and, 74
  immune response types, 73, 28
  incidence, 71
  macromolecules and, 73
  parasites and, 73
  pathophysiology, 72
  PMN (polymorphonuclear
    leukocytes), 74
  RAST, 80
  respiratory, 75
  shellfish and, 71

279

[Adult food allergy]
  skin, 75, 139
  skin tests, 79
  thrombocytopenia, 76, 134
  treatment, 78
    diet diary, 78
    elimination diet, 78
  urticaria 139, 75
Adverse reactions to foods, 125,
    126 (see also Food allergy)
Alcohol (ethanol)
  asthma and, 76, 141
  migraine and 76, 107
  triggers of reactions, 130
Allergenicity
  altered, 18, 212
  digestion and 18, 212
  enzymes and 18, 212
Allergens, 13 (see also Antigens)
  absorption, 19
  altered, 18, 275
  differences between, 1
  food's role, 13
  hidden, 234, 275
  ingestant, 1
  inhalant, 1
  purified, 212
Allergy (see Adult food allergy,
    Food allergy, and Pediatric
    food allergy)
  delayed, 2
  development steps, 6
  IgE, 2
  immediate, 2
  obvious, 2
  occult, 2
Amaranth
  wheat substitute, 239
American Academy of Allergy and
    Immunology
  controversial techniques and, 218–
    223
  position papers, 218, 219, 222, 223
Amines, 72
  histamine and, 72
    cheese and, 72

[Amines]
  pork and, 72
  sauerkraut and, 72
  strawberry and, 72
  tomato and, 72
  tuna and, 72
  phenylethylamine idiosyncracy
    and, 72
Anaphylaxis
  adult food allergy and, 77
  adverse reaction symptoms, 133
  angioedema and, 77
  bisulfites and, 130
  in gut, 28
  immediate reactions and, 127
  urticaria, angioedema and, 77
Anaphylotoxin, 74
Anemia
  cow's milk allergy and, 59
  gastrointestinal bleeding and, 59
  Heiner's syndrome and, 59, 135
  pediatric allergy and, 59
Angioedema, 75
  adverse reaction, 132, 135
  anaphylaxis and, 77
  azo dyes and, 75
  egg and, 263
  glottis, 75
  immediate reactions and, 127
  salicylates and, 75
Anti–
  antibodies produced in gut, 6, 17
  antihistamines, 4, 188, 272, 273
  anti-interleukin, 4
  antikinins, 4, 273
  antilymphokines, 4
  antiprostaglandin, 4, 273
Antibodies
  adults and, 19
  antibody-dependent absorption,
    19, 28
  in children, 19
  foods and, 17, 125, 130
  opsonizing, 19
  precipitating, 17
  Reaginic, 163, 164

Antigens, 13 (*see also* Allergens)
  absorption, 19
  ACTH (adrenocorticotrophic
    hormone), 14
  altered, 18, 275
  antibodies induced by, 16, 22, 274
  eczema and, 85, 86
  food diagnosis antigen, 79
  foods as 16, 17, 125
  foreignness, 14
  high/low dose presentation, 16
  immunodeterminants, 14
  immunology of, 13
  molecular size, 13
  presentation to immune system, 18
  priming, 21
  properties of, 17
  response to, 15
  route of administration, 16
  thymus and, 15
  tolerance, 15, 20, 21
  triggers of reactions, 130
Antihistamine, 188, 272
  H_1 and H_2, 276
Aphthous stomatitis, 140
APT-activated disk, 172
  DASA and, 172
Arthritis
  adult food allergy and, 76, 77
  cow's milk and, 87, 119
  food allergy and, 115, 117
  5-HIAA (hydroxyindoleacetic acid)
    and, 87
  IgA deficiency and, 118
  IgE and, 87
  jejunoileal bypass and, 118
  palindromic rheumatism, 116, 119
  rheumatoid, 87, 120
  type III reaction, 130
Arthus phenomenon, 130, 173
Aspirin (*see also* Salicylates)
  -free diet, 183
  migraine and, 110
  nonsteroidal anti-inflammatory
    drug, 273
  trigger of reactions, 130

Asthma, 74, 130, 132, 140
  alcohol and, 76
  baker's, 75
  eosinophilic gastritis and, 74
  fish smell and, 75
  green coffee bean, 75
  neutralization therapy and, 129,
    218
Atopy
  eczema, 83, 84, 265
  prevention, 263
Autologous urine injection, 223
  (*see also* Controversial
    diagnostic tests)
  Goodpasture's syndrome and, 223
Avoidance
  treatment and, 271, 272
Azo dyes, 75
  diet, 93
  urticaria and, 86

B

Baker's asthma, 75
  castor bean and, 75
  cereal dust inhalation and, 75
  coffee and, 75
  cotton seed and, 75
  fish odor and, 75
  flax and, 75
  flour and, 75
  potato and, 75
  soy and, 75
Barrier loss, 4, 5
  immaturity, 4
  inheritance, 4
  injury, 4
Beer
  migraine and, 140
Benzoates
  attention deficit disorder and, 224
  diet, 93, 183
  hyperactivity and, 224
  trigger of reactions, 130
  urticaria and, 86

Beverages, 250
  recipes, 250
Bisulfites
  anaphylaxis and, 130
  trigger of reactions, 130
Blast transformation, 17 (*see also*
    Diagnosis, tests)
B-lymphocyte, 5, 15
  antibody production, 5
Bread
  corn, 251
  oatmeal, 252
  recipes, 251
Breast feeding
  diet (*see* Diets)
  eczema and, 84
  enteritis from, 50
  gluten-sensitive enteropathy and, 44
  maternal diet and, 271
  pediatric cow's milk allergy and, 57
  prevention and, 265, 271
Buckwheat
  wheat substitute, 239

C

Caffeine
  withdrawal headache, 72
Cardiovascular diseases, 140
Casserole
  recipes, 253
Catsup, 257
  recipe, 257
Celiac disease, 132, 140 (*see also*
    Gluten-sensitive enteropathy
    (GSE))
Cell-mediated immunity (*see also*
    Immunity, Gell-Coombs)
Central nervous system
  children and adults, 139
  migraine (*see* Migraine headache)
  psychoneurotic, 141
  symptoms of food allergy, 135, 212
  tension-fatigue syndrome, 138
Cerebral blood flow
  migraine and, 101

Challenge
  double-blind, 144, 145, 184, 186
  eczema and, 138
  elimination diet and, 184
  food color, 186
  irritable bowel syndrome and, 87
  metabisulfite, 187
  monosodium glutamate (MSG),
    187
  open, 144
  rheumatoid arthritis and, 87
Challenge testing
  additive, 186
  blind, 17, 143
  coloring, 186
  cow's milk enteropathy, 49
  diagnosis, 143
  double-blind, 186
  metabisulfite, 187
  monosodium glutamate, 187
Cheese
  food idiosyncrasy and, 72
  histamine and, 72
  migraine and, 76, 140
Chinese cooking
  migraine and, 72
  monosodium glutamate and, 72
Chocolate
  migraine and, 76, 104, 107, 140
  pharmacological action, 76
Cinnarizine
  cromolyn-like, 273
Clinical features
  adverse reactions to foods, 132
  delayed reactions, 129
  eczema, 83
  irritable bowel syndrome, 87
  laboratory test application, 170
  migraine, 99
Cluster headache
  migraine, 100, 140
  migrainous neuralgia and, 100
Cod
  purified food allergen, 212
Coffee
  caffeine-withdrawal headache, 72

[Coffee]
green-bean asthma, 75
migraine and, 107
Cola
caffeine-withdrawal headache, 72
migraine and, 107
Colon
adult colitis and, 74, 140
cow's milk enteropathy and, 47
eosinophilic gastroenteritis and, 51
inflammatory bowel disease, 75
irritable bowel syndrome, 87,
140
ulcerative colitis, 140
Complement activation, 132, 173
Complexes, immune (*see* Immunity,
response types, III)
Compliance
dietary organization and, 236
elimination diet and, 233
master grocery list, 237
notebook, 237
Condiments
cooking and, 255
Controversial diagnostic tests, 80,
141, 211
American Academy of Allergy's
position paper, 218, 222, 223
autologous urine injection, 223
cytotoxic (Bryan), 80, 142, 221
end-point titration, 214
diagnosis and, 214
results, 216
treatment and, 215, 216
hyperactivity and, 226
leukopenic index, 221
provocation neutralization, 80, 147,
217
subcutaneous, 80, 147, 217, 274
sublingual, 80, 147, 217, 274
symptoms, 217
treatment, 147, 223, 274
Cooking
allergy and, 235
breads, 251
casserole, 253
catsup, 257

[Cooking]
condiments and, 255
corn-free, 242
dessert, 257
egg-free, 244
master grocery list, 237
meat dishes, 253, 254
milk-free, 245
pancakes, 253
salad, 258, 259, 260
substitutes and, 235
vegetable, 259
wheat-free, 239
Corn
bread, 251
cooking, 242
eczema and, 86
foods, 243
hidden ingredients, 234, 243
label substitutes, 234
pone, 197
Cortisone
eosinophilic gastroenteritis and,
51, 274
food allergy and, 189, 274
gluten sensitivity and, 42
Cow's milk
allergy prevention and, 271
arthritis and, 118
breast feeding and, 57, 271
clinical, 47, 49
colon involvement, 46
eczema and, 75, 84
eosinophilic infiltration and, 46
-free cooking, 245
goat's milk substitute, 58
hidden, 234
intrauterine sensitization, 56, 271
migraine and, 103, 105
pediatric, 55, 76, 145, 261, 262
pediatric food allergy and, 55, 57,
63, 134, 135
protein hydrolysate substitute, 57,
145
protein sensitivity, 46, 55, 75, 84
pulmonary hemosiderosis and, 76

[Cow's milk]
  soybean substitute and, 57, 145
  substitutes, 246
  thrombocytopenia and, 61, 130
  treatment, 49
Crohn's disease, 41
Cromolyn
  eczema and, 137
  eosinophilic gastroenteritis and, 52
  inflammatory bowel disease and, 74
  -like drugs, 273
  migraine and, 102, 110, 140
  prophylaxis and, 262, 268, 272, 273
  treatment, 146, 189, 272, 273
Crypt
  enteropathy and, 35
  flat-gut syndrome and, 36
  hypertrophy, 36, 40
  villus-crypt ratio, 35
Cyclic 3, 5-adenosine monophosphate
    (cAMP), 165

D

DASA
  APT disk and, 172
  diagnosis and, 170
Defense
  barrier loss, 4, 7
  causes of loss, 4
  interleukin, 4
Definition
  allergy, 163, 211
  antigens, 13
  food allergy, v, 163
  migraine, 99
Delayed reactions, 128
  diagnosis, 141
  DMSO (dimethyl sulfoxide), 142
  incidence, 128
  symptoms, 129
  triggers, 129, 130
Denatured diet, 183
  altered allergenicity, 212
  protein food allergen, 212

Dermatitis herpetiformis, 45
  GSE (gluten-sensitive enteropathy)
    and, 45
Dessert
  recipes, 257
Diagnosis
  antigen-induced blast transforma-
    tion, 17
  basophil histamine release, 80
  blind challenge, 17, 143
  controversial tests, 80, 142
  delayed food reactions, 141
  diagnostic criteria, 213, 214
  diagnostic difficulty, 211
  diets, 143
    diary, 78
    elimination, 78 (see also
      Elimination diet)
  DMSO (dimethyl sulfoxide), 142
  Dimsoft, 10, 142
  double-antibody assay, 172
  drugs and, 188
  inaccuracies, 3
  laboratory tests, 168-170
  Langerhans' cell, 10
  migraine, 99, 102, 109
  RAST (radio allergosorbent test),
    17, 102 (see also RAST)
  skin testing, 17, 142, 185
  skin tests (adult), 79, 142, 185
  tests, 3, 8, 17, 167-169, 172
Diazo allergen-specific assay (DASA),
    170
Diets
  additive-free, 183
  arthritis and, 116
  azo dyes, 93
  benzoic acid, 93
  breast feeding and, 271
    enteritis, 50
    GSE, 44
    milk allergy, 57
  denatured, 183
  diary, 78, 143, 182
  eczema and, 85, 266

[Diets]
  egg-free, 183, 208, 244
  fructose, 92
  history for diagnosis, 181
  maternal and prevention, 265, 271
  migraine and, 103, 107, 108
  milk-free, 89, 183, 207, 245
  notebook, 237
  prevention and, 266, 271
  restriction, 182
  rotation, 95, 144
    food families and, 95-98
  Rowe, 183, 196, 199
  tartrazine, 93
  treatment, 146, 182
  wheat-free, 183, 206, 239
  yeast-free, 91
Dimsoft, 6, 7, 10
  diagnostic test, 9, 10, 142, 176, 177
  immunology, 9, 10, 176
Disaccharidases, 37-39 39
  lactase, 39
Disodium cromoglycate (*see* Cromolyn)
DMSO (dimethyl sulfoxide), 6, 7, 10
  diagnosis, 142
  Dimsoft, 6, 10
  test, 176
  type IV, 176
Double-antibody assay, 172
Double-blind challenge (*see* Challenge)
Doxantrazole
  cromolyn-like, 273
Drugs
  antihistamine, 188, 272
  cortisone, 189, 274
  cromolyn, 189, 272
  diagnosis and, 188
  epinephrine, 188
  theophylline, 188
  treatment and, 188, 275
Dyes, 130 (*see also* Additives)

E

E. coli (*Escherichia coli*)
  IgA and, 269

Eczema, 75, 83, 131, 263
  additives and, 75, 86
  antigen avoidance and, 85, 86
  atopic, 83, 137
  breast feeding and, 50, 84
  diet and, 85, 266
  egg and, 75, 85
  endogenous, 83
  exogenous, 83
  features, 83
  IgE and, 83, 84
  immediate reactions and, 127
  immunology, 84
  incidence, 83
  mast cells and, 84
  photosensitivity and, 84
  prevention and, 268
  staphylococcus infection and, 84
  T-lymphocytes and, 84
  yeast and, 75
Edema
  adult food allergy and, 74
  angioedema (*see* Angioedema)
Egg, 56, 84
  eczema and, 75, 84, 85, 266
  -free cooking, 244
  -free diet, 183, 208
  hidden, 234, 244
  migraine and, 103, 108
  pediatric food allergy and, 56, 262
  prophylaxis, 262, 263
  substitutes, 245, 256
Electroencephalogram (EEG)
  migraine and, 101
Elemental diet, 57
  diagnosis, 143
  eczema and, 137
  pediatric cow's milk allergy and, 57
  treatment, 188
Elimination diet, 62, 78
  challenge, 62, 78, 143
  compliance, 233
  diagnosis, 143
  difficulties, 233
  forbidden foods, 206-208
  migraine and, 105, 107, 140
  pediatric food allergy and, 62

[Elimination diet]
  recipes, 192–196
  Rowe, 183, 196, 199
ELISA (enzyme-linked immuno-
    assay), 73, 80, 170
  clinical correlation, 170
Endogenous eczema, 83
End-point titration (see Contro-
    versial diagnostic tests)
  and IgE, 214
  immunotherapy and, 215
  placebo and, 215
  RAST and, 215
  results, 216
Enteropathy, 35
  breast feeding, 50
  causes, 41
  celiac disease (see Gluten-sensitive
    enteropathy)
  cow's milk protein sensitivity, 46
  Crohn's disease, 41
  development, 37
  disaccharidases, 39
  eosinophilic (allergic) gastroenteritis, 51
  flat-gut syndrome, 38
  gluten-sensitive enteropathy, 39
  GSE (see Gluten-sensitive enteropathy)
  immunodeficiency and, 41
  lactase deficiency, 39
  soy protein sensitivity, 49
  villus-crypt ratio, 37
  Whipple's disease, 41
  Zollinger-Ellison syndrome, 41
Enuresis, 60, 61, 132
  pediatric food allergy and, 60
Environment
  IgE expression and, 275
Enzyme, 18, 72
  altered antigenicity and, 18, 212, 279
  deficiency, 72
  favism and, 72
  food idiosyncrasy and, 72
  galactosemia and, 72
  glucose 6-phosphate dehydrogenase
    and, 72
Eosinophilic chemotactic factor of
    anaphylaxis (ECF–A), 165

Eosinophilic (allergic) gastroenteritis,
    50, 74
  adult food allergy and, 74
  asthma and, 74
  clinical, 50
  diagnosis, 50
  RAST and, 50
  treatment, 51
Eosiniphilic gastroenteropathy, 40,
    45, 50, 74
  adult food allergy and, 74
  asthma and, 74
  cow's milk protein sensitivity and,
    45
  mediator and, 131
Epilepsy
  adult food allergy and, 76
  migraine and, 100
Epinephrine, 188
Ergot
  migraine, 110
Ethanol (see Alcohol)
Exogenous eczema, 83

F

Families
  food, 96, 181
Family history
  migraine, 100
Fasting
  arthritis and, 119
  diagnosis, 143
  immune changes and, 117
Fava bean
  G-6-PD and, 172
  type II reaction and, 172
Feingold, 224, 225
  attention deficit disorder, 224
  benzoate and, 224
  diet, 224
  hyperactivity and, 224
  salicylate and, 224
  sugar and, 225
  tartrazine and, 224

Fish, 56
  adult food toxicity and, 71
  asthma and fish smell, 75
  pediatric food allergy and, 56
Flat-gut syndrome, 38
  bile-salt loss and, 39
  Crohn's, 41
  crypt hypertrophy and, 41
  diarrhea and, 39
  disaccharidase deficiency and, 39
  eosinophilic gastroenteropathy, 41
  etiology, 41
  food hypersensitivity and, 41
  gluten-sensitive enteropathy and,
    39
  immunodeficiency syndromes, 41
  infection and, 41
  malabsorption and, 39
  milk-sensitive enteropathy, 41
  pathology, 42
  protein malnutrition, 41
  secretory hormone stimuli and, 39
  soy-sensitive enteropathy, 41
  sprue, 41
  Whipple's disease, 41
  Zollinger–Ellison syndrome, 41
Food
  adverse reactions to, 126
  alteration, 18
  antigenicity, 16
  challenges (*see* Challenge)
  coloring, 186
  in corn, 243
  diary, 182
  dislikes and allergy, 182
  families, 96, 181
  idiosyncrasy, 72
  labels, 234, 235
  manufacturers and suppliers, 248–250
  migraine and, 103, 108
  reaction timing, 212
  substitutes, 234
  toxicity, 71
  triggers of reactions, 129
Food allergy
  adult, 71 (*see* Adult food allergy)

[Food allergy]
  arthritis and, 115, 117
  control, 29
  cow's milk, 55, 145
  development, 5
  diagnostic tests, 3, 8, 163–177
  eosinophilic gastroenteritis and, 51,
    74, (*see also* Eosinophilic
    gastroenteritis)
  future needs, 30, 271
  immune structures, 5, 6, 7, 8
  incidence, 3, 55, 71 (*see also*
    Incidence)
  mechanism, 5
    turn-off/turn-on, 5
  migraine and, 103, 108
  non-IgE, 125
  pediatric, 55 (*see also* Pediatric
    food allergy)
  prevention, 21, 146, 261
  prophylaxis, 145, 146, 263, 271
  school meals and, 234
  shock organ, 212
  suppliers, 248–250
  toxicity, idiosyncrasy, and, 71
    (*see also* Food toxicity)
  travel and, 236
  treatment, 145, 275
  turn-on, 262, 271
  uterine sensitization, 56, 261, 271
Food idiosyncrasy, 72, 125, 132
  enzyme deficiency, 72
  migraine and, 72, 109
  monoamine oxidase, 72
  monosodium glutamate, 72
  tyramine, 72
    cheese and, 7, 72
    Chianti and, 72
    herring and, 72
    yeast and, 72
Food toxicity, 71, 132
  acetanilid, 71
  amines, 72
  caffeine and, 72
  fish, 71
  hexachlorobenzene, 71

[Food toxicity]
  migraine and, 102
  mushroom, 71
  porphyria and, 71
  rapeseed and, 71
  shellfish, 71
  urticaria and, 72
Forbidden foods
  egg-free, 208
  milk-free, 207
  wheat-free, 206
Foreignness
  adrenocorticotropic hormone
      (ACTH), 14
  amine acids and, 14
  collagen and, 14
Fructose diet (*see* Diets, fructose)

G

Gastrointestinal tract
  adult food allergy and, 74
  anemia and, 59
  bleeding and pediatric allergy, 59
  immediate reactions and, 127
  immunity, adult, 72
  inflammatory bowel disease, 75
  mucosal, 72
  pediatric food allergy and, 62, 135
  shock organ, 212
  symptoms, 135, 140
  type III reaction, 130
Gell-Coombs, 8, 9, 28, 29, 130, 163, 173
  DMSO and type IV, 176
  food allergy production, 8, 9, 130
  in gut wall, 8, 9, 24, 25, 28, 130
  types of immune reactions, 8, 9, 28,
      29, 130, 164, 174, 177
Genetics (*see* Heredity)
  predisposition of pediatric food
      allergy, 56
Genitourinary tract
  albuminuria and, 61
  enuresis and, 61
  nephrotic syndrome and, 61

[Genitourinary tract]
  pediatric allergy and, 61
Gingko fruit, 74
  perirectal burning and, 74
  pruritis and, 74
  stomatitis and, 74
  tenesmus and, 74
Gluten-sensitive enteropathy (GSE,
      celiac disease), 37, 40, 132
  ADCC and, 27
  bird-fancier's disease and, 43
  breast feeding and, 43
  clinical, 43
  cooking and, 239
  cortisone and, 42
  dermatitis herpetiformis and, 44
  histocompatibility and, 42
  immunology, 41
  intestinal biopsy and, 44
  organ culture and, 41
  pathology, 41
  personality and, 44
  sweat test and, 44
  treatment, 44
Goat's milk
  cow's milk substitute, 58
  pediatric allergy and, 58
G-6-PD (glucose-6-phosphate
      dehydrogenase), 172
GSE (gluten-sensitive enteropathy)
      (*see* Gluten-sensitive
      enteropathy)

H

Hageman factor, 132
Headache, 72 (*see* Migraine headache)
  caffeine withdrawal, 72
  food toxicity and, 72
  histamine, 100
  Horton's neuralgia, 100
Heiner's syndrome, 60, 134, 173
  anemia and, 59
  diagnosis, 142
  gastrointestinal, 135
  precipitating antibodies and, 59, 173

[Heiner's syndrome]
pulmonary changes, 59
HEPP (human IgE pentapeptide)
IgE-blocking peptide, 274
Heredity
IgE phenotypic expression, 271
IgE response and, 56, 271
peanut and, 261
pediatric food allergy and, 56, 261
Herpes simplex
eczema and, 84
Hexachlorobenzene
food toxicity and, 71
prophyria and, 71
Histamine
basophile release, 80
food idiosyncrasy and, 72
foods causing release, 72
headache, 100
urinary levels, 142
Histamine headache
Horton's neuralgia and, 100
History, 181
additives and, 182
diagnosis and, 181
family and migraine, 100
Histocompatibility complex, 16
in gluten-sensitive enteropathy, 43
Ir genes, 16
Horton's neuralgia, 99, 100
migrainous neuralgia and, 100
5-hydroxyindoleacetic acid (5-HIAA)
migraine and, 101
rheumatoid arthritis and, 87
Hyperactivity, 212, 224
attention deficit disorder, 224
Feingold hypothesis and, 224
food allergy and, 212
sublingual neutralization and, 226
sugar and, 225
Hypoallergenic foods, 183
cooking and, 235
ingredients, 234
meals in school, 234
meals in training, 236

I

Idiosyncrasy (*see* Food idiosyncrasy)
IgA, 6, 20, 35, 56, 72, 73
activity, 23
antigen-dependent cell-mediated
cytotoxicity (ADCC), 23
arthritis and, 118
breast feeding and, 268
cell-mediated cytotoxicity, 23
deficiency in pediatric allergy, 58
E. coli and, 268
enteropathy and IgA subtypes, 35,
268
formation, 22
gatekeeper, 134
gut barrier, 6
increase in gluten-sensitive
enteropathy, 42
migraine and, 102
opsonization and, 23
Sabin vaccine and, 21
in secretions, 22
secretory, 20, 22, 56
secretory piece, 24
serum, 22
transport, 22
IgE, 2, 17, 25, 28, 56, 58, 72, 73, 76,
130
activity, 26
adult food allergy and, 72
allergic genetic expression, 271
anaphylactic reactions in gut, 28
blocking peptides and, 272, 274
colic and, 26
cow's milk enteropathy, 49
discovery, 163
eczema, 83, 84
ELISA and, 73
gastrointestinal, 25
in gut, 26
intestinal infections and, 27
in vitro tests, 142
irritable bowel syndrome and, 88
local concentrations (gut), 26

[IgE]
mediator, 131
migraine and, 102
urticaria and, 86
IgG, 3, 8, 9, 17, 24, 25, 72
antibody-dependent absorption, 19
biological properties, 25
blocking antibody, 274
complement and, 25
cow's milk and, 263
(in) gut, 25
Heiner's syndrome and, 59
IgG4, 59, 142
immunotherapy and, 274
precipitating antibodies and, 59, 172
IgM, 8, 9, 17, 24, 72
complement and, 24
Heiner's syndrome and, 59, 174
IgA competition, 24
precipitating antibodies and, 59, 174
secretory piece, 24
Immediate reactions, 127 (see also IgE)
Immunity
cell-mediated, 174
cellular, 17
complexes, 29, 31, 73, 74, 88
control in gastrointestinal tract, 29
deficiency in pediatric allergy, 58
DMSO and, 176
double-antibody assay, 172
fasting and, 117
gastrointestinal, 25, 27
Gell-Coombs, 8, 164
M cells, 8
pathogenesis, 28, 125
presentation, 18
priming, 21
reaction
in bowel, 10
in skin, 10, 75
response types, 8, 9, 28, 29, 130, 164
I (IgE), 28, 164
II, 28, 171
III, 29, 172 (see also Arthus
phenomenon)

[Immunity]
IV, 29, 174
V, 164
Sabin vaccine, 21
structures
thymus-dependent, 15
thymus-independent, 15
T-lymphocytes, 84
eczema and, 84
tolerance, 20
adherence, IgE, 27
suppression, 21
Immunodeficiency syndrome, 41
disgammaglobulinemia, 41
flat-gut syndrome and, 41
pediatric food allergy and, 62
transient hypogammaglobulinemia
41
Immunodeterminants
amino acids and, 13
definition, 13
polysaccharides and, 13
protein, 15
T-cell-dependent, 15
Immunology
eczema, 84
gastrointestinal, 72
gluten-sensitive enteropathy, 42
migraine, 102
Immunotherapy
blocking IgG, 274
hyposensitization, 274
oral hyposensitization, 275
Incidence
adult food allergy, 71
delayed reactions and, 128
eczema, 83
food allergy, 3
irritable bowel syndrome, 87
pediatric, 55
soy-protein sensitivity, 50
urticaria and angioedema, 75
Infant (see also Pediatric food
allergy)
diet, 182

Inflammatory bowel disease (IBD) (*see* Colon and Gastrointestinal tract)
Interleukin, 5, 10
macrophage release of, 5, 10
Intestinal biopsy
gluten challenge, 46
gluten-sensitive enteropathy and, 45
Ir gene, 16
immune reaction and, 16
major histocompatibility complex, 16
Irritable bowel syndrome, 87
guilty foods, 88
IgE and, 88
immune complexes and, 88

K

K-cell, 27
Ketotifen
cromolyn-like, 273
migraine and, 110

L

Labels
corn terms, 234
substitutes by manufacturers, 234
Lactose intolerance, 132
Lamina propria, 21, 23, 35, 37, 42, 72, 75
cells, 27, 35, 42, 72
in GSE, 42
IgE and, 25
IgG and, 25, 72
IgM and, 24, 72
priming, 21
routes of administration and, 21
secretory IgA and, 23
Langerhans' cell
eczema and, 85
"Leaky" gut, 262, 263
Leukocytotoxic test (*see* Controversial diagnostic tests)
Leukopenic index, 221 (*see also* Controversial diagnostic tests)

Leukotrienes (also SRS–A), 165
Lodoxamide
cromolynlike, 277
Lymphocytes
adult allergy and, 72
food allergy and, 125
lymphokines, 142, 174
sensitization, 130, 142
T-lymphocytes (*see* T-lymphocytes)
type IV reactions, 174

M

Macromolecules, 13, 16, 18, 73, 134
absorption, 73
adult allergy and, 72
pediatric allergy and, 58, 134
Macrophage, 4, 10, 16, 30, 131
antigen-processing, 4
control of immune reactions in gut, 30
eczema and Langerhans' cell, 85
Ir gene and, 16
Langerhans' cell, 10
MHC (major histocompatibility complex) and, 16
T-lymphocyte-stimulating, 4
T-suppressor, 30
Malabsorption, 35, 37, 44, 45
Malt
wheat-free diet and, 206
Manufacturers
food allergy products, 248–250
MAO (monoamine oxidase) and migraine, 140
Mast cell
eczema and, 84
IgE, 26, 28
triggers of reactions, 131
urticaria and, 86
Master grocery list, 237
M cell, 9, 20
absorption, 20
adult food allergy and, 72

[M cell]
  gastrointestinal immunity, 72
  mucosal, 72
  Peyer's patch and, 72
Meal management, 238
Meat dish
  recipes, 253, 254
Menstrual cycle
  migraine and, 100
Metabisulfite
  challenge, 187
Migraine headache, 72, 99, 132, 212
  adult food allergy and, 76
  alcohol, 76, 107
  beer and, 140
  cerebral blood flow and, 101
  cheese, 76, 107
  Chinese cooking and, 72
  chocolate, 76, 107
  classification, 99
  clinical features, 99
  cromolyn and, 102, 110
  diagnosis, 99, 102, 109
  EEG and, 101
  epilepsy and, 100
  ergot, 110
  family history, 100
  5-HIAA and, 101
  food idiosyncrasy and, 72
  foods and, 103, 108
  IgA and, 102
  IgE and, 102, 130
  immunology and, 102
  Ketotifen and, 110
  MAO, 140
  menstrual cycle and, 100
  monosodium glutamate and, 72
  nitrite and, 72
  orange and, 107
  platelets and, 101
  prostaglandin and, 102, 110
  serotonin and, 101
  tomato and, 72
  toxicity (food) and, 102
  treatment, 110
  type III, 131
  tyramine and, 72

[Migraine headache]
  wheat allergy and, 101
Migrainous neuralgia, 100
  cluster headache, 100
  histamine headache, 100
  Horton's neuralgia, 100
Migration inhabitation (see
        Diagnosis and Tests)
Milk (see Cow's milk)
Milk-free diet, 89, 183, 207
  butter substitutes, 90
  cooking, 245
  sensitive enteropathy, 41
  substitutes, 90
Milk-sensitive enteropathy, 41
Modified RAST, 220, 221
Monosodium glutamate (MSG)
  Chinese cooking and, 72
  migraine and, 72
Mucosa
  adult immunity, 72
  bleeding and milk allergy, 59
  maturity and pediatric allergy, 56
  M cells (see M cell)
  permeability, 58
Muffins
  recipes, 252
Mushroom
  adult food toxicity and, 71

N

Nephrotic syndrome, 61, 132
Neutralization
  provocative testing and, 80, 147,
        217 (see also Controversial
        diagnostic tests)
Nitrite
  food idiosyncrasy and, 72
  migraine headache and, 72
  urticaria and, 72
NK (natural killer) cells, 27
Noncompliance (see Compliance)
Notebook
  dietary, 237, 238
  master grocery list, 237
  meal management, 238

O

Oats
bread, 252
Opsonization
IgA, 23
IgM, 24
IgG, 25
Oral hyposensitization, 275
Orange
migraine and, 107
Organ culture
gluten sensitivity and, 42

P

Palindromic rheumatism, 116, 119
Pancakes
recipes, 253
Paper radioimmunosorbent test
(PRIST), 166
Parasite
adult food allergy and, 73
Peanut
heredity and, 263
migraine and, 103
purified allergen, 212
Pediatric food allergy, 55
breast feeding
eczema and, 84
enteritis and, 49
GSE, 44
milk and, 57
cow's milk, 55, 56, 57, 262, 263, 271
dermatologic manifestations, 60, 62
diagnosis, 61, 62
laboratory, 163–176
egg and, 263
elemental diets, 57
elimination diet and, 62
enuresis, 60
allergic cystitis, 61
gastrointestinal manifestations, 58, 59
gastrointestinal maturity, 56
goat's milk, 58

[Pediatric food allergy]
Heiner's syndrome, 58, 134, 142, 173
pulmonary hemosiderosis, 60
heredity and, 56, 271
immunodeficiency and, 62
incidence, 55
intrauterine sensitization, 56, 263, 268, 275
"leaky" gut, 263
macromolecules and, 58, 134
nephrotic syndrome, 61, 132
predisposing factors, 56, 271
prevention, 261, 266, 271
prognosis, 63
protein hydrolysates, 57, 268
respiratory manifestations, 58, 62
soybean, 57
thrombocytopenia, 61
twins and, 56
viral infections and, 58
Peptides
IgE-blocking, 276, 278
Personality change
gluten-free diet and, 45
gluten-sensitive enteropathy and, 45
Peyer's patch, 9, 20, 27, 29, 72
control of food reactions, 29
IgE and, 25
M cell, 9, 20, 27, 72
priming and, 21
Photosensitivity
eczema and, 84
Plasma cell, 72
Platelet
aggregation, 131
migraine and, 101, 102
Polymorphonuclear leukocyte, 74
Potato, 140
flour and wheat, 239
tobacco family, 140
Prevention
asthma and, 264, 265
breast feeding and, 265, 267
casein hydrolysate and, 268

[Prevention]
  diet and, 266
  egg, 262
  food allergy, 261, 271
  IgE expression, 271
  "leaky gut," 262, 263
  milk, 262
PRIST, 166
Procedures
  laboratory tests, 167–174
Prostaglandins
  arthritis and, 116, 117, 118
  irritable bowel syndrome (IBS) and, 87
  mediators, 132
  migraine and, 102, 110
  nonsteroidal anti-inflammatory drugs,
    273
  urticaria and, 86
Protein hydrolysates, 57
  pediatric milk allergy and, 57
  prevention and, 268
Provocation testing, 185 (see also
    Controversial diagnostic tests)
  neutralization therapy and, 80, 147,
    217
    American Academy of Allergy's
      position paper, 218, 219
    asthma and, 219
    subcutaneous, 217, 218
    sublingual, 217, 218
PRU (Phadebas RAST units)
  RAST scoring, 168, 169
Pruritis
  gastrointestinal manifestations, 74
  gingko fruit and, 74
Psychiatric disorders, 77
  adult food allergy and, 77

R

Radioimmunosorbent test (RIST), 165
Rapeseed oil
  acetanilid and, 71
  pneumonopathy and, 71

RAST (radioallergosorbent test),
    2, 17, 167, 185
  adult food allergy diagnosis, 80
  asthma and, 76
  cow's milk enteropathy, 49
  diagnosis, 176, 185, 219
  DMSO and, 176
  immediate reactions and, 127
  migraine and, 108
  modified, 169, 220
  pediatric allergy diagnosis and, 61
  PRU, 169
  scoring systems, 168
  skin-test titration and, 215
Reactions (see also Immunity,
    Gell-Coombs)
  fava bean, 172
  shock organ, 212
  timing, 212
  types, 8, 9, 28, 29, 130, 164
    I, 164
    II, 171
    III, 172
    IV, 174
Reaginic antibody, 163, 164 (see
    also IgE)
Recipes
  beverages, 250
  bread, 251
  casseroles, 253
  catsup, 257
  condiments and, 255
  dessert, 257
  egg-free, 245
  elimination diet, 192–196
  meat dishes, 253, 254
  milk-free, 246
  muffins, 252
  pancakes, 253
  rice, 191
  Rowe, 183, 196, 199
  salads, 258, 259, 260
  side dishes, 258
  vegetables, 259
  wheat-free, 240

Respiratory
  symptoms of food allergy, 135, 137
Restriction
  dietary, 182, 238
  infant diet, 182
  technique, 184
Reticuloendothelial
  system, 16
Rheumatoid arthritis, 87, 120 (*see
    also* Arthritis)
  dairy products and, 87
  5-HIAA and, 87
  food allergy and, 116
  joint pains, 76
Rhinorrhea
  adult food allergy, 76
Rice
  recipes, 191
  wheat substitute, 239
Rinkel technique, 215, 216 (*see also*
    Controversial diagnostic tests)
RIST, 165, 166
Rotation diets, 95, 144, 146
Rye
  wheat substitute, 239

S

Salad
  recipes, 258, 259, 260
Salicylates
  angioedema and, 75
  free-diet, 183
  hyperactivity and, 224
  triggers of reactions, 130
  urticaria and, 75
School meals, 235
Scoring systems
  PRU (Phadebas RAST units), 169
  RAST, 168
Secretory IgA, 20, 22, 56, 72 (*see
    also* IgA)
  biological activity, 23
  complement and, 23
  deficiency, 29

[Secretory IgA]
  E. coli and, 267
  function, 22
  hormone control, 29
  structure, 22
  transport, 22
Serotonin
  migraine and, 101
Shellfish
  adult food toxicity and, 71
Shock organ
  food allergy and, 212
Skin tests
  adult food allergy and, 79
  antigen, 79
  diagnosis, 79, 142, 185
  immediate reactions and, 127, 142
  immunotherapy and, 215
  migraine and, 103, 104
  prick test, 79
  RAST and, 219
  titration end-point, 214, 215
Slow-reacting substance of
      anaphylaxis (SRS-A), 165
    (*see also* Leukotrienes)
Soy
  Baker's asthma and, 75
  enteropathy, 41
  incidence, 50
  milk protein sensitivity and, 49
  pediatric food allergy and, 57, 182
  protein sensitivity, 50, 57
  soy flour as a wheat substitute,
      239
Sprue, 41
Staphylococcus aureus and eczema,
      84, 263
Stomatitis
  gingko fruit and, 74
Sublingual drops (*see* Controversial
      diagnostic tests)
Substitutes
  cooking and, 235
  egg-free diet and, 245
  manufacturers and, 234
  milk, 235

[Substitutes]
  milk-free diet and, 246
  ingredients, 234
  school meals, 235
  wheat-free diet and, 239
Subtypes IgA, 35
Sugar
  hyperactivity and, 225
Suppliers
  special allergy foods, 248–250
Sweat test
  cystic fibrosis and, 45
  gluten-sensitive enteropathy and, 45
Symptoms
  adverse reactions to foods, 132
  delayed allergy, 3
  provocation/neutralization testing
    and, 217
  tension-fatigue syndrome, 138,
    223, 224
  timing of, 1

T

Tapioca
  wheat substitute, 239
Tartrazine
  asthma and, 130
  diet, 93, 183, 186
  hyperactivity and, 224
Tension-fatigue syndrome, 138, 223, 224
Tests
  controversial (*see* Controversial
    diagnostic tests)
  diagnostic (*see* DASA, Diagnosis,
    Immunity, and RAST)
  laboratory, 3, 8, 17, 167–176
  procedures, 167–174
Thrombocytopenia
  adult food allergy and, 76, 134
  milk-induced, 130
  pediatric food allergy and, 61
Thymus, 15
  antigens
    thymus-dependent, 15
    thymus-independent, 15

Timing
  food reactions, 212
T-lymphocytes, 15, 27, 58, 174
  bowel barriers and, 4, 6, 9
  control of immunologic reactions
    of the gut, 30
  cytotoxic, 4, 27
  eczema and, 84, 137
  eosinophilic gastroenteritis and,
    50
  gluten-sensitive enteropathy and,
    42
  helper, 5, 16, 23
  histocompatibility and, 16
  Langerhans' cell and, 10
  lymphokines, 174
  nonspecific, 5
  NK cells, 27
  prevention and, 264
  suppressor, 5, 30, 73
  turn-on/turn-off, 5, 262
Tobacco, 140
  family
    eggplant, 140
    potato, 140
    tomato, 140
Tolerance, 20, 21
Tomato
  food idiosyncrasy and, 72
  histamine and, 72
  migraine headache and, 72
  tobacco and, 140
Toxicity, food (*see* Food toxicity)
Treatment (*see also* Food allergy)
  antihistamines, 272
  avoidance, 271
  blocking peptides and, 272, 274
  cortisone, 274
  cromolyn (*see* Cromolyn,
    treatment)
  drug, 188, 272
  epinephrine, 188
  IgE-blocking peptides, 274
  immunotherapy, 274
  oral hyposensitization, 275
Triggers
  food reactions and, 125, 126

[Triggers]
immunologic, 126, 128
nonimmunologic, 129
types, 129
additives, 130
foodstuffs, 129
T-suppressor, 72 (*see also* T-lymphocytes)
Turn-off, 271
T-lymphocyte and, 5
Turn-on, 262
Types (*see also* Immunity)
immune (Gell-Coombs) reactions, 8, 9, 28, 29, 130, 164
Tyramine, 72
cheese and, 72
Chianti and, 72
food idiosyncrasy and, 72
herring and, 72
histamine and, 72
migraine headache and, 72
monoamine oxidase and, 72
phenolsulfatransferase and, 72
platelets and, 72
yeast and, 72

U

Unproven diagnostic test, 213 (*see also* Controversial diagnostic tests)
Unproven treatments (*see* Controversial diagnostic tests)
Urine
autologous injection, 223
Urticaria, 72, 75, 86, 130
additives and (*see* Additives)
adult food allergy and, 75, 139
azo dyes and, 75, 86, 139
benzoates and, 86
IgE and, 86
mast cells and, 86
nitrites and, 72
preservatives and, 75, 139
prostaglandin and, 86
salicylates and, 75, 130, 139
yeast and, 75

Uterine sensitization, 56, 261, 266
pediatric food allergy, 56
prevention of food allergy, 261, 266, 271

V

Vasculitis, 134, 139
Vegetable
recipes, 259
Villus
compensatory hypertrophy, 38
-crypt ratio, 37
disaccharidases and, 37
enteropathy and, 37
Viral infections
pediatric allergy and, 58

W

Wheat
-free cooking, 239
-free diet, 183, 206
malt and, 206
migraine and, 100, 103, 107
recipes, 240
substitutes, 239
Whipple's disease, 41

Y

Yeast, 72, 91
angioedema and, 75
diet, 91
eczema, 86
food toxicity and, 72
urticaria and, 75

Z

Zinc
T-cell response and, 117
Zollinger-Ellison syndrome, 41